Investigating Reproductive Tract Infections and other Gynaecological Disorders

Reproductive tract infections and other gynaecological disorders among women represent an enormous global health burden. This significant new book will help focus research on an important though neglected area. The primary aims of the book are to provide an overview of reproductive tract infections and other gynaecological disorders, to highlight the conceptual and methodological challenges associated with undertaking research on this subject, and to serve as a reference for future research in this area. The book focuses on developing country settings, and recognises that gathering this sort of information requires a multidisciplinary and culturally sensitive approach. Findings from the research described in this book will undoubtedly assist physicians, social scientists, epidemiologists and public health practiners in evaluating the magnitude of this problem within the community at large and in identifying new potentially effective medical and behavioural interventions to address this problem.

Investigating Reproductive Tract Infections and other Gynaecological Disorders

A Multidisciplinary Research Approach

Edited by

Shireen Jejeebhoy
The Population Council, New Delhi, India

Michael Koenig
Johns Hopkins University, Baltimore, USA

and

Christopher Elias
Program for Appropriate Technology in Health (PATH), Seattle, USA

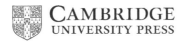

CAMBRIDGE
UNIVERSITY PRESS

CAMBRIDGE UNIVERSITY PRESS
Cambridge, New York, Melbourne, Madrid, Cape Town, Singapore, São Paulo

Cambridge University Press
The Edinburgh Building, Cambridge CB2 2RU, UK

Published in the United States of America by Cambridge University Press, New York

www.cambridge.org
Information on this title: www.cambridge.org/9780521818124

First published 2003
This digitally printed first paperback version 2006

A catalogue record for this publication is available from the British Library

Library of Congress Cataloguing in Publication data

Reproductive tract infections and other gynaecological disorders : research into
prevalence, correlates, and consequences / 2002.
    p. ; cm.
  Includes bibliographical references and index.
  ISBN 0 521 81812 5 (hardback)
    1. Generative organs, Female – Infections. 2. Sexually transmitted diseases. 3.
  Reproductive health. 4. Women – Diseases. 5. Gynecology. I. Jejeebhoy, Shireen J. II.
  Koenig, Michael Alan. III. Elias, Christopher.
    [DNLM: 1. Genital Diseases, Female. 2. Reproductive Medicine. 3. Sexually
  Transmitted Diseases. WP 140 R4247 2002]
  RG218 .R468 2002
  618.1–dc21   2002023388

ISBN-13 978-0-521-81812-4 hardback
ISBN-10 0-521-81812-5 hardback

ISBN-13 978-0-521-03194-3 paperback
ISBN-10 0-521-03194-X paperback

Contents

Contributors

Dr Abhay Bang
SEARCH
PO & District Gadchiroli
Maharashtra 442 605
India

E-mail: search@mah.nic.in

Dr Rani Bang
SEARCH
PO & District Gadchiroli
Maharashtra 442 605
India

E-mail: search@mah.nic.in

Dr Aysen Bulut
Institute of Child Health
University of Istanbul
Cocuk Hastanesi
Millet Cad. 34390 Capa
Istanbul
Turkey

E-mail: kbulut@superonline.com

Professor John Cleland
Director
Centre for Population Studies
London School of Hygiene and Tropical
    Medicine
49–51 Bedford Square
London WC1B 3DP
UK

E-mail: john.cleland@lshtm.ac.uk

Dr Ruth Dixon-Mueller
SJO 566
1601 NW 97th Ave. Unit C-101
PO Box 025216
Miami
FL 33102-5216
USA

E-mail: dixonmueller@yahoo.com

Dr Christopher Elias
President
Program for Appropriate Technology in
    Health (PATH)
1455 NW Leary Way
Seattle
WA 98107
USA

E-mail: celias@path.org

Dr Veronique Filippi
Maternal and Child Epidemiology Unit
Maternal Health Programme
Department of Infectious and Tropical
    Diseases
London School of Hygiene and Tropical
    Medicine
Keppel Street
London WC1E 7HT
UK

E-mail: veronique.filippi@lshtm.ac.uk

Dr Joel Gittelsohn
Associate Professor
Division of Human Nutrition
Department of International Health
Bloomberg School of Public Health
Johns Hopkins University
615 North Wolfe Street
Baltimore
MD 21205-2179
USA

E-mail: jgittels@jhsph.edu

Dr Ronald Gray
Bloomberg School of Public Health
Johns Hopkins University
615 North Wolfe Street
Baltimore
MD 21205-2179
USA

Dr Siobán Harlow
Associate Professor of Epidemiology
University of Michigan
109 Observatory St
Ann Arbor, MI 48109
USA

E-mail: harlow@umich.edu

Dr Graham Hart
Associate Director
MRC Social and Public Health Sciences Unit
University of Glasgow
4 Lilybank Gardens
Glasgow G12 8RZ
UK

E-mail: Graham@msoc.mrc.gla.ac.uk

Dr Sarah Hawkes
85 Pearl Street
New Haven
CT 06511
USA

E-mail: sarahhawkes99@hotmail.com

Dr Shireen Jejeebhoy
The Population Council
Zone 5-A Ground Floor
India Habitat Centre
Lodi Road
New Delhi 110003
India

E-mail: sjejeebhoy@vsnl.net

Dr Hind Khattab
Delta Consultants Ltd
12 Dr Mahmoud Hefny Street
Garden City
Cairo
Egypt

E-mail: espsrh@starnet.com.eg

Dr Michael Koenig
Associate Professor
Department of Population and Family
    Health Sciences
Bloomberg School of Public Health
Johns Hopkins University
615 North Wolfe Street
Baltimore
MD 21205-2179
USA

E-mail: mkoenig@jhsph.edu

Dr Jane Kuypers
University of Washington
4014 University Way NE
Seattle
WA 98105-6203
USA

E-mail: kuypers@u.washington.edu

Dr Nicola Low
Department of Social Medicine
University of Bristol
Canynge Hall
Whiteladies Road
Bristol BS8 2PR
UK

E-mail: nicola.low@bristol.ac.uk

Dr Tom Marshall
Maternal Health Group
Infectious Diseases Epidemiology Unit
London School of Hygiene and Tropical
    Medicine
Keppel Street
London WC1E 7HT
UK

E-mail: tom.marshall@lshtm.ac.uk

Dr Mary Meehan
Centre for Population and Family Health
SPH/POP B-2
Columbia University
2960 Broadway
New York
NY 10027-6902
USA

E-mail: mjmeehan@infocom.co.ug

Dr André Meheus
Department of Epidemiology and
    Community Medicine
University of Antwerp
Universiteitsplein 1
B-2610 Antwerp
Belgium

E-mail: engelen@uia.ua.ac.be

Dr Nandini Oomman
5620 Oak Place
Bethesda
MD 20817
USA

E-mail: noomman@erols.com

Dr Pertti Pelto
Wellington Mews
Wing 5 Flat 102
North Main Rd
Sangamwadi
Koregaon Park
Pune 411 001
India

E-mail: peltob@satyam.net.in
        perttipelto@hotmail.com

Dr Thomas Quinn
Professor of Medicine
Johns Hopkins University
1159 Ross Research Building
11th Floor, Room 1159
720 Rutland Avenue
Baltimore
MD 21205-2196

Dr David Serwadda
Associate Professor
Institute of Public Health (Room 219)
Mulago Hospital Complex
PO Box 7051
Kampala
Uganda

E-mail: dserwada@imul.com

Dr Mary Shepherd
Department of Population and Family
    Health Sciences
Bloomberg School of Public Health
Johns Hopkins University
615 North Wolfe Street
Baltimore
MD 21205-2179
USA

E-mail: mshepher@jhsph.edu

Dr Janneke van de Wijgert
Population Council
One Dag Hammarskjold Plaza
New York
NY 10017
USA

E-mail: jvandewijgert@popcouncil.org

Dr Maria Wawer
Clinical Professor of Public Health
Department of Population and Family
    Health
Columbia University
2960 Broadway
New York
NY 10027-6902
USA

**World Health Organization Regional
    Office for the Western Pacific**
PO Box 2932
Manila 1099
Philippines

Dr Huda Zurayk
Professor and Dean
Faculty of Health Sciences
American University Beirut
Beirut
Lebanon
E-mail: hzurayk@aub.edu.lb

Foreword

Until the 1990s, interest in exploring women's experiences of reproductive and other gynaecological disorders was limited. The pioneering works of Abhay and Rani Bang in India, Judith Wasserheit in Bangladesh and Huda Zurayk, Hind Khattab and Nabil Younis in Egypt were among the handful of community-based studies that had attempted to explore this subject using both self-reported as well as clinically-diagnosed and laboratory-detected measures of morbidity. The 1994 International Conference on Population and Development marked a radical change in global interest in the topic – it argued for a more comprehensive focus on women's reproductive health, including, specifically, reproductive tract infections and other gynaecological morbidities, and boosted interest in filling gaps in what is known about the prevalence and patterns of reproductive tract infections and what they mean for women's health and well-being.

As a result, there has been a rapidly expanding number of research studies on the prevalence and correlates of reproductive tract infections, or gynaecological morbidity more generally. The experiences of these studies have raised a number of concerns. An analytic framework to guide research was missing. Hugely variable estimates of morbidity were reported both between studies in similar settings and even within a single study depending on the methodology used, making interpretation difficult. Factors underlying morbidity and the health-seeking patterns of symptomatic women remained unexplored, and serious ethical issues were raised. Despite the interest in conducting multidisciplinary research on the topic, the field has thus far lacked a clear and systematic set of guidelines for the planning and conduct of research that addresses the clinical as well as behavioural and social aspects of women's gynaecological disorders, the contexts in which these occur, their antecedents and consequences, and the insights they provide for programme development.

It was the recognition of these gaps and limitations in the current state of evidence on women's reproductive tract infections and other gynaecological disorders that prompted a partnership between the UNDP/UNFPA/WHO/World Bank Special Programme of Research, Development and Research Training in Human Reproduction (HRP), the Ford Foundation and the Rockefeller Foundation to undertake a multidisciplinary project intended to shed light on optimal research approaches to the study of this complex topic. This volume is the culmination of that effort.

Investigating Reproductive Tract Infections and Other Gynaecological Disorders fills an important need. It disentangles the complexities of conducting research on this topic, and offers researchers a sound, evidence-based assessment of optimal research approaches to the study of reproductive tract infections and other gynaecological disorders. Recognizing the need for a multidisciplinary nature of any investigation on women's reproductive morbidity, the book incorporates the perspectives of different disciplines, with representation from the social, biomedical and statistical spheres. It presents comprehensive strategies and methods for the design of multidisciplinary research and makes researchers aware of the advantages and limitations of, and complementarities between, various research methods and the imperative of involving the communities being studied in the research. It sets out definitions of the reproductive tract infections and other types of gynaecological morbidity that are usually studied, and it describes methodological approaches that enable more refined estimates of the prevalence of self-reported, clinically-diagnosed and laboratory-detected morbidity. The book also offers a conceptual framework for the study of behavioural determinants and consequences for women's lives, gender issues and the special obstacles impeding women from seeking timely and appropriate care, and for future explorations of the role of men. It highlights the need to go beyond numbers and use qualitative methods to enrich what is known about the context in which women's gynaecological morbidity occurs. Importantly, it discusses analytical approaches that assist the reader in assimilating and interpreting the findings from data collected from a multitude of different sources (qualitative and quantitative, clinical and laboratory). Finally, the volume draws out implications arising from the emerging research agenda for programmes and interventions.

Rigorously researched, the book conveys the complexities required of solid research and dispels any misconceptions that research on reproductive tract infection and other gynaecological disorders is simple, quick or easy to conduct. It is clear that this volume is not intended to be an introductory research text. Rather, it is intended for those with formal training in the social, bio-medical or epidemiological sciences and for those who are experienced in the conduct of health research and are interested in engaging in multidisciplinary research on women's health.

The volume clearly represents a new and important contribution to a rapidly-growing field. It appears at a time when the field of sexual and reproductive health is asking new and difficult questions on factors underlying risk behaviours that require explanations that go beyond the confines of a single discipline. It provides researchers the tools with which to obtain sound estimates of the health burden that reproductive tract infections and other gynaecological disorders impose on women in resource-poor settings, to interpret estimates from different sources of data, and to explore the factors underlying these reproductive ill health conditions and the ways in which the experience of them impinges on women's lives.

The 28 authors bring together a range of strengths and experiences that have been synthesized into a cogent and instructive, elegantly and clearly written discourse on approaches to studying this topic. *Investigating Reproductive Tract Infections and Other Gynaecological Disorders* is essential reading for researchers interested in measuring and explaining women's gynaecological morbidity. I am confident that the volume will contribute to a generation of new and sound information on the measurement of reproductive tract infections, and on explanations of reproductive choice, risk and protection, gender relations, obstacles to timely care and other critical areas related to women's health and disease.

Paul F.A. Van Look

Acknowledgements

The need to review research approaches to the study of reproductive tract infections and other gynaecological disorders among women in developing countries is evident. Despite the considerable interest in conducting research on this topic, questions arose concerning the ideal study – topics that needed to be addressed, appropriate designs and community engagement, the kinds of clinical and laboratory examinations required, ways of interpreting findings from different sources of data and implications for programmes and policies. It was the need to address these questions that culminated in this multidisciplinary effort.

This work would have been impossible without the insights, co-operation and support of many.

Iqbal Shah, Senior Social Scientist and Paul Van Look, Director, Department of Reproductive Health and Research, World Health Organisation (Geneva) have been pivotal in this endeavour. They responded enthusiastically to the idea of assembling a consultative group, documenting research approaches, and basing this project at the World Health Organization (WHO) in Geneva. We owe them a special debt of gratitude for this and for their valuable guidance and insights in shaping the volume both in terms of its content and its implementation.

We are also grateful to them and other members of an informal working group at WHO – Olusola Ayeni, Sarah Bott, Jane Cottingham, Catherine d'Arcangues, Olav Meirik, Denise Roth – who provided valuable input at the formative stage of the project. Many colleagues and friends, all over the world, have given of their time peer reviewing and discussing various chapters of this volume. Their insights and comments, incorporated in the text, have helped shape the focus of the book and have enriched the comprehensiveness of many chapters. We are especially grateful to Ties Boerma, Isabelle DeZoysa, Judith Fortney, Michael Mbizvo, Olav Meirik, Paddy Rowe, Sagri Singh, Iqbal Shah and Kathryn Yount for their valuable comments and suggestions.

The administrative requirements attached to the production of a volume with 15 chapters and 28 contributors cannot be underestimated, and the assistance of Nicky Sabatini-Fox, Corinne Penhale and Maud Keizer in facilitating this is gratefully acknowledged. We are particularly indebted to Nicky Sabatini-Fox, who has been the backbone of this project, and has so ably co-ordinated its various phases, responding to concerns raised by editors, authors and management, and preparing many versions of the typescript.

Turning the collection of papers into a book required attention from many. We are grateful to Raju Khanna for his advice and assistance in securing this publication; to Deepika Ganju for her significant editorial contributions and careful attention to detail, which have made the volume more readable and precise; and to the publication team at CUP who so ably and painstakingly expedited its publication.

This project could not have been conducted without the generous financial support from three organisations: the Ford Foundation (New Delhi), the Rockefeller Foundation (New York) and the UNDP/UNFPA/WHO/World Bank Special Programme of Research, Development and Research Training in Human Reproduction (HRP), Department of Reproductive Health and Research, World Health Organization (Geneva) which housed the project. The support of these three organizations is gratefully acknowledged.

Finally, we are grateful to the authors themselves for agreeing to take on this ambitious project, and for responding so amiably to a host of requests, from incorporating suggestions from peer reviews on their own contributions to providing peer reviews of those of colleagues.

Shireen Jejeebhoy
Michael Koenig
Christopher Elias

Introduction and overview

Shireen Jejeebhoy,[1] Michael Koenig[2] and Christopher Elias[3]

[1] The Population Council, New Delhi, India; [2] Johns Hopkins University, Baltimore, USA; [3] PATH, Seattle, USA

Objectives

Since the late 1980s, several studies have highlighted the widespread prevalence of reproductive tract infections and gynaecological morbidities within community settings. Studies have been carried out in Egypt (Younis et al., 1993; Zurayk et al., 1995), India (Bang et al., 1989; Bhatia et al., 1997; Latha et al., 1997; Oomman, 1996), Nigeria (Brabin et al., 1995), Bangladesh (Wasserheit et al., 1989; Hawkes, 2002) and Turkey (Bulut et al., 1997), among others. These findings have spurred a great deal of interest among the research and NGO (non-governmental organizations) communities on the prevalence, correlates and consequences of reproductive tract infections, and gynaecological morbidity more generally, using both self-reported as well as clinically diagnosed and laboratory detected measures of morbidity.

The experience of studies so far has also raised a variety of methodological concerns and complexities, and offers a rich source of methodological lessons for future work (Koenig et al., 1998). These lessons become especially important to document in the light of the rapidly expanding number of ongoing or planned research studies on the prevalence and correlates of reproductive tract infections or gynaecological morbidities. Substantial sums of money are likely to be invested in the coming years in knowledge, attitudes and practice (KAP) surveys of reproductive tract infections, both by large investigations such as the Demographic and Health Surveys, and by smaller in-country investigations.

The objective of this volume is to draw upon this considerable experience in order to provide a synthesis of research approaches to the study of reproductive tract infections and other gynaecological disorders. Recognizing the multidisciplinary nature of any investigation on women's reproductive morbidity, contributors to this volume come from different disciplines, with representation from the social, biomedical and statistical spheres. In synthesizing approaches, the volume focuses not only on defining reproductive tract infections and other gynaecological morbidities that are usually studied, and ways of measuring their prevalence, but also provides a conceptual framework for the study of behavioural determinants and consequences for women's lives, and for future explorations of the role of men; methodological approaches for the study of self-reported, clinically diagnosed and laboratory detected morbidities; and analytical approaches to the synthesis and interpretation of data from a multitude of sources (qualitative and quantitative, clinical and laboratory). Finally, the volume draws out implications arising from the emerging research agenda for programmes and interventions.

Priority areas covered

This volume begins by defining the gynaecological morbidities that can be studied by the approaches discussed herein. As indicated by van de Wijgert and Elias (Chapter 2), these cover a variety of conditions such as reproductive tract infections (including those that are sexually transmitted, endogenous and iatrogenic). It also includes gynaecological cancers, endocrine disorders, genital prolapse, infertility, sexual dysfunction and menopausal symptoms. Their chapter defines each of these, including the symptoms that most often characterize them for those conditions that are not asymptomatic.

Several critical methodological issues are raised that must be addressed in any future studies.

Social and contextual influences: building a framework for analysis

The primary objective of studies thus far has been to estimate the prevalence of gynaecological morbidity within the communities studied. Comparatively less emphasis has been placed on understanding the social, behavioural and biomedical antecedents of such morbidity. In particular, the roles of potentially key but difficult-to-research determinants, such as sexual behaviour and practice, and iatrogenic factors, such as unsafe abortion and delivery practices, in influencing women's vulnerability to gynaecological morbidity, remain largely unexplored.

Jejeebhoy and Koenig (Chapter 3) provide, on the basis of an extensive review of the available literature, a conceptual framework describing immediate and background determinants of morbidity and health seeking. They also shed light on what is known about the consequences and implications of gynaecological morbidity for women's daily lives. Their review addresses how such morbidity impacts women's ability to fulfil a diverse and wide range of expected domestic and familial roles – economic productivity, domestic responsibilities, marital and sexual relationships – as well as on their own mental health and psychological well-being.

Also highlighted by Hawkes and Hart (Chapter 4) is the role of male partners, in terms of their own sexual and reproductive health, their importance as a source of transmission of sexually transmitted infection to other partners and their role in assisting or impeding women's ability to address and resolve reproductive health problems.

Study approaches: community-based studies and alternatives

Several approaches can be considered for studying reproductive tract infections and other gynaecological morbidities. Community-based studies, discussed by Zurayk (Chapter 5), have most commonly been used. Zurayk explains that these studies generally involve simultaneous consideration of self-reported experiences, as well as findings from clinical and laboratory examinations, and are preferred, clearly, for their representative samples. However, as Zurayk cautions, conducting such studies is generally complex and expensive. Community-based studies, for instance, generally require a multitude of data collection methods – qualitative and quantitative assessments of symptoms, correlates and consequences, along with clinical and laboratory investigations. Significant sample loss and self-selection because of women's refusal or reluctance to undergo clinical examination represent serious methodological problems in community-based studies of gynaecological morbidity. The significant sample loss experienced in many studies for the clinical component occurs for a number of reasons, including negative community attitudes, especially among husbands, and cultural sensitivity regarding gynaecological examination. By far the most significant reason for non-compliance, however, is that women who have no apparent symptoms of reproductive morbidity are unwilling to consent to a clinical examination. These results suggest that the overall prevalence of gynaecological morbidity may be biased upward as a result of sample selectivity, with the bias most pronounced in studies with higher rates of sample loss.

Given the frequently formidable challenges faced by community-based studies of reproductive tract infections, as outlined by Koenig and Shepherd (Chapter 6), alternative study designs may frequently need to be considered. The authors review studies that have used various facility based samples – women seeking sterilization services, women attending family planning clinics or those attending facilities for other non-gynaecological reasons – and discuss the relative advantages and disadvantages of studies using these designs.

Fostering close interaction with the community

As contributions from Khattab, Bang and Bang, and Serwadda and Wawer (Chapter 7) underscore, a high level of community rapport and interaction is essential for studies of this nature. One way of achieving this is by conducting the studies in co-ordination with voluntary organizations with a long-standing record of service to the communities. Even so, careful and exhaustive preparatory efforts and engagement with communities are nonetheless required in order for researchers to gain community cooperation and active support. Given the asymmetric nature of gender relations in many settings, convincing male community and family members of the rationale and need for such studies assumes paramount importance in successfully enlisting the participation of women.

In a number of settings, it will be necessary to include appropriate medical treatment or referral to respondents as a component of the study, since for many women this may represent the only opportunity to address their reproductive health problems. The inclusion of medical treatment as a component of the study of women's reproductive health problems may be a prerequisite in settings where few poor women have access to high-quality gynaecological care. This is important not only from an ethical perspective, but also to enlist women's cooperation and participation in studies of this nature. It is unlikely that many women would willingly acknowledge sensitive problems or agree to submit to what for many constitutes an invasive and embarrassing examination, if effective treatment was not provided.

Methodologies for clinical and laboratory components of studies

An additional source of variability, which may have contributed to widely divergent estimates of clinically diagnosed morbidity, is the lack of consistency across studies in clinicians' diagnoses of gynaecological morbidity. Elias, Low and Hawkes (Chapter 8) discuss the limitations of defining and observing reproductive tract morbidity in community-based research, and make recommendations for future practice. Their chapter illustrates the problems of inter-observer variation and variation in diagnostic criteria across studies. It also underscores the importance of using standardized definitions of clinically diagnosed morbidity, and proposes a core set of terms and definitions that are both well-supported by evidence from the literature and readily applied in clinical practice. Moreover, given the lack of consistent correlation between clinically diagnosed morbidity and the presence of laboratory diagnosed reproductive tract infections, it is important that laboratory testing is included for a core group of reproductive tract pathogens, and that it be considered an essential component of all community-based studies of gynaecological morbidity.

Laboratory testing has faced a variety of difficulties, including difficulties of diagnosis, women's reluctance to undergo pelvic examinations, the consequent selectivity of the populations studied and the requirement of sophisticated laboratory facilities which is unrealistic in most resource-poor settings. Kuypers and WHO Regional Office for the Western Pacific (Chapter 9) summarize feasible laboratory methods that are useful for the detection of 11 reproductive tract infections using sophisticated molecular biology techniques. Their chapter highlights that not all organisms can be detected using all types of assays, nor can all laboratories perform all types of assays. For each organism discussed, a table is provided that describes the sensitivity and specificity, the advantages and disadvantages, and the appropriate level of use of each method. The chapter provides a technical overview of the kinds of tests that can be performed in existing laboratory facilities in resource-poor settings. A major disadvantage is that the biological samples required can only be obtained through genital and/or pelvic examination.

The recent development of new diagnostic technologies has enabled researchers to bypass the requirement of pelvic examination and has greatly enhanced the feasibility of conducting field studies of sexually transmitted infections, reproductive tract infections and other selected reproductive conditions. Meehan, Wawer, Serwadda, Gray and Quinn (Chapter 10) describe these new technologies. A major advantage is that many of these methods avoid provider-dependent specimen collection (urine, self-administered vaginal swabs) permitting application in diverse settings, including the home. While these tests have been successfully administered in selected research studies, notably by the authors, their wider use is currently constrained by the need for sophisticated laboratory facilities and by cost. The authors note, however, that costs are likely to decline over time, as is the complexity of some assay techniques.

Approaches for exploring women's perceptions and experiences

Cleland and Harlow (Chapter 11) and Oomman and Gittlesohn (Chapter 12) discuss quantitative and qualitative approaches for exploring women's perceptions and experiences of gynaecological morbidity, respectively. As Oomman and Gittlesohn indicate, in-depth qualitative research is critical for several reasons. It enables a better understanding of women's perceptions of morbidity, and local terms and expressions used to describe gynaecological complaints; such an understanding enables investigators to pick up the subtle and more indirect ways in which women describe some gynaecological problems. In-depth research also allows the investigator to explore women's attitudes to discussing or revealing certain kinds of morbidities, and provides an idea of morbidities that are likely to be underreported by a single question in conventional surveys; as well as beliefs regarding the causes of morbidity, the types of treatment considered appropriate for different reproductive health problems, treatment-seeking decision-making and behaviour, and their consequences for women's lives. And, finally, it offers the opportunity to corroborate the findings obtained from standard survey techniques on the magnitude of various gynaecological morbidities. The chapter also highlights the importance of triangulation (the use of different techniques to collect information on the same topic), iteration (a sequence of activities in which each informs the next), flexibility and contextualization (detailed analysis of the social setting in which the study takes place), and outlines a methodologically rigorous and systematic use of qualitative methods to investigate specific dimensions of gynaecological morbidity.

Cleland and Harlow focus on appropriate designs for survey research, and the need for framing questions that are specific. They include detailed probing and address issues of severity. Such a focus can address many of the significant response biases, which may lead women to underreport or overreport actual morbidity. For example, underreporting of gynaecological morbidity can result from the widespread perception among many women that such conditions are normal, and therefore merit neither acknowledgement nor complaint. In the light of this, special efforts are required to elicit such information from women. Questions need to be specific, and they need to probe beyond respondents' initial responses in ascertaining the true extent of gynaecological morbidity among women. At the same time, poorly framed questions can lead to the possibility of overreporting of some gynaecological morbidities. One reason for this is the effect of omitting questions on severity when querying about morbidity. A more general and problematic issue is that questions have often tended to be vague and open to subjective interpretation – for example, 'scanty' periods or 'excessive/abnormal' vaginal discharge. A serious concern in many studies is the omission of direct questions on severity, on the level of discomfort or pain, and on the extent to which reported morbidity interfered with women's daily routines and responsibilities. The authors present specific case studies on the application of survey research methods to the study of vaginal discharge and menstrual problems.

Integrating findings from multiple sources of information

The various approaches described for the study of reproductive tract infections and other gynaecological morbidities is likely to generate a vast amount of data drawn from a variety of sources. Two chapters in this volume address the ways in which these data can be analysed and interpreted. Pelto and Cleland (Chapter 13) examine the ways in which qualitative and quantitative methods have been used together in reproductive health research. A variety of approaches to integrating qualitative and quantitative data are outlined, ranging from qualitative and quantitative approaches used in a single instrument to designs that field a qualitative component preceding and following a survey. The chapter outlines the ways in which data from these different approaches have been analysed and the ways in which the triangulation of different types of data can be effectively presented and interpreted.

Marshall, Filippi, Meheus and Bulut (Chapter 14) explore the ways in which morbidity drawn from different sources – self-reports, clinical examination and laboratory testing – can be interpreted. This chapter points out that findings from these three sources of data are often inconsistent. They highlight that only in exceptional circumstances is there likely to be a good fit between self-reported and medically diagnosed morbidities, and that sensitivity and specificity are generally low. Their chapter concludes that illness and disease – as reflected in self-reported and medically diagnosed conditions – should always be considered as logically separate. The measurement of each should be separately considered, and the findings, collectively, interpreted as complementary approaches to understanding reproductive health.

Drawing the links from research to action

The final chapter, by Dixon-Mueller (Chapter 15), highlights the relevance of studies measuring gynaecological morbidity and its causes and consequences, for informing programmes and policies and turning research into action. She reiterates six basic needs that can be satisfied by the research arising from this volume. They can: assist in prioritizing prevention and control of reproductive tract infections in public health agendas; direct programmes on the need to integrate information, screening and services into ongoing programmes already serving women, and highlight mechanisms of doing so; point out lacunae in provider skills and argue for increasing investments in training, supervision and basic supplies; argue for increased attention to partner notification and services in sexually transmitted infection programmes; enhance understanding of behavioural factors promoting infection and devise cost-effective and culturally acceptable interventions; and suggest modifications in multiple sectors to enable women and men to protect their sexual and reproductive health. Dixon-Mueller argues that while researchers need not play the role of activists, it is their responsibility to disseminate their findings in ways that can act as tools for action, that are accessible to the broader community of health care providers, educational institutions, the media and policy makers and programme administrators, and that make succinct and practical suggestions for action.

Findings can be turned into action in a variety of ways. They can feed into training materials for providers at various levels – materials can extend, if appropriate, to guidelines for diagnosis and testing, for taking medical histories and assessing risk behaviours, counselling and so on – ideally including both technical and social aspects of service delivery. Secondly, findings can be translated into locally relevant information materials for outreach workers and community members – research findings can inform the development of these materials, for example, by identifying locally relevant terminology and ways of discussing sensitive topics, as well as by suggesting how best to impart information (on symptom recognition, signs or consequences of infection) and identifying and dispelling common misperceptions or fears of treatment. Thirdly, the media are another effective way of transmitting research findings, whether it is the print media that can expose educated and urban populations to the topic, or local entertainment mechanisms for harder to reach groups. Fourthly, findings can feed sexuality education and group counselling forums in schools, workplaces and other settings in which women and men gather.

Finally, findings must reach governments in order that a positive policy and programme environment for addressing women's reproductive tract infections and gynaecological morbidity can be created. In short, well-conducted research must be well-disseminated, and its messages tailored to meet the needs of the diverse actors that are required in the prevention and treatment of reproductive tract infections and other gynaecological morbidity.

Lessons learned

The chapters in this volume offer a number of insights for researchers. Above all, they reiterate the complexity involved in conducting community-based studies of reproductive tract infections and other gynaecological morbidity, and suggest that such studies be conducted infrequently, using multidisciplinary research teams, and only when financial and infrastructural resources are in place. Other lessons emerging from this volume include:

- It is imperative that studies go beyond documenting morbidity prevalence and focus equally on proximate and background factors placing women at risk of acquiring such morbidity; treatment seeking behaviours adopted by women and the constraints they face in acquiring appropriate and timely care; and if possible, the consequences for women's lives.
- The association between self-reported, clinically diagnosed and laboratory tested morbidity remains poor, and studies limited to self-reported morbidity need to recognize the limitations of their findings. Such studies need to focus on potential risk factors, behaviours exposing women to risk of morbidity and health seeking behaviours of women experiencing a morbidity.
- Careful planning is required for the effective conduct of such studies, and it is inadvisable to consider a community-based study if the percentage of sample women expected to comply with clinical and laboratory examinations is below 75.
- Where community-based studies are not feasible, alternative study designs need to be explored – notably those drawing their samples from among women attending health facilities for family planning or other health services.
- Study designs need to be imaginative. Qualitative designs continue to provide depth on women's perceptions and experiences of morbidity and health seeking, but ideally they must be pursued using such methods as triangulation, contextualization and iteration. Survey methods, on the other hand, are central in providing estimates of the prevalence of women's perceived illness, and probing the kinds of symptoms experienced, treatments sought and obstacles faced.
- Finally, the volume points to the ethical imperative of involving communities in studies of reproductive tract infections and other gynaecological morbidity. Since

poor women the world over have few opportunities to undergo gynaecological investigations in their lives, participation in a research project on the topic should provide women, as far as possible, with opportunities for treatment or referral, and for information on behaviours facilitating prevention.

Studies of reproductive tract infections and other gynaecological morbidities thus far have yielded widely varying prevalence rates. The different methodologies employed and the varying quality of approaches used has led many to question the magnitude of the problem suggested in several studies. This volume seeks to contribute to a more uniform and rigorous approach to the study of reproductive tract infections and other gynaecological morbidities, and lay out the kinds of limitations and complexities implied in research on this topic. More precise and detailed information on cause-specific gynaecological morbidity would go a long way in convincing governments of the need to integrate services relating to gynaecological morbidity into primary health care agendas, shaping programmes that enable women to overcome barriers in accessing care, and outlining misperceptions that need to be dispelled and appropriate and acceptable messages that raise awareness of prevention and promotion among women and communities more generally. The contribution of this volume is in providing research approaches to the study of reproductive tract infections and other gynaecological disorders that are robust enough to enable meaningful programmatic and policy responses.

REFERENCES

Bang RA, Bang AT, Baitule M et al. (1989) High prevalence of gynaecological diseases in rural Indian women. *Lancet*, 1(8629): 85–87.

Bhatia JC, Cleland J, Bhagavan L et al. (1997) Gynaecological morbidity in south India. *Studies in family planning*, **28**(2): 95–103.

Brabin L, Kemp J, Obunge OK et al. (1995) Reproductive tract infections and abortion among adolescent girls in rural Nigeria. *Lancet*, **345**(8945): 300–304.

Bulut A, Filippi V, Marshall T et al. (1997) Contraceptive choice and reproductive morbidity in Istanbul. *Studies in family planning*, **28**(1): 35–43.

Hawkes S, Morison L, Chakraborty J et al. (2002). Reproductive tract infections: prevalence and risk factors in rural Bangladesh. *Bulletin of the World Health Organization*, **80**(3): 180–188.

Koenig M, Jejeebhoy S, Singh S et al. (1998) Investigating gynaecological morbidity in India: not just another KAP survey. *Reproductive health matters*, **6**(11): 84–97.

Latha K, Kanani SJ, Maitra N et al. (1997) Prevalence of clinically detectable gynaecological morbidity in India: results of four community-based studies. *Journal of family welfare*, **43**(4): 8–16.

Oomman NM (1996) *Poverty and Pathology: Comparing rural Rajasthani women's ethnomedical models with biomedical models of reproductive behaviour.* Ph.D. Thesis, Johns Hopkins University.

Wasserheit JN, Harris JR, Chakraborty J et al. (1989) Reproductive tract infections in a family planning population in rural Bangladesh. *Studies in family planning*, **20**(2): 69–80.

Younis N, Khattab H, Zurayk H et al. (1993) A community study of gynaecological and related morbidities in rural Egypt. *Studies in family planning*, **24**(3): 175–186.

Zurayk H, Khattab H, Younis N et al. (1995) Comparing women's reports with medical diagnoses of reproductive morbidity conditions in rural Egypt. *Studies in family planning*, **26**(1): 14–21.

2

Defining reproductive tract infections and other gynaecological morbidities

Janneke van de Wijgert[1] and Christopher Elias[2]

[1] Population Council, New York, USA; [2] PATH, Seattle, USA

The 1994 United Nations International Conference on Population and Development (ICPD) stressed the importance of women's health, and reproductive health in particular, to stabilize population growth and promote sustainable development (United Nations, 1994). A rights-based approach to sexual and reproductive health was adopted, which was re-affirmed and extended at the Fourth World Conference on Women in Beijing in 1995, and again at the ICPD + 5 review in 1999. In line with the ICPD Programme of Action, many governments and organizations have expanded their activities in women's health in recent years. In addition to fertility regulation and child survival, a growing number of research agendas now include maternal health, reproductive tract infections, adolescent reproductive health, harmful traditional practices (such as female genital cutting), unsafe abortion and violence against women.

In the ICPD Programme of Action, reproductive health is defined as 'a state of complete physical, mental and social well-being and not merely the absence of disease or infirmity, in all matters relating to the reproductive system and to its functions and processes.' It explicitly includes sexual health, which is defined as 'the enhancement of life and personal relations, not merely counselling and care related to reproduction and sexually transmitted diseases' (United Nations, 1994: 45, 46). These definitions are far broader than the World Health Organization (WHO) definition of reproductive morbidity, discussed later in this chapter (World Health Organization, 1990). For the first time, governments and organizations agreed to go beyond the narrow emphasis of women as mothers, and include gender issues and sexuality during the various stages of women's lives as important components of reproductive health.

To address this new agenda in reproductive health, much research is needed to fill information gaps in the areas of women's health that have been neglected in the past. One such area is gynaecological morbidity. While HIV/AIDS and other sexually transmitted infections (STIs) have received much attention since the advent of the AIDS pandemic, the importance of research on other gynaecological and sexual health problems is only slowly gaining international recognition. Approximately 30 population-based studies since the late 1980s have shown that many women worldwide have gynaecological problems (reviewed in Chapter 8), but that a 'culture of silence' surrounds their suffering (Dixon-Mueller and Wasserheit, 1991; Khattab, 1992). Additional population-based studies (as opposed to clinic-based studies) are needed to document the prevalence of gynaecological morbidity in communities that have not yet been studied, to explore the determinants and social context of disease, and to collect background information for the design and evaluation of community-based interventions aimed at improving the quality of women's lives. In this book, researchers share what they have learned from implementing population-based studies on gynaecological morbidity in developing countries, and what they consider to be current research priorities. This chapter provides a framework by defining the different types of morbidity that can occur among women.

Defining women's morbidity

Morbidity has been defined as a 'diseased condition or state', or the 'incidence of disease in a population' (Academic Medical Publishing, 1997). Although the definition of morbidity is much narrower than the earlier definition of health, it makes morbidity more measurable and amenable to intervention than health. Frequently used concepts to measure morbidity are: the occurrence of a disease condition or symptoms of a disease condition, impairment, disability or handicap; and perceptions of ill health and quality of life (see Chapters 5 and 14). Other morbidity dimensions that may be measured include severity of the condition, duration, time of onset, accumulation and sequelae of specific conditions, demographic, behavioural and other risk factors for morbidity, and the social context in which the morbidity occurs (see Chapter 3).

Women's morbidity includes all morbidity afflicting women, and is often categorized as reproductive or non-reproductive (Fortney, 1995). Reproductive morbidity refers to diseases that affect the reproductive system, although not necessarily as a consequence of reproduction. Non-reproductive morbidity refers to all other categories of disease, including diseases that afflict only women, diseases that affect women differentially compared to men because of differences in exposure, susceptibility, treatment and consequences, and diseases that afflict both women and men.

Reproductive morbidity can be subdivided into obstetric/maternal morbidity, gynaecological morbidity and contraceptive morbidity (see Figure 2.1). WHO has defined these categories as follows: *obstetric morbidity* – morbidity in a woman (who has been pregnant, regardless of the site or duration of the pregnancy) from

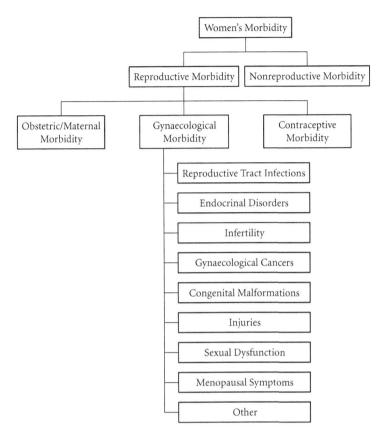

Figure 2.1   Types of morbidity in women.

any cause related to or aggravated by the pregnancy or its management, but not from accidental or incidental causes; *gynaecological morbidity* – any condition, disease or dysfunction of the reproductive system that is not related to pregnancy, abortion or childbirth, but may be related to sexual behaviour; *contraceptive morbidity* – conditions that result from efforts (other than abortion) to limit fertility, whether they are traditional or modern methods (World Health Organization, 1990).

Each of the three categories of reproductive morbidity can be further subdivided. As this volume focuses on gynaecological morbidity, subdivisions of only this category are listed in Figure 2.1. These include, for example, reproductive tract infections, endocrinal (hormonal) disorders, infertility, gynaecological cancers, congenital malformations or birth defects, injuries, sexual dysfunction and menopausal symptoms (Fortney, 1995). As will become clear, there is considerable overlap between the subcategories of gynaecological morbidity, obstetric/maternal morbidity and contraceptive morbidity. Infertility, for example, can have an obstetric cause, but could also be the result of a sexually transmitted disease, endocrinal disorder or congenital malformation. While the guidelines in this volume are useful for the study of most gynaecological morbidities, they focus on reproductive tract infections, endocrinal disorders, infertility and two common conditions that are generally classified as obstetric morbidity (genitourinary prolapse and vesicovaginal fistulae).

Reproductive tract infections

Reproductive tract infections refer to three different types of infections that affect the reproductive tract: sexually transmitted infections caused by viruses, bacteria or other microorganisms that are transmitted through sexual activity with an infected partner; endogenous infections that result from an overgrowth of organisms normally present in the vagina; and iatrogenic infections that are caused by the introduction of microorganisms into the reproductive tract through a medical procedure (see Figure 2.2). In addition, reproductive tract infections are often categorized according to the site of infection. Infections that cause inflammation of the external genital area and lower reproductive tract in women are referred to as vulvovaginitis or vaginitis, inflammation of the cervix as cervicitis,[1] and infection of the upper reproductive tract as pelvic inflammatory disease (PID). Vaginal infection is most commonly caused by endogenous infections (such as candidiasis or bacterial vaginosis) but can also be caused by certain STIs (such as trichomoniasis). Cervical infection is most commonly caused by STIs (such as gonorrhoea and chlamydia), but can be caused by a variety of pathogens. Both vaginal and cervical infections can spread to the upper reproductive tract, but cervical infections are more prone to such progression (Cates, Rolfs and Aral, 1990). Transcervical procedures (such as menstrual regulation, abortion and the insertion of intrauterine devices – IUDs) may facilitate infection of the upper reproductive tract.

The significance and prevalence of reproductive tract infections among women in the third world was first documented in the late 1980s (Dixon-Mueller and Wasserheit, 1991; Wasserheit, 1989). An exhaustive review of the available literature showed that reproductive tract infections were common among women who were not acknowledged sex workers in almost all developing countries where data were available, even in asymptomatic populations (Wasserheit, 1989). Prevalence was higher in African populations than those of Asia and Latin America, but there were no consistent prevalence patterns across countries, or even within the same continent. These early findings have been confirmed in subsequent studies (see, for

---

[1] For a full discussion see Chapter 8. The term cervicitis is increasingly falling out of favour because it has often been used in reference to conditions that do not necessarily indicate cervical infection, including common normal physiological variants.

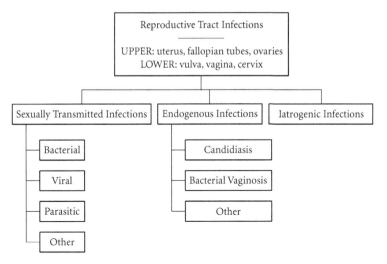

Figure 2.2   Reproductive tract infections.

example, Haberland et al., 1999). Women with lower reproductive tract infections experience considerable physical symptoms and emotional distress, but the potential spread of these infections to the upper reproductive tract, other long-term consequences, and the synergy between reproductive tract and HIV infections are even more worrisome. As will be discussed later, HIV/AIDS, PID and cervical cancer are major causes of severe morbidity and mortality among women in developing countries.

Sexually transmitted infections

These are caused by viruses, bacteria and other microorganisms (over 30 different organisms in all) that are transmitted sexually, and can enter a person's urethra, vagina, mouth or anus. The basic characteristics of the most common STIs are listed in Table 2.1. STIs can cause a wide variety of symptoms (including genital ulcers, genital warts, abnormal genital tract discharge and pelvic pain), but are often asymptomatic. Long-term sequelae include infertility in both men and women, cervical cancer, ectopic pregnancy, spontaneous abortion, premature rupture of membranes, premature delivery and consequent low birth weight, neonatal blindness and infection, and death (Morse, Moreland and Holmes, 1996). The social, psychological and economic consequences of sexually transmitted infections are often devastating (see Dallabetta et al., 1996; Population Council, 1999). While STIs caused by bacterial and protozoal agents have been curable by appropriate antibiotics and chemotherapeutic agents for more than 40 years (Table 2.1), viral STIs at present cannot be cured.

According to WHO estimates, there are over 340 million new cases of curable

Table 2.1. Basic characteristics of some prevalent sexually transmitted infections

Sexually transmitted infection	Microorganism	Symptoms & signs in women	Symptoms & signs in men	Cure?	Consequences if untreated
Trichomoniasis	Protozoa	Vaginitis Foamy discharge with fishy odour	Watery, white or greenish fluid from penis Discomfort during urination Often no symptoms	Yes	**Neonatal complications:** premature delivery low birth rate
Gonorrhoea	Bacteria	Greenish/yellow discharge with unpleasant odour Frequent/uncomfortable urination Cervical infection Urethral infection Bartholin's abscess Often no symptoms	Pain during urination Pus-like discharge from penis Occasionally no symptoms	Yes	Pelvic inflammatory disease Infertility in men and women **Maternal–fetal complications:** premature rupture of membranes premature delivery potentially blinding neonatal conjunctivitis
Chlamydia	Bacteria	Cervical infection Urethral infection Frequent/painful urination Bartholinitis Majority are asymptomatic	Pain during urination Pus-like discharge from penis Often no symptoms	Yes	Pelvic inflammatory disease Peri-hepatitis **Neonatal complications:** conjunctivitis pneumonia
Syphilis	Bacteria	**Primary:** painless ulcers at site of inoculation (genital area, rectum, mouth) **Secondary:** 4–8 weeks after ulcers, generalized lesions on skin and mucous membranes, fever, malaise **Latent:** no symptoms or signs; tertiary syphilis will develop in about a third of untreated cases and has numerous systemic manifestations.		Yes	**Late complications:** neurological problems that can lead to paralysis and blindness; cardiovascular disease; severe lesions in skin, mucous membranes, bones, viscera; death **Maternal–fetal complications:** stillbirth; congenital syphilis

Chancroid	Bacteria	Soft, painful sore on vagina, penis or anus Swollen lymph glands in groin area Women notice ulcer less often than men	Yes	Scarring, fibrosis Formation of fistula
Lymphogranuloma venereum (LGV)	Bacteria	Primary lesion (usually an ulcer) is mainly asymptomatic; large tender inguinal nodes	Yes	Inflammation and swelling of inguinal lymph nodes; nodes rupture and can ulcerate and suppurate
Herpes simplex virus	Virus	Recurrent episodes of painful blisters on vulva, vagina, penis or anus	No	Can be transmitted to neonates resulting in infection and death of infant
Hepatitis B	Virus	Acute infection; often no symptoms or signs	No (vaccine available)	Liver damage, sometimes leading to cancer after several decades; possible transmission to neonate
Human papilloma virus	Virus	Genital warts	No	Association with development of anogenital cancers, including cervical cancer
HIV/AIDS	Virus	Vulnerability to many opportunistic infections, especially tuberculosis	No	Prolonged illness and death; transmission to infant through pregnancy, delivery and breastfeeding in up to 40% of cases

Source: Adapted from Population Council (1999).

STIs each year (170 million cases of trichomoniasis, 89 million cases of chlamydia, 62 million cases of gonorrhoea, 12 million cases of syphilis and 7 million cases of chancroid) (WHO/UNAIDS, 1997). The largest absolute number of new infections are thought to occur in South and South east Asia (46 per cent), followed by sub-Saharan Africa (20 per cent), Latin America and the Caribbean (11 per cent). PID, which can be caused by chlamydia, gonorrhoea or bacterial vaginosis-associated organisms, has long been recognized as the major cause of morbidity and mortality among women in the Third World, and has been associated with severe long-term sequelae such as infertility, ectopic pregnancy and chronic pelvic pain (Muir and Belsey, 1980; Westrom, 1980).

Viral STIs for which no cure is available, constitute an even bigger problem. UNAIDS estimates that 40 million people were living with HIV and AIDS in December 2001 (of whom over 90 per cent were in developing countries), 5 million people were newly infected with HIV in 2001 and 20 million people had died of AIDS since the beginning of the epidemic (UNAIDS, 2001). Sub-Saharan Africa carries the major burden of HIV and AIDS, with close to 70 per cent of the global total of people living with HIV in this area. Herpes and papilloma virus infections are also believed to be common in developing countries, but population-based prevalence data are scarce (Bosch et al., 1995; Mindel, 1998).

It has been well documented that both ulcerative and non-ulcerative STIs greatly facilitate the transmission and acquisition of HIV (Cohen, 1998; Wasserheit, 1992). Recent evidence suggests that endogenous infections may also be associated with enhanced HIV transmission (Martin et al., 1999; Taha et al., 1998). A 1995 community-based randomized trial in Mwanza district, rural Tanzania shows that treating individuals for STIs using the syndromic approach reduced the incidence of HIV in the study population by 38 per cent (Grosskurth et al., 1995). Prevention and management of STIs have, therefore, become a critical strategy to minimize the impact of the HIV/AIDS pandemic.

Recommendations have been published for the prevention and control of STIs aimed at Ministry of Health officials in resource-poor countries (WHO/UNAIDS, 1997). Because so many STIs are undiagnosed or cannot be treated, primary prevention of their transmission is crucial, and should be integrated with related efforts for the primary prevention of HIV. Primary prevention strategies include reducing the exposure to sexually transmitted disease pathogens by promoting sexual abstinence and a delay in coital debut, and reducing the number of sexual partners and by having mutually monogamous relationships. It is also important to reduce the efficiency of transmission by promoting and enabling safer sex practices, such as non-penetrative sex and condom use. Secondary prevention, consisting of shortening the duration of infectivity by identification and prompt treatment of infected persons, should include the promotion of health care seeking behaviour, screening to identify asymptomatic infections, effective, accessible and acceptable clinical services, and support and counselling services, including partner notification.

STIs can be diagnosed clinically or by laboratory testing. Although the latter is most accurate, it is not feasible in many parts of the world. WHO and UNAIDS, therefore, recommend the adoption of syndromic diagnosis and treatment of STIs in resource-poor settings (World Health Organization, 1997; WHO/UNAIDS, 1997). Syndromic case management is based on classifying the main causative agents that give rise to a particular syndrome (genital ulcers in men and women, urethral discharge in men, vaginal discharge in women, and lower abdominal pain in women), using a combination of symptoms reported by the client and signs observed by the clinician. It then uses flowcharts that help the health care provider reach a diagnosis and decide on the treatment. The recommended treatment is effective for all the pathogens that could have caused the identified syndrome. The syndromic approach, sometimes in combination with risk scoring, has been tested and implemented in a variety of countries. It was found to be effective for genital ulcers in men and women and urethral discharge in men, but less effective for vaginal discharge (particularly the management of cervical infections) and lower abdominal pain in women (Dallabetta et al., 1996; Haberland et al., 1999). However, this method is not useful for identifying asymptomatic infections, which disproportionately affect women.

Although sufficient knowledge and expertise on HIV/AIDS and STIs have been gathered in the last decade to establish prevention and care interventions, further research is needed. For example, the search continues for effective vaccines and female-controlled methods of HIV/STI prevention, simple low-cost screening and diagnostic tests for STIs, less costly therapeutics, and optimum strategies for case-finding and targeting of services. Furthermore, interventions aimed at behaviour change, the syndromic case management approach, and integration of family planning and HIV/sexually transmitted disease management services must continue to be evaluated and improved.

Endogenous infections

The normal vaginal flora of healthy women of childbearing age is dominated by lactobacilli (Eschenbach et al., 1989). However, in the case of endogenous infections, an overgrowth of other organisms occurs. Candidiasis is caused by an overgrowth of the fungus *Candida*, often as a result of the recent use of antibiotics, the use of progesterone-containing oral contraceptives or immune suppression (Morse, Moreland and Holmes, 1996). There is no evidence that *Candida* is transmitted by sexual intercourse. Some women appear to be prone to candidiasis for reasons that are not well understood. Symptoms of candidiasis include thick, curd-like discharge, vulvovaginal inflammation and painful sexual intercourse.

Bacterial vaginosis is also an imbalance of the normal vaginal ecology and often results in an increase in vaginal pH (>4.5). Among women with bacterial vaginosis, the normally dominant lactobacilli are replaced by *Gardenerella vaginalis*, Gram-negative rods and *Peptostreptococcus* species. A homogeneous discharge and vaginal inflammation may be present, but bacterial vaginosis often remains asymptomatic. Its occurrence is associated with sexual activity (although it is not clearly sexually transmitted) (Hooton, Roberts and Stamm, 1994), IUD use (Cates and Stone, 1992), douching (Onderdonk et al., 1992) and the use of vaginal 'drying' or 'tightening' agents (van de Wijgert et al., 2000).

The diagnosis of bacterial vaginosis is usually made on the basis of a set of clinical criteria (the Amsel criteria) rather than the detection of the fore-mentioned organisms (Amsel et al., 1983). Since even experienced clinicians cannot often reliably distinguish between vaginal discharge caused by various organisms, and not all women with vaginal infections develop an abnormal discharge, microscopy can be used to aid in the diagnosis. *Candida* is best seen by adding potassium hydroxide to vaginal fluid on a glass slide, which is then viewed under a light microscope. Bacterial vaginosis is often characterized by the presence of clue cells (epithelial cells covered with bacterial vaginosis-associated microorganisms) on Gram stain (dried and stained vaginal fluid on a glass slide), or by scoring Gram stains according to the Nugent criteria (Nugent, Krohn and Hillier, 1991).

Worldwide, endogenous infections are the most common cause of reproductive tract infections among women. It has been estimated that approximately 75 per cent of all American women will experience at least one episode of vaginal candidiasis during their lifetime (National Institute of Allergy and Infectious Diseases, 1992). Studies in Zimbabwe, Malawi, Kenya and elsewhere in Africa suggest that up to 50 per cent of healthy African women have bacterial vaginosis or intermediate flora (Martin et al., 1999; Mason et al., 1989; Taha et al., 1998). Many women believe that the symptoms caused by vaginal infections are normal and part of the female experience and, consequently, do not seek care due to shame or lack of information. Furthermore, the discharge associated with endogenous infections is often misdiagnosed as discharge produced by STIs, such as trichomoniasis, gonorrhoea and chlamydia. Aggressive syndromic management of vaginal discharge may therefore result in considerable over-use of antibiotics, especially if women are routinely treated for suspected cervical infection.

Endogenous infections can be prevented by reducing risk behaviours (for example, avoiding vaginal douching, and using low-dose rather than high-dose oral contraceptive pills). These infections can be treated with oral antimicrobials or topical intravaginal creams. Although they are usually not sexually transmitted, male partners may experience some discomfort associated with candidiasis. Consequently, men are sometimes treated, mainly to prevent re-infection among women with frequent recurrence of this condition. If not treated, endogenous infections have the potential to cause severe complications, such as premature rupture of the membranes and premature birth during pregnancy (Morse, Moreland and Holmes, 1996). Bacterial vaginosis can lead to PID, and there is growing evidence that it is associated with increased heterosexual and perinatal transmission of HIV (Martin et al., 1999; Taha et al., 1998).

Iatrogenic infections

Iatrogenic reproductive tract infections are the result of bacteria being introduced into the normally sterile environment of the upper reproductive tract through a medical procedure, such as the insertion of an IUD, induced abortion or during delivery. Unsafe abortions are a particularly common cause of iatrogenic infections. According to WHO estimates, 20 million unsafe abortions take place every year (World Health Organization, 2000), of which the vast majority take place in developing countries. Complications occur after 10–50 per cent of unsafe abortions (Safe Motherhood Interagency Group, 1998). The causal bacteria either originate from improperly sterilized examination or medical instruments (such as vaginal specula) or from endogenous infections or STIs already present in the lower reproductive tract. Iatrogenic infections can involve the uterus, endometrium, fallopian tubes and ovaries, and can therefore result in very serious consequences. Warning symptoms include pain in the pelvic region, sudden high fever, chills, menstrual disturbances, unusual vaginal discharge and pain during intercourse.

Iatrogenic infections are preventable by improving the quality and accessibility of good medical services, including family planning and abortion services. When they do occur, they can often be successfully treated with antibiotics. Unfortunately, many such infections are treated only after they have already caused irreparable harm, such as scarring or blockage of the fallopian tubes, or severe tissue damage.

Endocrinal disorders and infertility

Endocrinal or hormonal disorders can affect several aspects of reproduction, from menstrual function to infertility. Menstrual disorders are frequently reported in studies on gynaecological morbidity, and include problems with the regularity, frequency, volume and duration of menstrual bleeding as well as painful menstruation and premenstrual syndrome (Bang et al., 1989; Bhatia and Cleland, 1995). Amenorrhoea, or the absence of menstruation, is a disturbing symptom for many women and a common reason for seeking care. Pregnancy must always be considered as a cause of amenorrhoea. In developing countries, it is also often associated with breastfeeding or the use of hormonal methods of contraception (such as DMPA injections). Other menstrual disorders include oligomenorrhoea (regular or irregular bleeding at intervals of more than 40 days), polymenorrhoea (regular or irregular bleeding at intervals of less than 22 days), menorrhagia (bleeding that is excessive in both amount and duration), intermenstrual bleeding (bleeding that occurs between regular menstrual periods), dysmenorrhoea (painful menstruation) and premenstrual syndrome (severe premenstrual symptoms during the luteal phase of the menstrual cycle). While most menstrual disorders are caused by hormonal dysfunction, other causes include adnexal and uterine cysts or masses, and infection of the endometrium.

Infertility can be caused by endocrinal disorders, long-term sequelae of STIs, puerperal sepsis, post-abortion sepsis and congenital malformations. It is estimated that 50–80 per cent of infertility in sub-Saharan Africa can be attributed to prior upper reproductive tract infections (Belsey, 1976), and between 1990 and 1995, that 60–80 million couples worldwide were infertile (World Health Organization, 2000). In many societies, the social and psychological consequences of infertility are severe. Infertility is, therefore, a component of many population-based studies of gynaecological morbidity (Bang et al., 1989; Klouman et al., 1997).

Genitourinary prolapse and vesicovaginal fistula

Genitourinary prolapse (the abnormal downward displacement of the vaginal walls or uterus from their normal anatomic position within the pelvis) and vesicovaginal fistula (an opening between the bladder and the vagina that causes urine leakage through the vagina) are classified as obstetric morbidity. However, they are often reported in population-based studies of gynaecological morbidity because they remain present in women after pregnancy and childbirth (Koenig et al., 1998; Younis et al., 1993). Both conditions are usually the direct result of multiple pregnancies and prolonged or obstructed labour. Vesicovaginal fistula can also be caused by crude attempts at induced abortion, female genital cutting and accidental injury during obstetric surgery (Bello, 1995; Jackson and Smith, 1997). These conditions, therefore, occur mostly in developing countries, where women have multiple pregnancies and inadequate access to good quality obstetric and abortion care.

Symptoms of genitourinary prolapse include feeling a lump within the vagina, coital difficulty (pain during sex, loss of vaginal sensation), constipation, backache, and if the prolapse resulted in kinking of the urethra, difficulty with urination and recurrent urinary tract infections (Jackson and Smith, 1997). Prolapse can be prevented by reducing the number of pregnancies, appropriate management of labour, and possibly by (postnatal) pelvic exercises and hormone replacement therapy (if the vaginal epithelium is atrophic). Mild prolapse is often asymptomatic and does not need treatment other than counselling. More severe cases can be managed with the treatment of exacerbating factors (such as chronic coughs), vaginal pessaries in the shape of a ring (to provide tissue support), oestrogen cream (to reduce discomfort and erosion) and surgical repair.

Women with vesicovaginal fistula suffer from urinary incontinence which, if not managed properly, causes a number of problems (Bello, 1995). This continuous urine leakage makes them vulnerable to urinary tract infection and chronic vulval skin irritation. Vesicovaginal fistula sometimes leads to a narrowing of the vagina, amenorrhoea and inability to carry a pregnancy to term. The social consequences are often severe. Many women with persistent vesicovaginal fistula lose their husbands and are outcasts in society because they smell. Vesicovaginal fistula can be prevented by reducing the number of pregnancies and abortions, appropriate management of labour, and avoiding female genital cutting. Treatment consists of surgical repair. The success of the repair depends on the extent of damage and duration of the condition before medical care was sought, but is generally successful.

Gynaecological cancers

Gynaecological cancers are cancers of the cervix, breast, endometrium, ovary, vagina, vulva and (rarely) the fallopian tube. Cervical cancer, commonly caused by HPV (human papillomavirus) subtypes 16, 18, 31, 33 and 35, is the most common cancer among women in the developing world and is often fatal if not diagnosed early (Bosch et al., 1995; Ponten et al., 1995). According to WHO estimates, there are 450 000 new cases of cervical cancer each year, of which some 80 per cent occur in developing countries (World Health Organization, 2000). Factors thought to be associated with increased risk of cervical cancer include young age at first sexual intercourse, multiple sexual partners, having a male partner who has multiple sexual partners, smoking, poor nutritional status, hormonal factors (such as delayed age at birth of first child) and the use of hormonal contraception (Ponten et al., 1995). Women who are infected with both HIV and HPV are more likely to develop cervical cancer than HIV-negative women (Cu-Uvin et al., 1996).

Primary prevention consists of reducing high-risk behaviours, particularly high-risk sexual behaviours. Secondary prevention consists of identification of pre-cancerous lesions and early treatment. Effective therapy is available and includes cautery, loop excision, cryotherapy, laser therapy, cone biopsy and hysterectomy. All procedures, with the exception of hysterectomy, can be performed in outpatient clinics, and cryotherapy does not necessarily require electricity. However, identifying women with pre-cancerous lesions in a timely fashion has proved to be difficult.

Ideally, screening should be performed every three years, which is not feasible in most resource-poor settings. Women who have mild dysplasia on screening should be re-screened after 6 months, and women with moderate to severe dysplasia should be referred to a gynaecologist.

Currently available screening methods include Papanicolaou (Pap) smears and visual inspection of the cervix with acetic acid (VIA) and, possibly, magnification (VIAM) (Nene et al., 1996; University of Zimbabwe/JHPIEGO Cervical Cancer Screening Project, 2000). Pap smears require trained cytotechnologists and pathologists, and there is often a delay between sample collection and reporting results. VIA, on the other hand, is fairly non-specific and may result in significant overtreatment. Research has recently been accelerated to identify effective, affordable and acceptable screening and treatment methods for pre-cancerous lesions in resource-poor settings (Cullins et al., 1999).

Other gynaecological morbidities

Congenital malformations

Congenital malformations, or birth defects of the genital organs, occur in almost infinite variations and are often not apparent until an adolescent fails to menstruate or a sexually active woman fails to conceive. They are usually not measured in studies of gynaecological morbidity because they are relatively rare, and often not recognized as a congenital malformation.

Injuries

This category includes injuries caused by traditional practices (such as female genital cutting), sexual abuse or accidents. Female genital cutting has been practised worldwide for a variety of reasons, including ensuring virginity, securing fertility, and securing the social and economic future of daughters. In a 1998 comprehensive review of the available data, it was estimated that as many as 137 million women in Africa had undergone some form of female genital cutting (Toubia and Izett, 1998). Complications of female genital cutting include haemorrhage, urinary tract infections, tetanus, fistula and infertility. Other traditional cultural practices that may harm women, even though they are often intended to benefit them, include traditional treatment of medical and social problems, and vaginal drying and tightening practices.

Recently, sexual abuse and violence against women have gained recognition as major causes of reproductive morbidity (Heise, Pitanguy and Germain, 1994). Statistics from around the world suggest that sexual coercion and domestic violence are common in the lives of women and girls. They not only cause physical injury and profound emotional trauma, but are also associated with other reproductive health problems (for example, many women will not confront a partner about his unsafe sexual behaviour for fear of abuse).

Sexual dysfunction

This can be caused by a wide variety of factors including infertility, childhood sexual abuse, rape, female genital cutting, fistula, genitourinary prolapse, vaginal infections, congenital malformations, adhesions from injuries or inconsiderate partners. Symptoms of sexual dysfunction that are sometimes measured in studies of gynaecological morbidity include dyspareunia (pain during sex), vaginismus (a painful spasmodic contraction of the vagina, often rendering penetration impossible) and frigidity (see, for example, Bang et al., 1989).

Menopausal symptoms

Menopausal symptoms include hormone-related gynaecological problems that occur during menopause, post-menopausal uterine bleeding and atrophic vaginitis (inflammation of the vaginal mucosa secondary to thinning and decreased lubrication of the vaginal walls, often caused by a decrease in oestrogen). However, the majority of women in studies of gynaecological morbidity in developing countries are of reproductive age (even when there is no age limit to study participation), and menopausal symptoms are therefore uncommon.

Other gynaecological morbidities

This broad category includes endometriosis, ovarian cysts, uterine fibroids, polyps, and non-inflammatory and inflammatory diseases of the pelvic organs not attributable to STIs (for example, female genital tuberculosis and genital tract schistosomiasis). While cervical ectopy (also referred to as cervical erosion or ectropion) is often reported as a gynaecological abnormality, many researchers and clinicians would argue that it is a normal physiological finding (see Chapter 8).

Interaction between gynaecological morbidity and family planning

Gynaecological morbidity and family planning interact in numerous ways. Symptoms of reproductive tract infections, for example, may be attributed to contraceptive methods and might thus change attitudes toward contraception. IUD insertion and tubal ligation may induce iatrogenic infections if implements are not properly sterilized, or induce PID if lower reproductive tract infections are present at the time of the procedure (Cates and Stone, 1992; Wasserheit et al., 1989). Hormonal contraceptives, particularly high-dose pills, may disturb the balance of the vaginal environment and cause endogenous infections (Haukkamaa et al., 1986). On the other hand, they may decrease the risk of PID (Cates and Stone,

1992). Research is ongoing to determine whether hormonal contraceptive methods are in any way associated with HIV transmission.

Unfortunately, the methods that best prevent pregnancy (hormonal methods, IUDs and sterilization) are not the same methods that best prevent transmission of STIs (male and female condoms). Dual protection (protection from both unwanted pregnancy and sexually transmitted infections, including HIV) can be achieved through, for example, the use of another contraceptive in conjunction with male or female condoms. An alternative is the use of condoms as the principal method of contraception, with the use of emergency contraception in the event of condom slippage or breakage. The interaction between gynaecological morbidity and family planning methods, strategies for dual protection and the development of new methods of HIV/sexually transmitted disease prevention (such as vaginal microbicides) will continue to be important areas of research in the next decade.

Studying gynaecological morbidity

Studies on gynaecological morbidity can be very broad and cover the entire category, or cover a subcategory (such as reproductive tract infections) or smaller subsets (such as bacterial vaginosis). Sometimes, related obstetric morbidity (such as genitourinary prolapse and vesicovaginal fistula), contraceptive and non-reproductive morbidities (such as anaemia, hypertension and urinary tract infections) are also measured (Younis et al., 1993). A researcher's perspective of the importance or usefulness of a category may differ from that of a health care provider or policy maker, and there may be good reasons to integrate categories rather than separate them. It is, however, important that researchers frame their questions carefully and define clearly what kind(s) of morbidity they are addressing.

REFERENCES

Academic Medical Publishing (1997) *The online medical dictionary*. London, Academic Medical Publishing and CancerWEB.

Amsel R, Totten PA, Spiegel CA et al. (1983) Nonspecific vaginitis: diagnostic criteria and microbial and epidemiologic associations. *American journal of medicine*, 74(1): 14–22.

Bang RA, Bang AT, Baitule M et al. (1989) High prevalence of gynaecological diseases in rural Indian women. *Lancet*, 1(8629): 85–88.

Bello K (1995) Vesicovaginal fistula (VVF): only to a woman accursed. In: Roberts JH, Vlassoff C, eds. *The female client and the health-care provider*, pp. 19–41. Ottawa, International Development Research Center.

Belsey MA (1976) The epidemiology of infertility: a review with particular reference to sub-Saharan Africa. *Bulletin of the World Health Organization*, **54**: 319.

Bhatia JC, Cleland J (1995) Self-reported symptoms of gynecological morbidity and their treatment in south India. *Studies in family planning*, **26**(4): 203–216.

Bosch FX, Manos MM, Munoz N et al. (1995) Prevalence of human papillomavirus in cervical cancer: a worldwide perspective. *Journal of the National Cancer Institute*, **87**: 796–802.

Cates W, Rolfs RT, Aral SO (1990) Sexually transmitted diseases, pelvic inflammatory disease, and infertility: an epidemiological update. *Epidemiology reviews*, **12**: 199–220.

Cates W, Stone KM (1992) Family planning, sexually transmitted diseases and contraceptive choice: a literature update – part II. *Family planning perspectives*, **24**(3): 122–128.

Cohen MS (1998) Sexually transmitted diseases enhance HIV transmission: no longer a hypothesis. *Lancet*, **351**(Suppl. III): 5–7.

Cullins VE, Wright TC, Beattie KJ et al. (1999) Cervical cancer prevention using visual screening methods. *Reproductive health matters*, **7**(14): 134–143.

Population Council (1999) *Reproductive tract infections: a set of fact sheets*. Bangkok, Population Council, South and East Asia–Thailand Office.

Cu-Uvin S, Flanigan TP, Rich JD et al. (1996) Human immunodeficiency virus infection and acquired immunodeficiency syndrome among North American women. *American journal of medicine*, **101**(3): 316–322.

Dallabetta G, Field ML, Laga M et al. (1996) STDs: global burden and challenges for control. In: Dallabetta G, Laga M, Lamptey P, eds. *Control of sexually transmitted diseases: a handbook for the design and management of programs*, pp. 1–22. Arlington, AIDSCAP/Family Health International.

Dixon-Mueller R, Wasserheit J (1991) *The culture of silence*. Washington, DC, International Women's Health Coalition.

Eschenbach DA, Davick PR, Williams BL et al. (1989) Prevalence of hydrogen peroxide-producing lactobacillus species in normal women and women with bacterial vaginosis. *Journal of clinical microbiology*, **27**(2): 251–256.

Fortney JA (1995) *Reproductive morbidity: a conceptual framework*. Research Triangle Park, Family Health International.

Grosskurth H, Mosha F, Todd J et al. (1995) Impact of improved treatment of sexually transmitted diseases on HIV infection in rural Tanzania: randomised controlled trial. *Lancet*, **346**: 530–536.

Haberland N, Winikoff B, Sloan N et al. (1999) *Case finding and case management of chlamydia and gonorrhea infections among women: what we do and do not know*. New York, Population Council.

Haukkamaa M, Stranden P, Jousimies-Somer H et al. (1986) Bacterial flora of the cervix in women using different methods of contraception. *American journal of obstetrics and gynecology*, **154**(3): 520–524.

Heise LL, Pitanguy J, Germain A (1994) *Violence against women*. Washington, DC, World Bank.

Hooton TM, Roberts PL, Stamm WE (1994) Effects of recent sexual activity and use of a diaphragm on the vaginal microflora. *Clinical infectious diseases*, **19**(8): 274–278.

Jackson S, Smith P (1997) Fortnightly review: diagnosing and managing genitourinary prolapse. *British medical journal*, 314(7084): 875–880.

Khattab HAS (1992) *The silent endurance*. Cairo, UNICEF, Regional Office for the Middle East and North Africa.

Klouman E, Masenga EJ, Klepp K-I et al. (1997) HIV and reproductive tract infections in a total village population in rural Kilimanjaro, Tanzania: women at increased risk. *Journal of acquired immune deficiency syndromes*, 14(2): 163–168.

Koenig M, Jejeebhoy S, Singh S et al. (1998) Investigating gynaecological morbidity in India: not just another KAP survey. *Reproductive health matters*, 6(11): 84–97.

Martin HL, Richardson BA, Nyange PM et al. (1999) Vaginal lactobacilli, microbial flora, and risk of human immunodeficiency virus type 1 and sexually transmitted disease acquisition. *Journal of infectious diseases*, 180(12): 1863–1868.

Mason PR, Katzenstein DA, Chimbira THK et al. (1989) Microbial flora of the lower genital tract of women in labour at Harare Maternity Hospital. *Central African journal of medicine*, 35(3): 337–343.

Mindel A (1998) Genital herpes – how much of a public health problem? *Lancet*, 351(Suppl. III): 16–18.

Morse SA, Moreland AA, Holmes KK, eds. (1996) *Atlas of sexually transmitted diseases and AIDS*. London, Mosby-Wolfe.

Muir DG, Belsey MA (1980) Pelvic inflammatory disease and its consequences in the developing world. *American journal of obstetrics and gynecology*, 138(7): 913–928.

Nene BM, Deshpande S, Jayant K et al. (1996) Early detection of cervical cancer by visual inspection: a population-based study in rural India. *International journal of cancer*, 68: 770–773.

National Institute for Allergy and Infectious Diseases (1992) *Fact sheet on sexually transmitted diseases; NIH Publication No. 92–909D*. Bethesda, NIAID Office of Communications.

Nugent RP, Krohn MA, Hillier SL (1991) Reliability of diagnosing bacterial vaginosis is improved by a standardized method of Gram stain interpretation. *Journal of clinical microbiology*, 29(2): 297–301.

Onderdonk AB, Delaney ML, Hinkson PL et al. (1992) Quantitative and qualitative effects of douche preparations on vaginal microflora. *Obstetrics and gynecology*, 80(1): 333–338.

Ponten J, Adami H-O, Bergstrom R et al. (1995) Strategies for global control of cervical cancer. *International journal of cancer*, 60: 1–26.

Population Council (1999) *Reproductive tract infections: a set of fact sheets*. Bangkok, Population Council South and East Asia–Thailand Office.

Safe Motherhood Interagency Group (1998) *Safe motherhood fact sheet: unsafe abortion*. New York, Family Care International.

Taha ET, Hoover DR, Dallabetta GA et al. (1998) Bacterial vaginosis and disturbances of vaginal flora: association with increased acquisition of HIV. *AIDS*, 12(13): 1699–1706.

Toubia N, Izett S (1998) *Female genital mutilation*. Geneva, World Health Organization.

UNAIDS (2001) *AIDS Epidemic Update: December 2001*. Geneva, UNAIDS.

United Nations (1994) *Programme of Action of the United Nations International Conference on Population and Development, Cairo, Egypt*. New York, United Nations.

University of Zimbabwe/JHPIEGO Cervical Cancer Project (2000) Visual inspection with acetic acid for cervical-cancer screening: test qualities in a primary-care setting. *Lancet*, 353(9156): 869–873.

van de Wijgert JHHM, Mason PR, Gwanzura L et al. (2000) Intravaginal practices, vaginal flora disturbances, and acquisition of sexually transmitted diseases in Zimbabwean women. *Journal of infectious diseases*, 181(2): 587–594.

Wasserheit JN (1989) The significance and scope of reproductive tract infections among third world women. *Supplement to International journal of gynecology and obstetrics*, 3: 145–168.

Wasserheit JN (1992) Epidemiological synergy interrelationships between human immunodeficiency virus infection and other sexually transmitted diseases. *Sexually transmitted diseases*, 19(2): 61–77.

Wasserheit JN, Harris JR, Chakraborty J et al. (1989) Reproductive tract infections in a family planning population in rural Bangladesh. *Studies in family planning*, 20(2): 69–80.

Westrom L (1980) Incidence, prevalence, and trends of acute pelvic inflammatory disease and its consequences in industrialized countries. *American journal of obstetrics and gynecology*, 138(7): 881–892.

WHO/UNAIDS (1997) *Sexually transmitted diseases: policies and principles for prevention and care*. Geneva, UNAIDS.

World Health Organization (1990) *Measuring reproductive morbidity: report of a technical working group*. Geneva, World Health Organization.

World Health Organization (1997) *Management of sexually transmitted diseases*. Geneva, World Health Organization, Global Program on AIDS.

WHO (2000) *The dimensions of reproductive ill-health, 1990–1995*. Geneva, World Health Organization.

Younis N, Khattab H, Zurayk H et al. (1993) A community study of gynaecological and related morbidities in rural Egypt. *Studies in family planning*, 24(3): 175–186.

3

The social context of gynaecological morbidity: correlates, consequences and health seeking behaviour

Shireen Jejeebhoy[1] and Michael Koenig[2]

[1] The Population Council, New Delhi, India; [2] Johns Hopkins University, Baltimore, USA

Background and conceptual framework

Although, over the last decade, several studies have highlighted the widespread prevalence of reproductive tract infections and other gynaecological morbidities within community settings, few have explored the social context of gynaecological morbidity: its behavioural antecedents; the consequences of morbidity for women's lives; and/or women's health seeking patterns surrounding it. The objective of this paper is to shed light on what is known on each of these issues and to suggest a set of research questions to be explored in subsequent studies on the behavioural context of gynaecological morbidity.

A review of available evidence reveals that our understanding of the range and importance of the determinants of gynaecological morbidity – biomedical, behavioural, environmental and iatrogenic – remains at a very rudimentary stage. The roles of potentially key determinants, ranging from sexual behaviour and practice and iatrogenic factors, to behavioural norms for women and men, to misperceptions regarding healthy practices, to constraints on women's access to information and services, and the role of male partners, are undoubtedly difficult to research.

Studies conducted thus far also collectively shed relatively little light on the ways in which women seek treatment for gynaecological problems, or on the consequences and implications of gynaecological morbidity for women's daily lives. Little is known about *whether* women seek treatment, *what types* of care are sought and, in particular, the actual or perceived *barriers* faced by women in seeking care. Similarly, little is known about how such morbidity affects women's ability to fulfil a diverse and wide range of expected roles – economic productivity, domestic responsibilities, marital and sexual relationships – as well as their own psychological well-being. Moreover, gynaecological problems include a continuum of conditions, which range from inconvenience to disability or even death, and in the

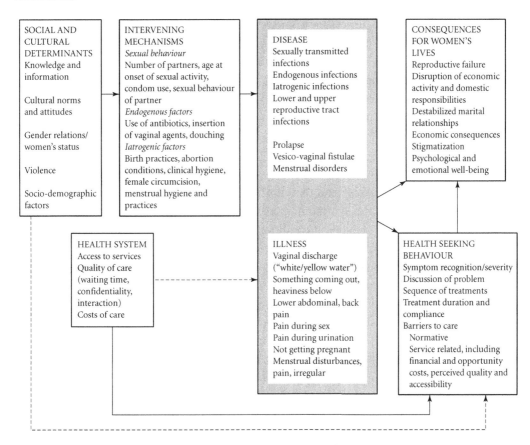

Figure 3.1   Gynaecological morbidity and its consequences – a framework.

absence of more detailed research on severity, there has been a tendency to view all such conditions as equivalent. It is clear, however, that from the perspectives of both individual women and public health priorities, these conditions have widely different implications in terms of severity, priority and required intervention. A review of the literature does, however, suggest a variety of immediate and background factors that put women at risk of gynaecological morbidity as well as consequences for women arising from such morbidity. Drawing upon this evidence, Figure 3.1 presents a conceptual framework for exploring the determinants and consequences of reproductive tract infections and other gynaecological disorders, and associated health seeking behaviour. This framework guides the discussion in this chapter.

This chapter is intended to highlight leading substantive issues that future studies of women's reproductive morbidity will need to address. The following sections discuss the main themes related to the immediate and background determinants of morbidity, consequences for women's lives and treatment seeking behaviour. These sections suggest a multiplicity of concerns, all of which may not be possible to address in a single study. Corresponding to each section, we provide a summary table highlighting the main themes, the study design most commonly used to explore each theme and, where possible, examples of the kinds of questions that may be posed to obtain information on each issue.

Determinants

Our framework recognizes that morbidity is both perceived and observed. While *illness* connotes the symptoms perceived by the sufferer and attributed by the sufferer to a gynaecological condition, *disease* is defined as clinically observed or laboratory confirmed malfunction (Kleinman, 1980). In the case of gynaecological disorders, illness and disease do not always tap the same aspect of morbidity, and hence there is not always a one-to-one correspondence between perceived and observed morbidity. Typically, perceived morbidities or illnesses include menstrual disturbances, lower backache and abdominal pain, 'a feeling of something coming out' or 'heaviness below' (symptoms of prolapse), infertility, pain during urination or sex, and, most often, vaginal discharge.

Disease, in contrast, includes both reproductive tract infections and certain other aspects of gynaecological ill health. The principal types of morbidities have been identified in Chapter 2 and in Figure 3.1, and are outlined below. To recapitulate, these include the following reproductive tract infections:
- *Sexually transmitted infections* (chlamydial infection, gonorrhoea, trichomoniasis, syphilis, chancroid, genital herpes, genital warts and HIV).
- *Endogenous infections* (bacterial vaginosis, candidiasis caused by overgrowth of microorganisms normally present in the vagina).
- *Iatrogenic infections*, which are associated with invasive medical procedures. For instance, poor delivery or abortion practices can be responsible for gynaecological morbidities such as prolapse (Elias, 1996; Wasserheit and Holmes, 1992).
- *Other factors.* Studies have indicated that several non-infectious gynaecological conditions that are considered reproductive are associated with sexual and reproductive behaviours and, as a result, also tend to be silently borne by women. These include such conditions as prolapse, menstrual disturbances, vesicovaginal fistulae, dyspareunia or pain during sexual intercourse, and urinary tract disorders.

The framework recognizes that these morbidities are determined by a multiplicity of factors, both immediate and more distal (see Figure 3.1). Intervening factors are the risk behaviours and conditions that are immediately responsible for the morbidity. Background factors, in contrast, refer to the factors underlying these risk behaviours and conditions, and include norms and other socio-cultural and demographic factors that shape gynaecological morbidities and the ways in which they do so. The pathways for each major type of gynaecological morbidity are distinctive and different.

Intervening mechanisms

Intervening mechanisms listed in Figure 3.1 make clear that risk factors vary for each type of morbidity considered, and range from sexual behaviour to intra-uterine device (IUD) insertion, unsafe abortion, childbirth and female circumcision. Table 3.1 summarizes the main risk factors studied, and offers examples of questions that have been used to obtain relevant information. It must be acknowledged, however, as suggested in Chapter 11, that questions of this nature may have limited relevance in measuring risk factors or causes because causal analysis requires a specific and well-defined outcome variable, a criterion that is not always possible in the case of stand-alone community surveys of gynaecological morbidity. Ideally, causal approaches are most appropriate where they are accompanied by a laboratory component.

Sexual transmission

Exposure to reproductive tract infections classified as sexually transmitted infections (STIs) is closely related to the age at onset of sexual activity, the number of partners over a lifetime and at a given point in time, the sexual behaviours of partners, the pattern of condom use, and possibly certain sexual practices, including intercourse during menstruation.

Early onset of sexual activity

Early sexual activity is more likely to be spontaneous and unprotected than later onset, hence placing the individual at higher risk of STI exposure. In some settings, very young females are married to older, possibly infected men. Moreover, the vaginal epithelium is thin and unprotected during adolescence and hence more susceptible to infection. For all these reasons, age at initiation of sexual activity is a risk factor (Aral and Wasserheit, 1998; Brabin, Raleigh and Dumella, 1992; Newton and Keith, 1985).

Multiple partners

This often implies casual sex practices, including sexual relations with sex workers. There is considerable evidence that the number of partners with whom an individual has sexual relations in a given period, especially when partners are sex workers or casual contacts, increases exposure to STIs.

Table 3.1. Core risk factors and illustrative examples of questions used in selected studies

Core items	Method used	Questions	Source
General			
Perceived causes of symptoms	Qualitative		
Sexual Transmission			
Age at sexual debut	Survey	Now I need to ask you some questions about sexual activity in order to gain a better understanding of some family life issues: How old were you when you first had sexual intercourse?	World Health Organization (WHO), 1998
Condom use in last x months and consistency of condom use	Survey	Now I need to ask you some questions about sexual activity in order to gain a better understanding of some family life issues: The last time you had sexual intercourse, was a condom used? Did you use a condom always, occasionally or only at the beginning of the relationship?	WHO, 1998
Number of partners in last x months	Survey	What is your relationship to the man with whom you last had sex? For how long have you had a sexual relationship with this man? Have you had sexual intercourse with anyone else in the last 12 months? Have you ever had a sexual relationship that lasted for one night or a very short time? Have you ever had sex with anyone other than a regular partner? If yes, how long ago was the most recent time something like that happened? Have you ever had sexual intercourse with someone other than your partner? How many different sexual partners have you had?	WHO, 1998 Phan thi Lien et al., 1999
Sexual intercourse during menstruation	Survey	Do you ever have intercourse during menstruation? If so, how frequently? Do you have intercourse during menses (frequently, at least every other month, sometimes, never)?	WHO, 1990 Kaufman et al., 1996

Sexual behaviour of partners	Survey	Do any of your partners have genital symptoms? If yes, what symptoms? Has your partner ever had sexual intercourse with someone other than you? If yes, can you estimate how many different sexual partners he has had in the past 3 months, past year, with bar girls or prostitutes? Some infections of the reproductive tract are acquired through sexual intercourse. A person can get a sexually transmitted infection if one's partner has had previous exposure to an infection through sexual activity with another partner and has not had the appropriate treatment. Do you think that you could possibly be at risk of getting an infection in this way?	Phan thi Lien et al., 1999
Endogenous factors			
Antibiotic resistance	Survey	Have you used any medications before coming (to the facility)? Are you currently taking antibiotics?	Phan thi Lien et al., 1999
Douching	Survey	Do you sometimes use vaginal douching? Do you sometimes use powder for vaginal cleansing?	Khattab et al., 1997
Inserting vaginal agents, practices	Survey	Do women place objects or substances in the genital or anal area? If so, which objects or substances? When? With what frequency? For what purpose?	WHO, 1990
		Do you ever use preparations in the vagina? Vaginal suppositories? Herbal or traditional medication? Why do you use these vaginal preparations (for relief from symptoms, for cleansing after menstruation, for treatment)?	Kaufman et al., 1996
Inserting vaginal agents, morbidity		Do these product produce lesions, irritation or symptoms of infection?	WHO, 1990
Iatrogenic factors			
Obstetric experiences	Survey	Where did you give birth?	IIPS, 1998
Conditions at delivery		Who assisted with the delivery of your (last, second last . . .) child?	
Obstetric problems relating to the last pregnancy	Survey	At any time during the 2 months after the delivery of your last child, did you have massive vaginal bleeding? Very high fever?	IIPS, 1998

Table 3.1 (*cont.*)

Core items	Method used	Questions	Source
Abortion experience	Survey, open-ended questions	Sometimes women have a pregnancy that did not finish. Have you ever had a pregnancy which ended before 6 months? How many weeks pregnant were you at the time the loss occurred? Did the pregnancy end by itself or did you or someone else do something to end it? What was used to end your pregnancy?	Graham et al., 1995
Post-abortion complications		Did you face any problems after the abortion? Did you have any bleeding? Inflammation/infection?	
Clinical contraception: IUD, tubal ligation; experience	Survey	Who inserted the IUD? Where did you go to get the IUD inserted? Where did you get sterilized? How would you rate the care you received during or immediately after the operation/IUD insertion? What improvements would you suggest in the care you received?	IIPS, 1998
Complications	Survey	Do you think there are any health problems related to this method? What is the problem? Have you ever experienced a health problem with this method? What was this health problem?	Graham et al., 1995
Experience of circumcision	Survey	Have you ever been circumcized? How old were you when you were circumcized? Who performed the circumcision? Where was the circumcision performed? Do you know what tool was used in the circumcision (sharp blade, scalpel, scissors)? Was the vaginal area sewn closed or almost closed?	El-Zanaty et al., 1996
Complications associated with circumcision		Did the vaginal area have to be cut open when you began menstruating or first married? Did you have any complications at the time of the circumcision or afterwards? What were these (severe pain at wound, bleeding, infection/fever, difficulty in passing urine, swelling, shock)?	

Other factors

Menstrual hygiene, genital hygiene, practice	Survey	What type of sanitary protection do you use during menstruation? Do you do paddy field work when menstruating? Do you wash the vulva (genitals) during menstruation? Bathe during menstruation?	Kaufman et al., 1996
		What is the protection you use during menstruation? How do you wash during menstruation? How do you wash these things (if not using disposable)? Where do you hang them out to dry?	Khattab et al., 1997
		What type of sanitary protection do you use? How often do you wash the genital area? What do you use when washing?	Phan thi Lien et al., 1999
Quality of surface water for bathing	Survey	Where and how frequently do you bathe? What is the source of water for family use? Does the family use the same basin for washing the face and feet? Which way do you wipe after using the toilet?	Kaufman et al., 1996

Sexual behaviour of partners

Multiple partner status and exchange of sex for money by partners are reasons for higher risk of infection. In a study of 18 countries participating in a standardized World Health Organization (WHO) survey, the proportion of men reporting five or more sex partners in the past year ranged from 0 per cent in Sri Lanka to 11 per cent in Thailand; for women the level never exceeded 3 per cent (Carael et al., 1995; see also Aral and Wasserheit, 1998). Studies in India have observed an association between pelvic inflammatory disease (PID) among women and husbands' extra-marital contacts (Brabin et al., 1998; Gogate et al., 1998). An in-depth study in Zimbabwe of 60 clinic patients with repeated STIs observed that while almost all men perceived that they had been infected during a sex worker contact, almost all women reported that they had been infected by their husbands (Pitts, Bowman and McMaster, 1995).

Extent of condom use and consistency of use

What happens during sexual relations is equally important. Although barrier methods, including male and female condoms, do indeed protect against exposure to the risk of infection, and although use has been increasing, condom use remains limited and often inconsistent. For example, a major risk factor for HIV in pregnant women in a Harare maternity hospital is reported use of condoms in casual relationships, but no condom use with the husband or regular partner (Mbizvo, Mashu and Chipato, 1996).

Sexual intercourse during menstruation

A study of women in southern Iran reports that the risk of cervicitis increases with the practice of sexual relations during menstruation. The evidence also suggests that there is a higher proportion of women with moderate and severe cervicitis among those reporting intercourse during menses, although the factors underlying this association remain unclear (Keshavarz et al., 1997). A US study found frequency of sex during menstruation to be significantly associated with women's self-reported history of chlamydial infection (Foxman, Aral and Holmes, 1998). At least one other study has reported an association between sex during menstruation and gynaecological infection (Kaufman et al., 1996).[1]

Endogenous factors

Endogenous infections are caused by behaviours that alter the vaginal environment in such a way as to promote the excessive growth of organisms that are present naturally. These include the following:

---

[1] At the same time, available evidence suggests that the practice of sexual relations during menstruation may be relatively infrequent in many developing countries. Only 6 per cent of women in China reported engaging in sexual relations during menstruation (Kaufman et al., 1996).

Antibiotic resistance

Studies suggest that inhabitants in some parts of Africa, Latin America, and South and Southeast Asia have developed high levels of antibiotic resistance, probably because of the unrestricted use of over-the-counter antibiotics (Wasserheit, 1989; Wasserheit et al., 1989).

Douching

Douching has been associated with higher rates of self-reported or clinically diagnosed genital tract infection (Foxman, Aral and Holmes, 1998; Roddy, 1993; Wolner-Hanssen et al., 1990). In one multivariate study, douching during the past two months was associated with an adjusted relative risk of 1.7 (95 per cent confidence interval 1.04–2.82), with the risk of PID increasing with frequency of douching (Wolner-Hanssen et al., 1990). A study in China found douching to be associated with a significantly higher risk of cervicitis (Kaufman et al., 1996). A study of pregnant women from the Ivory Coast reported no relationship between douching with soap and water and genital infection, but a significant association between douching with antiseptics and chlamydial infection (La Ruche et al., 1999). A study of pregnant women attending a prenatal clinic in Surabaya, Indonesia reported significant associations between the likelihood of a medically diagnosed STI and regular douching with soap and water (relative ratio = 2.7), betel leaf or commercial agents (relative ratio = 9.4) (Joesoef et al., 1996).

Inserting vaginal agents

Studies point to intravaginal preparations used to increase the male partner's pleasure during sex as a common practice in some African countries (Brown, Ayowa and Brown, 1993; Dallabetta et al., 1995), and as a practice that may potentially facilitate the transmission of HIV and other sexually transmitted infections (Wasserheit, 1989). The Ivory Coast study found a significant association between the use of vaginal agents and both candidiasis and *Ureaplasma urealyticum,* a bacterium found most frequently in the genital tract (La Ruche et al., 1999).

Iatrogenic factors

Iatrogenic infections are acquired through a number of routes, including unhygienic delivery conditions and procedures such as pregnancy termination, menstrual regulation, IUD insertion, sterilization procedures and circumcision.

Obstetric experience

There is considerable evidence that relates reproductive tract infections to birth and contraceptive practices. For one, a strong association between age, parity and morbidity has often been observed. A study of young married women aged 16–22 years in rural south India finds a strong link between marital duration, parity and the experience of reproductive tract infections. The chances of having a reproductive tract infection were 1.5 times higher among women who had experienced two or more pregnancies as those who had experienced fewer pregnancies, and 2.6 times higher among those married for 5 or more years compared to the recently married (Prasad et al., 1999). These findings are attributed to a combination of factors such as the sexual behaviour of husbands of these women, but mainly to iatrogenic infections linked to pregnancy and abortion experiences.

A study of factors influencing self-reported morbidity among recently delivered women in south India concluded that obstetric problems play an important role in affecting such conditions as menstrual problems, lower reproductive tract infections and acute PID. For example, the experience of obstetric problems during the most recent birth was a strong predictor of all three types of symptoms, with odds ratios ranging from 2.2 for menstrual problems to 4.8 for lower abdominal pain/discharge with fever (Bhatia and Cleland, 1995).

Unsafe delivery conditions have been singled out as an important factor underlying subsequent gynaecological morbidity. For example, in the study discussed earlier, delivery at home (or in a government institution) was also a significant risk factor as compared to delivery in a private facility (Bhatia and Cleland, 1995). In Pakistan, 72 per cent of infections could be traced to unsafe childbirth conditions (Wasserheit, 1989). In Nigeria, Adekunle and Lapido (1992) identify such practices as unhygienic birth conditions, unskilled birth attendants and the insertion of caustic herbs into the birth canal as factors contributing to reproductive tract infections. A study of nomadic women in southern Iran suggests a direct association between the number of deliveries and cervicitis; moreover, women whose births were attended by a neighbour were significantly more likely to experience cervicitis than other women (Keshavarz et al., 1997). Finally, studies in Africa in particular have noted a close association between untreated prolonged obstructed labour and the development of obstetric or vesicovaginal fistulae (Arrowsmith, Hamlin and Wall, 1996).

Several studies have linked recent deliveries with other types of gynaecological morbidity. In the Giza study in Egypt, age and the number of previous pregnancies were closely related to uterine prolapse: each additional year of age increased the risk of prolapse by 7 per cent and each additional delivery more than doubled that risk (Younis et al., 1993). A study in south India that assessed long-term morbidities following delivery found that among 3844 women who delivered up to 24 months prior to the study, 3 per cent experienced uterine prolapse and urinary incontinence, respectively, and two women reported rectovaginal fistulae (Srinivasa et al., 1997).

Post-abortion complications

Few studies have assessed the link between induced abortion and gynaecological morbidity. Yet, pelvic infection is a common complication of abortion (Stevenson and Radcliffe, 1995). Wasserheit estimates that in Southeast Asia, post-abortion infection is a leading cause of PID (60–80 per cent of women hospitalized for this condition), and in Pakistan, 23 per cent of infections relate to unsafe abortion (Wasserheit, 1989). A study of women presenting to clinics in Mumbai, India for pelvic pain found that 26 per cent with confirmed PID reported having undergone an abortion, compared to 2 per cent of women without PID (Gogate et al., 1998). A study from rural China found that women who reported having undergone an induced abortion at a county-level facility were significantly more likely to have a diagnosed reproductive tract infection compared to women who did not undergo an abortion or had obtained one in a more sophisticated facility (Kaufman et al., 1996).

Contraceptive use

Gynaecological morbidity has also been associated, in a number of studies, with tubal ligation and IUD use.[2] In fact, in some settings (such as urban India) PID appears to be linked more closely to invasive procedures such as clinical contraception (and abortion) than to STIs (Brabin et al., 1998; Gogate et al., 1998).

Evidence of the links between morbidity and IUD use comes from studies conducted in several countries. A study in Bangladesh reported that IUD users were almost seven times more likely to develop PID as women who were not using a contraceptive method (Wasserheit, 1989). The Giza study in Egypt observed that women currently using an IUD had 1.8 times higher risk of reproductive tract infections compared to other women (Younis et al., 1993). Similarly, a study of factors influencing reported morbidity among recently delivered women in south India indicates that IUD users report significantly higher rates of PID than women who did not practise any form of contraception (2.5 times as high) (Bhatia and Cleland, 1995).[3] In addition, studies in Bali, Indonesia and Yunnan Province, China, indicate that IUD users reported higher rates of morbidity than users of other methods (Kaufman et al., 1996; Patten and Susanti, 1998). In contrast, a study from Turkey found that IUD users have a higher risk of menstrual disorders but not reproductive tract infections (Bulut et al., 1997).

Wasserheit (1989) attributes the association between IUD use and reproductive tract infections to three mechanisms: IUDs may alter the cervicovaginal milieu and predispose users to bacterial vaginosis; the IUD tail may facilitate ascent of

---

[2] The link between PID and the use of other contraceptive methods is more tenuous but has also been observed. For example, the consistent use of mechanical and barrier methods has been associated with decreased risk of cervical infection in some studies but not in others. Oral contraceptives appear to increase the risk of cervical chlamydial infection, although a recent study suggests that it has a protective effect on PID (Aral and Wasserheit, 1998). It has been suggested that smoking and douching increase the risk of PID infection (Aral and Wasserheit, 1998).

[3] A subsequent study based on laboratory and clinically diagnosed conditions found no significant association between IUD use and gynaecological morbidity (Bhatia et al., 1997). Other studies in India report relatively low rates of PID among IUD users (Brabin, Raleigh and Dumella, 1992). However, a study from the US also identified as risk factors, 'medical procedures breaking the cervical barrier' (for example, IUD insertion) and induced abortion (Roddy, 1993).

organisms into the endometrial cavity for women with a lower reproductive tract infection; and IUDs may compromise host defences against the pathogens that reach the upper tract. Clearly, the role of IUD insertion conditions and their potential to cause infection also need to be assessed.

Many of the studies examining the association between tubal ligation and gynaecological morbidity are from South Asia. In the previously cited study of south India, for example, sterilized women were more likely than women who had not undergone sterilization to report lower reproductive tract infections (relative ratio = 1.57) and acute PID (relative ratio = 2.50) (Bhatia and Cleland, 1995). In their Bangladesh study, Wasserheit et al. (1989) also found that women who had undergone tubal ligation were seven times more likely to have a diagnosed reproductive tract infection compared to non-contracepting women. The clinical study in Mumbai, India reports that 22 per cent of women who had undergone a laparascopy were diagnosed with PID, compared to 2 per cent from the control group (Gogate et al., 1998).[4] A link between female sterilization and reproductive tract infections was also reported in a study from western Rajasthan (Oomman, 1996).

A study by Hawkes et al. (1999) of women complaining of vaginal discharge and seeking care at maternal/child/family planning centres in Matlab, Bangladesh finds that women with an IUD or who have had a tubectomy are more likely to have an endogenous infection than those using no contraception. Infections were observed among 53 per cent of IUD users and 45 per cent of sterilized women, compared to 32 per cent of non-users and 12 per cent of condom users. These relationships persisted in multivariate analyses: relative ratios were 2.43, 1.72 and 0.28, respectively, for IUD users, tubectomized women and condom users (Hawkes et al., 1999).

Other factors

A number of other factors reportedly influence gynaecological morbidity.

Menstrual hygiene

Menstrual hygiene practices have been found to be a significant risk factor for menstrual disorders (Bulut et al., 1997) or symptoms of lower reproductive tract infections (Bhatia and Cleland, 1995). A study in Bangladesh found that women who used rags prepared at home to absorb menstrual blood were almost twice as likely to have bacterial vaginosis as were those who used nothing (Wasserheit, 1989). The

---

[4] In a cross-sectional study, women presenting for infertility and PID were compared to a control group of fertile, healthy women attending facilities for tubal ligation. Questionnaires covered marital status, religion, migrant history, education and income, as well as contraceptive use and the sexual history of the woman and her partner. A clinical module also covered information on gynaecological histories (including menstruation, and symptoms of genital and urinary tract infections) and obstetric, medical and surgical histories. Unfortunately, information on the situation during delivery, abortion, IUD insertion and tubal ligation was not solicited (Brabin et al., 1998; Gogate et al., 1998).

Giza study in Egypt found that women who did not use disposable cotton or napkins, and who did not boil cloths used to absorb menstrual blood, had a significantly higher risk of reproductive tract infections (OR = 1.66) (Younis et al., 1993).

Personal hygiene

The study from south India found that good personal hygiene practices by women (bathing, washing) were associated with a lower risk of self-reported reproductive tract infections (Bhatia and Cleland, 1995). A study of rural China similarly reported that women who used unhygienic surface water and shared bathing facilities were at increased risk of reproductive tract infections. At the same time, infrequent bathing was also found to be associated with increased risk of bacterial vaginosis (Kaufman et al., 1996). A study of rural and urban Mexico observes that a larger proportion of women perceive poor hygiene to be the leading cause of reproductive illness, rather than sexual contact, inconsistent condom use or multiple sex partners (Miranda et al., 1999).

Previous experience of infection

PID is also related to recurrent infections of the cervix. Compared to women with one documented chlamydial infection, women with two chlamydial infections are four times more likely to be hospitalized for PID. Ectopic pregnancy was also related to infection with both chlamydia and gonorrhoea. Studies suggest that such social contextual factors as age, ethnicity and residence are more powerful risk factors for recurrent cervical infection than factors related to sexual behaviour (Aral and Wasserheit, 1998).

Finally, female circumcision or infibulation in countries such as the Sudan and Ghana have similarly been hypothesized to contribute to PID and infertility due to endogenous pathogens (Wasserheit, 1989; Wasserheit et al., 1989). Studies in the Sudan suggest that between 20 and 25 per cent of infertility may be attributable to female circumcision (Mahdi Al Dirie, n.d.).

Social and cultural determinants of reproductive tract infections/gynaecological morbidity

By and large, studies of gynaecological morbidity have not systematically explored the factors underlying unsafe sexual behaviours or unsafe pregnancy, abortion and contraception. The factors for which evidence is most plentiful are reviewed in this section. Unfortunately, not all the background determinants of reproductive tract infections and other gynaecological morbidities described in Figure 3.1 have received due attention. Table 3.2 summarizes the main determinants and offers examples of questions that studies have used to obtain relevant information, where these are available.

Table 3.2. Summary of core social and cultural determinants of reproductive tract infections/gynaecological morbidity, and illustrations of questions used in selected studies

Core items	Method used	Questions	Source
Lack of information and misperceptions			
What is considered 'normal'?	Survey	In a man, what signs and symptoms would lead you to think that he has an infection?	Macro
Perceptions of typical symptoms		In a woman, what signs and symptoms would lead you to think that she has such an infection?	International, 1999
Perceptions of seriousness of problems	Focus group discussions	How serious a problem is STD/HIV for women/men in this area? What are the main causes? How should one avoid these symptoms?	World Health Organization (WHO), 1998
Perceived aetiology, modes of transmission	Semi-structured	What are possible causes of . . .? Probe 'heat', witchcraft, body, weakness, contraceptive method, delivery and abortion, diseases of the uterus, food, tension.	Bang and Bang, 1994
Is the link between sexual behaviour and certain symptoms perceived?	Survey	Is there anything a person can do to avoid getting AIDS or the virus that causes AIDS?	Macro International, 1999; IIPS, 1998
		In your view, is a person's chance of getting AIDS influenced by the number of sexual partners he or she has?	
		If a person has sex with only one partner, does this person have a greater or a lesser chance of getting AIDS than a person who has sex with many partners?	
		In your view, is a person's chance of getting AIDS affected by using a condom every time he or she has sexual intercourse? (If yes): If a person uses a condom every time he or she has sexual intercourse, does this person have a greater or a lesser chance of getting AIDS than someone who doesn't use a condom?	
		Is it possible for a healthy-looking person to have the AIDS virus?	
	Survey	What diseases occur as a result of sexual relations? What are their most common signs or symptoms? What do they look like? Feel like? Smell like? Do they cause pain?	WHO, 1990
		What kinds of treatment are available for these diseases?	
		Who performs these treatments?	

Attitudes

Acceptability of multiple partners	Survey	Say whether you agree, disagree or have mixed feelings about the following statements: A man needs to have more than one partner, etc.	WHO, 1998
	Survey	What are your opinions about the following sexual relationships (always wrong; to not wrong at all): A married person having sexual relations with someone other than his/her partner, etc.	Wellings, 1996
Double standards	Survey	Is the sexual conduct of men treated differently from that of women? If so, what are the most important differences? Are there differences in the occasional partner relations of men as opposed to women?	WHO, 1990
Condom acceptability	Survey	Say whether you agree, disagree or have mixed feelings or no opinion about the statements: Using a condom is an effective way of preventing STD/HIV; condoms encourage promiscuous behaviour; the only reason to use a condom is because you don't trust your partner.	WHO, 1998

Constraints on women's autonomy, unequal gender relations

Decision-making authority	Survey	Who in your family usually has the final say on the following decisions: Your own health care?, Making large household purchases?, etc. Are you usually allowed to go to the following places alone? Local market, local health centre or doctor?, etc. Who takes this decision (when you want to see a physician)? Who accompanies you?	El-Zanaty et al., 1996
Control over resources	Survey	Who pays the physician's fees?	Khattab et al., 1997
Sexual negotiation	Survey	Husbands and wives do not always agree on everything. Please tell me if you think a wife is justified in refusing to have sex with her husband when: She knows her husband has sex with other women?, She knows her husband has a sexually transmitted disease?, etc. Who usually has the most influence over whether or not to use a condom: the man, the woman or both equally? Say whether you think it is acceptable or unacceptable for a married woman to ask her husband to use a condom?	Khattab et al., 1997

Table 3.2 (*cont.*)

Core items	Method used	Questions	Source
	FGDs	Now I have an example of a married couple. The woman is having injections to space between births. The husband travels away from home for long periods of time for work. The wife fears that he is having affairs while away, and especially fears that he will bring a sexually transmitted infection or, even worse, HIV home. If this happened in this community, what could she do to protect herself? Can she ask him to use a condom? Can she refuse to have sex with him? Can she talk about it with him?	WHO, 1998
	Survey	Imagine that you and your partner decide to have sex, but he will not use a condom. You do not want to have sex without a condom. How sure are you that you could keep from having sex until your partner agrees it is OK to use a condom?	Mathai et al., 1997
	Survey	Responses in the following situations: Asking a boyfriend about his previous sexual experiences; telling someone you know who has multiple partners that you don't want to have sex with them; talking about condom use; telling a casual friend that you don't want to have sex at present; refusing sex if the partner won't agree to use condoms	Lahai-Momoh and Ross, 1997
Men's roles: Physical and sexual violence			
Physical, sexual	Survey	Sometimes a husband is annoyed or angered by things that his wife does. In your opinion, is a husband justified in hitting or beating his wife in the following situations: If she goes out without telling him? If she refuses to have sex with him?, etc.	El-Zanaty et al., 1996
		From the time you were married, has anyone ever beaten you? If yes, can you tell me who has done this to you since you were married? Approximately how many times were you beaten in the past one year? Have you ever been beaten when you were pregnant?	

| | | | How often have you been beaten or physically mistreated in the last 12 months? | International Institute for Population Sciences, 1998 |

Adolescence

| Informed choice, self-esteem | | Which birth control method did you or your partner use at the first intercourse? Who made the decision to use contraception at that time?/ in the last intercourse? Have you ever asked a partner to wear a condom? Has any of the following ever happened because you asked a partner to wear a condom?: Partner refused/threatened/made you have sex anyway without a condom, etc. | Serbanescu and Morris, 1998 |

Now I am going to read you a series of statements . . . tell me whether you agree: My life is chiefly controlled by people with more power than me; it is not always wise to plan too far ahead because many things turn out to be a matter of good or bad luck, etc.

Husband/partner occupation

| Occupation and co-residence patterns | Survey | What is your husband's/partner's occupation? That is, what kind of work does he mainly do? | DHS, 1999 |

Has your husband ever travelled away from home for one night or more in the last 12 months? — WHO, 1998

Does his job ever take him away from home for more than one night at a time? — Wellings, 1996

Notes: FGD, focus group discussion; STD, sexually transmitted disease.

Incomplete information and misperceptions

Incomplete information and misinformation abound in the area of gynaecological morbidity, and are compounded by the culture of silence. There is evidence that women and men are poorly informed not only about behaviours and conditions that influence gynaecological morbidity, but also about the symptoms of morbidity in themselves and in their partners, the fact that symptoms can be treated and where they can be treated. Because there is little agreement in many settings on what characteristics are 'normal', there is also very little agreement on which symptom should warrant treatment (see, for example, Olukoya and Elias, 1996). A qualitative study in Vietnam observes that women do perceive vaginal discharge as illness, but only when it has a strong odour or is any colour but white (Gorbach et al., 1997). It is important, then, that studies explore knowledge about normal and abnormal symptoms or how severe a symptom must be before it is perceived as morbidity.

Studies also need to explore local beliefs and knowledge regarding the prevention of symptoms. For example, in two studies of Nigeria, a wide range of home remedies were recommended to prevent discharge and infertility, such as reducing the number of sexual partners, adhering to expectations regarding abstinence, and using herbal drinks and douches. Antibiotics and 'injection' were recommended only if herbs were ineffective (Erwin, 1993; Olukoya and Elias, 1996).

A number of studies have focused on knowledge and perceptions of HIV/AIDS, its modes of transmission and possible preventive measures. Yet, the questions posed by standard surveys are limited in conveying the depth of awareness. The evidence suggests a general awareness of AIDS but not necessarily of other STIs or reproductive tract infections, and considerable misinformation concerning modes of transmission. For example, in a study of women in Kampala, AIDS was reported as a major disease in the community by 71 per cent of women interviewed. In contrast, STIs were reported by only 3 per cent (Wallman, 1996). In this study, women appeared to be well informed about STI symptoms, but obtaining such information required careful probing. Probing also highlighted, however, that a description of symptoms and an awareness of modes of transmission were not always complete or accurate (Kaharuza et al., 1996). Although sparse, there is some evidence that safer sexual behaviour, for example, is influenced by the level of specific information on STI risk, patterns of transmission, methods of prevention and sources of health care (Aral and Wasserheit, 1998).

Although awareness of the multiplicity of factors causing reproductive tract infections is limited, even among symptomatic women, women do recognize some of the risk factors. For example, a study in Nigeria observed that 41 per cent of symptomatic women attributed their condition to such natural causes as diet and impure blood, and 13 per cent to using unclean toilets; 17 per cent could not identify a cause, but 22 per cent made the link to sexual activity (13 per cent to their husband's other partners and 9 per cent to their own extra-marital partners) (Erwin, 1993). In the qualitative study in Vietnam, women attributed symptoms of gynaecological morbidity to 'harmful winds', weather changes, hard work or difficult times; but in a second interview, some women did indeed indicate a link to sexual behaviour or IUD use (Gorbach et al., 1997). While women residing in an urban slum in India did not appear to be aware of sexual risk factors, they did recognize the association of frequent pregnancies and sterilization experiences with one symptom of reproductive tract infections – discharge (Kanani, Latha and Shah, 1994). Similarly, poor Indian women were aware that 'mishandling at the time of delivery' could lead to prolapse (Patel et al., 1994).

Unequal gender relations and sexual negotiation

Gender power imbalances and women's relative lack of autonomy are leading background factors underlying their vulnerability to sexual risk behaviours. Unbalanced power relations have inhibited women from adopting behavioural strategies that would protect them from acquiring STIs and some non-sexually transmitted infections, although the strength of the relationship varies by context (see, for example, Aral, 1992; Carael, 1997; Gupta, Weiss and Whelan, 1996; Wasserheit, 1989).

Women's lack of autonomy influences their risk of infection and other gynaecological morbidities in a number of important ways. In many settings, women have limited decision-making authority surrounding their own lives and health. In those settings, it is unlikely that they make decisions on whether or not to engage in sex, can insist on condom use or make decisions on pregnancy and delivery care. Limited control over resources among women in many settings compounds their lack of decision-making – it makes them socially and economically dependent on their husbands or partners, including in the sexual and reproductive arenas, and in the area of health care, including care during pregnancy and childbirth, or at the time of abortion. Yet another barrier is the lack of intimacy or partner communication, which makes talking about sex, pregnancy and safe practices virtually impossible. Cultural norms emphasizing female chastity impede women's adequate access to knowledge about sexuality, fertility control and disease.

Even where women and men know the protective influence of condoms and the risks associated with multiple partners, few women have the power to insist on condom use among their husbands and partners. For example, in an in-depth study of STI among clinic patients in Zimbabwe, despite fairly high levels of awareness of risk behaviours, women report powerlessness in negotiating sexual matters and lack of control in areas relating to sexuality. One-third of all women were unable to persuade their husbands to use condoms; and correspondingly, few men indicated that they would desist from having multiple partners or would use condoms in future (Pitts, Bowman and McMaster, 1995). In Mexico, women acknowledged the importance of faithfulness to one's partner in preventing infection but recognized that 'sometimes men run around and a wife has no way of making sure he is protecting himself'. Despite knowledge of the causes of infection and awareness of partner behaviour, women disclosed that they still found themselves with little recourse for protection (Miranda et al., 1999). The limited sexual autonomy of women is evident from a study of rural Tamil Nadu, India: two-thirds of symptomatic women who attempted to refuse the sexual advances of their husbands were rebuffed, and verbally or physically abused (Santhya and Dasvarma, 1998).

On the other hand, where women have decision-making authority, they are better able to protect themselves. In Ekiti, Nigeria, over 90 per cent of Yoruba women – well known for their economic independence – were involved in the decision to seek treatment for themselves in case of sickness. Nearly all women indicated that they would refuse to have unprotected sexual relations if their husbands had a STI (Orubuloye, Oguntimehin and Sadiq, 1997).

Sexual negotiation skills among women appear to have an influence on safer sex. While difficult to measure, several studies have used the AIDS social assertiveness scale. This scale comprises a series of 33 items, including seven that relate to negotiation, scored on a five-point Likert scale (Lahai-Momoh and Ross, 1997; Ross, Caudle and Taylor, 1991; Venier, Ross and Akande, 1998). Questions on sexual negotiation include whether respondents would ask their boyfriend/girlfriend about previous sexual experiences, tell a casual or close boyfriend/girlfriend with whom they are thinking about having sex that they want to delay it at present, refuse to have sex unless condoms are used, tell someone who has multiple partners that they would not have sex with them or talk about condom use. This scale was administered to adolescents in several settings (Sierra Leone: Lahai-Momoh and Ross, 1997; Kenya, Nigeria, Zimbabwe: Venier, Ross and Akande, 1998; South Australia: Ross, Caudle and Taylor, 1991). Results across three countries suggest that this scale is robust across cultures (Venier, Ross and Akande, 1998). The study of adolescent females in Sierra Leone was unable to link skill levels with chances of having sex or intercourse, but was able to establish that those who were less anxious about negotiating were more likely to have used a condom (Lahai-Momoh and Ross, 1997). Similar findings were reported in a study of young African–American women in the United States (US), where regular condom use was significantly determined by assertiveness, communication skills and sexual self-control over condom use (Wingood and DiClemente, 1998).

Men's roles are important from several perspectives: their own risk taking and the extent to which they assume responsibility for protecting their partners from STIs as well as the extent to which they share the responsibility for healthy practices in general, and those surrounding delivery and abortion among their partners, in particular their wives. A study of rural Tamil Nadu reports that over two-fifths of men reported that they disapproved of sexual denial by their symptomatic wives. A similar proportion expressed their right to sexual gratification, irrespective of the wife's consent (Santhya and Dasvarma, 1998).

Unequal gender norms and sexual risk-taking behaviours

In many settings, community attitudes facilitate and reinforce risk behaviours. Gender norms and sexual double standards intensify female vulnerability and limit their skills for negotiating safer sex outcomes. Strong cultural prohibitions in many settings make it impossible for women to deny sex to partners (see, for example, de Zoysa, Sweat and Denison, 1996; George and Jaiswal, 1995; McDermott et al., 1993). Cultural double standards, moreover, condone multiple sexual partners or casual sex among men; females who are the regular partners of these men have limited power to change this practice or even insist on condom use in their own relations with their regular partners (see Isarabhakdi, 1995; Rugpao, 1995; Tangchonlatip, 1997; Wasserheit, 1989). For example, studies from many settings report that both females and males agree that premarital sexual activity and having multiple partners are acceptable for males but not for females (Isarabhakdi, 1995; Rugpao, 1995); multiple partners and even symptoms of STIs among men are seen as signs of masculinity (Aral, 1992). In Thailand, despite the onset of the HIV epidemic, cultural norms permitting married men to have relations with sex workers are so strong that the practice continues, and wives do not feel entitled to voice their concerns (see, for example, Tangchonlatip, 1997). Similarly, women in Mexico recognize that extramarital affairs are common among men, who then bring infection home to their wives or regular partners (Miranda et al., 1999).

In sum, studies of the determinants of gynaecological morbidity need to focus on women's autonomy, gender power relations and, in particular, sexual negotiation skills. This requires a mix of qualitative and quantitative approaches, and a mix of actual experience and responses in a hypothetical situation. For example, several studies (see for example El-Zanaty et al., 1996), including the Demographic and Health Survey (DHS), have attempted to operationalize female empowerment through a series of questions reflecting women's decision-making power, access to and control over household resources, mobility and freedom from the threat of violence. These can be expanded or re-framed to focus on sexual negotiation.

Physical and sexual violence

Physical and sexual violence represent major public health problems in developing countries. A recent review of population-based evidence suggests that generally between 20 and 50 per cent of women experience physical violence within their marriage from their husband or male partner (Heise, Pitanguay and Germain, 1994). The limited available evidence also suggests very high levels of coercive sexual relations and sexual abuse, both during childhood as well as within marriage. For example, 22 per cent of men in a north Indian survey reported having forced their wives to have sex against their will (EVALUATION Project, 1997) and half the women in a Sierra Leone survey reported that they had been forced by their husband/partner into sexual relations (Coker and Richter, 1998).

There is some evidence, primarily from Western countries, pointing to possible links between physical or sexual violence and gynaecological morbidity. A US-based study examined the influence of experiences of child abuse, violent crime victimization and spouse abuse on gynaecological morbidity (severe menstrual problems, STIs and urinary tract infections) (Plichta and Abraham, 1996). Its findings suggest that both childhood sexual abuse and having been a victim of violent crime almost doubled the odds of having a gynaecological problem, and spouse abuse tripled the odds, even after controlling for sociodemographic factors and access to care. A series of studies in Norway has documented the positive association between women's residence in a physically or sexually abusive relationship and reported gynaecological symptoms, chronic pelvic pain and/or medically treated PID (Schei, 1990; Schei and Bakketeig, 1989). Findings suggest that while 12 per cent of women in the general community reported PID, as many as 58 per cent of battered women did so (Schei, 1991). A US-based study of women with gynaecological morbidity observes very high rates of sexual violence: 32 per cent had been sexually assaulted, including rape (20 per cent) and/or other non-consensual contact (28 per cent); figures that are much higher than in the general population (Miranda et al., 1998).

Evidence is also emerging from developing countries. A study in Rwanda observed that HIV-positive women were more likely than other women to report coercive sex (van der Straten et al., 1995). Another study in Chiapas, Mexico observed that women who suffered violence were also likely to suffer illness, unwanted fertility and infections, including STIs (Glantz and Halperin, 1996). Finally, a study in Zimbabwe highlights the role of fear of violence in inhibiting women from negotiating sexual relations, including insisting on condom use or treatment for partners with symptoms of STIs (Njovana and Watts, 1996). Clearly, much more research is needed to determine whether the relationship between violence and gynaecological morbidity is causal, or if they are both co-determined by other factors.

Young age and vulnerability to infection

Inequalities of age interact with inequalities of gender to make young women particularly vulnerable to infection. Age is a central factor marking vulnerability to

STIs, and pregnancy- and contraception-related morbidities. Half of all STIs occur among youth aged 15–24 years, and in some countries 60 per cent of all new infections occur among individuals in these ages, with a female-to-male ratio of 2:1 (Brabin, 1996).

Numerous studies of STIs/HIV among pregnant women confirm that young women are particularly vulnerable. For example, a study of pregnant women in Nairobi revealed that a significant proportion of women suffered from STIs. Included among the significant correlates were young age, single marital status and number of sex partners, but not illiteracy, unemployment, parity or frequency of sexual intercourse (Okumu, Kamu and Rogo, 1993). A study of risk factors for HIV in pregnant women in a maternity hospital in Harare, Zimbabwe also emphasizes the importance of such factors as young age and single marital status (Mbizvo et al., 1996).

Several reasons account for the heightened risk that young women face. Biologically, their cervical mucus is less viscous and thus easier to penetrate (Roddy, 1993). Behaviourally, they are more likely than older women to engage in unsafe sex, or in sex with partners who engage in casual and unprotected sex (see, for example, Maggwa and Ngugi, 1992). Informed choice is particularly constrained among young women, and they are more vulnerable than older women to unwanted sex, coerced sex, early and poorly-attended pregnancies and deliveries, and consequently to both STIs and non-sexually transmitted infections. Early childbearing accompanied by poor care and unsafe delivery conditions are also responsible for other morbidities, including vesicovaginal fistulae – an injury occurring at childbirth as a result of unrelieved obstructed labour that leaves the woman incontinent and unable to bear additional children (Murphy, 1981). Adolescence is also a period during which female circumcision occurs in many settings, with attendant risks of infection to young women. Where unwanted pregnancies are terminated among adolescents, such concerns as the need for privacy, lack of resources and information often leads them to delayed action and unskilled providers, again increasing the possibility of infection (see, for example, Ganatra et al., 2000; Mundigo and Indriso, 1999). Others have attributed the high levels of STIs among adolescents to such behavioural factors as risky sexual activity, drug use and health care behaviour, and to psychological factors such as self-esteem and locus of control (Yarber and Parrillo, 1992).

Husband's/partner's occupation

An increasingly observed factor underlying sexually transmitted reproductive tract infections among women is the occupational status of the husband or partner. Long distance truck drivers have been recognized for their high-risk behaviours and infection levels, but what is becoming increasingly evident is the transmission of infection to their wives and regular partners. Several studies find that the wives and regular partners of men whose occupations take them away from home for long periods of time are more likely to suffer STIs than women who co-reside with their husbands or partners (see, for example, Maggwa and Ngugi, 1992 in Kenya). A study of young married women in rural south India reports that women whose husbands were drivers or in the army, and therefore resided away from them, were far more likely to have experienced a reproductive tract infection than women whose husbands were co-resident (Prasad et al., 1999). In Bali, Indonesia, it was found that women whose husbands often live elsewhere were more likely to report reproductive tract infection symptoms than women with non-migrant husbands. In comparison, age, education and occupation were insignificant correlates of morbidity (Patten and Susanti, 1998). An exception to this finding comes from the Giza study in Egypt, where co-residence with the husband was assumed to be a proxy for sexual activity, and availability of the husband almost doubled the risk of contracting a reproductive tract infection (Younis et al., 1993). Clearly, co-residence is a proxy indicator and needs to be supplemented by more direct information on husband's sexual practices and partners.

Social consequences of reproductive tract infections/gynaecological morbidity

As shown in Figure 3.1, gynaecological morbidity has implications and consequences for a range of interrelated aspects of women's lives, including reproductive failure, as well as such social consequences as the disruption of women's domestic activities and economic roles, verbal and physical abuse, fear of childlessness, abandonment and the threat of or actual divorce, or disruption of marital relations, and damage to psychological and emotional well-being. In extreme cases, gynaecological morbidity may even result in death. Few studies have to date explored these consequences in depth, and hence sample questions have not been collated as in other sections but, where available, are discussed below. The following section presents much of the limited available evidence and highlights the multiple consequences for women's lives.

Reproductive failure

Many health-related consequences of reproductive tract infections and gynaecological morbidities are now well known (Wasserheit, 1989). Lower reproductive tract infections, for example, if untreated, can lead to upper tract infections because social stigma inhibits timely health seeking, and appropriate information and care are unavailable. Other contributing factors are antibiotic resistance and such iatrogenic factors as poorly performed abortion procedures or IUD insertions. Wasserheit (1989) suggests that the prevalence of lower reproductive tract infections in most developing countries is so high that trans-cervical procedures (such as IUD insertion, and abortion and childbirth) are likely to result in upper tract infections. Reproductive tract infections in pregnancy also place women at increased risk of post-abortion or puerperal upper tract infection and sepsis (Elias, Leonard and Thompson, 1993; Wasserheit, 1989). Reproductive tract infections in pregnancy also place a burden on families, given their association with higher rates of fetal death, low birth weight and congenital infections (Wasserheit, 1989).

Reproductive tract infections are also associated with primary and secondary infertility. Elias et al. (1993) attribute 50–80 per cent of infertility reported in sub-Saharan Africa, 15–40 per cent in Asia, 30 per cent in Latin America and 10–35 per cent in the developed world to reproductive tract infections. Gonorrhoea, genital tuberculosis, post-abortion or postpartum sepsis and even obstetric difficulties contribute significantly to infertility, and syphilis significantly reduces women's chances of carrying a pregnancy to term (Bergstrom, 1992). The consequences of infertility are dire in many developing countries, resulting in social stigma, marital discord, abandonment, low self-esteem and potential exploitation by a host of practitioners from whom treatment is sought (see, for example, Unisa, 1999).

Disruption of economic activity and domestic responsibilities

Women perform a host of activities, both economic and domestic, and many of these are disrupted or difficult to complete as a result of gynaecological morbidities. Women observe that such morbidities as excessive discharge are physically exhausting, and associate them with health consequences like loss of appetite, body and back ache, dizziness and 'weakness' that make it difficult to conduct economic activities or perform domestic tasks (Ramasubban and Singh, 2001; Ross et al., 1998). Moreover, in some cultures such as South Asia, where daily routines like cooking or praying are prohibited during menstruation, intermenstrual spotting or other signs of discharge can also disrupt women's normal domestic responsibilities.[5]

Effect on marital relationships

Marital relationships can also be disrupted in several ways. For women, these include abandonment and rejection by the husband or partner, concern about breach of trust and difficulties in negotiating safe outcomes. For one, sexual relations may be disturbed ('Does the problem interfere in your sexual relationship with your husband?') (Graham et al., 1995). Moreover, studies have pointed out

---

[5] In order to explore these issues, surveys have asked general questions, such as 'Does this problem down below ever prevent you from carrying out your normal daily activities?' 'How much did your menstrual bleeding limit your day-to-day activities, such as employment, housework or social activities?' (Graham et al., 1995). Studies have also attempted to explore, through in-depth interviews, terms such as 'weakness', and the ways in which they limit women's lives.

that in cases where a condition makes sexual activity difficult or unpleasant (for example, vaginal discharge and vesicovaginal fistulae), affected women are often rejected by their sexual partners or verbally abused by them, even when the partner is the source of the infection (Faundes and Tanaka, 1992). In Kampala, Uganda, traditional healers report that such symptoms as rash, genital ulcers and discharge among women can result in rejection and divorce (Kaharuza et al., 1996). Vesicovaginal fistulae, similarly, frequently lead to desertion and abandonment by the husband (Arrowsmith, Hamlin and Wall, 1996; Inhorn, 1996; Murphy, 1981). In northern Nigeria, divorce and abandonment rates for women with vesicovaginal fistulae were significantly higher than in the general population (Murphy, 1981).

Infertility is also linked with abandonment and fear of desertion by the husband (Cain, 1986; Ross et al., 1998). It can threaten women's self-esteem and, indeed, their security within their family and community in settings in which women's prestige and security are linked with the number of children they bear (see, for example, Wasserheit and Holmes, 1992). A study of childless women in rural south India finds that although marital life was reported to be harmonious among 72 per cent of the sample, 12 per cent of husbands had taken a second wife, 4 per cent were having relations with other women, 4 per cent had sought a divorce and 16 per cent were reportedly considering taking a second wife. About two-thirds of the sample reported being beaten or fearing their husbands, and 26 per cent reported the experience of severe or very severe violence (Unisa, 1999).

Concerns about infidelity and breach of trust also disturb marital relationships (see, for example, Zurayk, forthcoming). Several studies report that the experience of reproductive tract infection symptoms leads women to doubt the fidelity of their partners (Pitts, Bowman and McMaster, 1995; Zurayk, forthcoming).

Relationships are also affected by the difficulties infected women face in securing safe outcomes for themselves. The study of STIs clinic attendees in Harare, Zimbabwe highlights this consequence. Here, although the roles of condoms and multiple partners were known by women and men, one-third of all infected women were unable to persuade their husbands to use condoms and, correspondingly, few men indicated that they would desist from having multiple partners or use condoms in future. At the same time, women reported a helplessness about their husband's behaviour, and a powerlessness to abandon the threatening relationship. Only two of 30 women interviewed in-depth intended to leave their husbands (Pitts, Bowman and McMaster, 1995).

Economic consequences

Economic consequences for the individual and the household – both perceived and actual – may also be substantial. Direct costs include those of diagnosing and treating the disease and preventing its spread. Potential indirect costs include the value of labour lost (women who experience severe symptoms are frequently unable to carry out economic activities, whether for wage work or in the family farm or business). By one estimate, the average annual number of discounted healthy or productive days lost per capita by women with sexually transmitted infections in an urban area in Africa were 0.25 days for chancroid and 15.9 days for syphilis (Piot and Rowley, 1992). In a study of childless women in south India, the high costs involved were observed to be the leading deterrent to seeking treatment, inhibiting some 43 per cent of those who sought no care. Indeed, among those who did seek care, costs were prohibitive: increasing from about US $25 for those who sought only one course of treatment (about one-quarter of the sample) to around US $500 for those who sought five or more courses of treatment (about one-fifth of the sample) (Unisa, 1999). At the same time, the economic consequences of leaving a husband who has outside sexual partners may be perceived as more serious than the health risks of remaining in that union (Gupta, Weiss and Whelan, 1996; Pitts, Bowman and McMaster, 1995).

Stigmatization

Reproductive tract infections, particularly STIs, have different social meanings for women and men. In some settings, STIs may actually be status enhancing for men (Aral, 1992; Pitts, Bowman and McMaster, 1995). In contrast, the social experience is acutely stigmatizing for women: far more so than for men in most settings. Even such symptoms as discharge, incontinence and intermenstrual bleeding, for example, can be cause for shame and embarrassment among women. In Mexico, the stigma attached to various STIs was so strong that rural women preferred to refer to them under the general label of 'vaginal infections' (Miranda et al., 1999). An extreme example is women in Nigeria who suffer vesicovaginal fistulae. They are treated, and expect to be treated, as outcasts and are not allowed to pray, cook or participate fully in social gatherings (Murphy, 1981).

Psychological and emotional distress

The experience of symptoms of gynaecological morbidity can provoke fear and anxiety, apart from shame and embarrassment, among women. There is considerable evidence from developed countries of a link between depression and gynaecological illness (see Patel and Oomman, 1999, for a review). A clinic-based study in San Francisco of young ethnically diverse women experiencing a variety of gynaecological problems observes that over one-fifth were currently experiencing major depression (compared to rates of 5–6 per cent in general samples of women), and 13 per cent reported anxiety disorders (compared to 2–4 per cent in a general sample). However, this article does not discuss possible sources of depression or anxiety (Miranda et al., 1998).

Evidence from developing countries is less common. A review of the literature in South Asia has, however, accumulated a considerable body of qualitative evidence linking gynaecological and psychological illness, specifically vaginal discharge, with mental stress and weakness (Patel and Oomman, 1999). In a case-control study in India, half of all women attending a gynaecology clinic for the first time were found to have a significant psychological disorder, as compared to 26 per cent of women who reported no physical health problem (Agarwala, Malik and Padubidri, 1990). A second study in a psychiatric clinic in India compared women reporting physical symptoms with women reporting good health: a third of the women reporting physical symptoms attributed the cause of their symptoms to vaginal discharge, compared to 13 per cent of the control group (Chaturvedi, Chandra and Isaac, 1993). The suggestion is that the experience of gynaecological symptoms has precipitated symptoms of psychological distress. In Vietnam, a qualitative study indicates that while women experiencing symptoms of gynaecological morbidity were reluctant to express emotions and consistently denied emotional consequences in the first interview, probed responses in the second interview uncovered feelings of depression, fear, sadness and anger (Gorbach et al., 1997).

Health seeking behaviour

Studies in such diverse settings as Egypt (Younis et al., 1993) and India (Bang et al., 1989) have shown that although morbidity levels are high, relatively few women have sought appropriate care. As suggested in Figure 3.1, a range of factors inhibits appropriate health seeking. This section discusses the main themes of interest in exploring health seeking behaviours, the various remedies and types of care sought, and factors underlying delays in treatment seeking. Table 3.3 summarizes the main themes of interest in exploring health seeking behaviours, and offers examples of questions that studies have used to obtain relevant information.

Symptom recognition

Many infections are asymptomatic and thus go unnoticed by women. For example, estimates indicate that 70–75 per cent of women infected with *Chlamydia trachomatis* are asymptomatic (Gerbase, Rowley and Mertens, 1998). Even if noticed, symptoms are often taken as normal and are thus ignored (see, for example, Gittelsohn et al., 1994; Kanani, Latha and Shah, 1994; Santhya and Dasvarma, 1998; Sharada et al., 1997). Hence, studies need to assess lay beliefs and practices relevant to symptoms of gynaecological morbidity and health behaviour (see, for example, Ward, Mertens and Thomas, 1997). Even when women recognize a symptom to be abnormal and causing discomfort, treatment seeking is often inhibited.

Table 3.3. Summary of core items on health seeking behaviours, and illustrative examples of questions used in selected studies

Core items	Method used	Questions	Source
Expressing the problem			
	Key informant interviews	How do people know when they have the disease/ condition? What do people look for?	World Health Organization (WHO), 1995
Communicating the problem			
	Qualitative	Why did you not mention your complaint of white discharge? Shy and scared, doubts would be cast on your chastity, it is normal, fear of beating	Bang and Bang, 1994
	Key informant interview/ FGD/in-depth interview	If someone thinks they have the above condition, who do they tell? What would the participant do if she had any condition? What symptom would she look for? Who would she tell?	WHO, 1995
	Open-ended questions	Who can you talk to about . . .	Pitts et al., 1995
	Survey	If someone thinks that (s)he has a sexually transmitted disease, would (s)he be likely to tell his/her sexual partner?	WHO, 1990
Actions taken (and inaction)			
Treatment and provider	Qualitative	Have you ever had a sexually transmitted disease? If so, do you know which one(s)? What kind of treatment did you use? Who treated you?	WHO, 1990
	Survey	Have you seen anyone for advice or treatment to help you with this problem? (list all providers, traditional/modern)	IIPS, 1998
	Key informant interview/FGD	If someone thinks they have the above condition, where do they go for help? What happens to people with these conditions who don't go for treatment? Where would the participant go for help?	WHO, 1995

Table 3.3 (cont.)

Core items	Method used	Questions	Source
	Survey	Have you seen anyone for advice or treatment for this problem? Whom did you see and where? (If no treatment sought) Why?	Graham et al., 1995
Sequence of health seeking			
What respondent did first, second, etc.	Qualitative	Pattern	Bang and Bang, 1994
	Survey	Did you do anything yourself regarding this discharge complaint? What did you do? From whom did you know this method? Did you consult a physician? Did you seek the advice of somebody else (pharmacy, nurse/nurse-midwife/traditional midwife/family/neighbours, friends/other)? What did they prescribe?	Khattab et al., 1997
Barriers to care, individual and family level			
Reluctance to undergo a physical examination		Not asked	
Lack of confidentiality/stigmatization		Not asked	
Female autonomy	Survey	Many different factors can prevent women from getting medical advice or treatment for themselves. When you are sick and want to get advice or treatment, is each of the following a big problem, a small problem or no problem for you? Knowing where to go, getting permission to go, getting money needed for treatment, etc. If you are ill and need to see a doctor, do you first have to ask someone's permission? Whose permission?	El-Zanaty et al., 1996

Barriers to care, facility level

Service quality and accessibility	Survey	Did the provider spend enough time with you? Did s/he talk to you nicely, somewhat nicely or not nicely? Did you receive the service that you went for? How long did you have to wait before being served? Did the staff respect your need for privacy? Would you say the health facility was very clean, somewhat clean or not clean?	IIPS, 1998
	Exit interviews	Were you told the following: how sexually transmitted infections are transmitted? About your symptoms, that you can be asymptomatic? Were you given any condoms? Were you seen in a private room? How long did you wait? What were the attitudes of the staff?	Harrison et al., 1998
Service-related costs	In-depth interview with client	How much has it cost you to come here (including have you had to take time off work, etc.)? How do you feel about your visit here? (Probe about attitudes, difficulties talking to staff about symptoms, confidentiality, privacy, embarrassment, shame)	WHO, 1995

Communication networks related to gynaecological morbidity

The first hurdle to women seeking appropriate treatment is the culture of silence. Many studies have shown that women consider any morbidity relating to the reproductive system a matter of shame and may not even communicate it within the family, let alone seek care for it (Bang et al., 1989; Oomman, 1996; SEWA-Rural, 1994; Younis et al., 1993). In Brazil, a study of gynaecological morbidity among women attending a hospital for non-gynaecological reasons showed that while 10 per cent had trichomoniasis, none of these women considered the symptom important enough to have sought treatment (Faundes and Tanaka, 1992). In parts of Africa such as Nigeria, discussion related to the reproductive tract is taboo (Adekunle and Lapido, 1992). In Tamil Nadu, India, women report apprehension about confiding in anyone. For example, 'How will I tell anyone about it [white discharge]: they will think that I have done something wrong' (Santhya and Dasvarma, 1998: 10).

When women do communicate the experience of symptoms, it is usually to family members and, to a lesser extent, to friends and providers. In Zimbabwe, for example, although women report few sources of social support and few felt able to discuss the issue with anyone, those that did, discussed it with a family member (Pitts, Bowman and McMaster, 1995). In South Asia, similarly, it is husbands to whom women first turn (see, for example, Gittelsohn et al., 1994; Oomman, 1996; SEWA-Rural, 1994; Visaria, 1997). An in-depth study from the Giza project in Egypt illustrates the critical role that husbands play in blocking or facilitating their wives' decisions to seek medical care for more serious gynaecological conditions (Khattab, 1992). In Vietnam, in contrast, women appeared to rely on their peers to discuss symptoms and possible treatments (Gorbach et al., 1997), as did men with STI symptoms in Zimbabwe (Pitts, Bowman and McMaster, 1995).

Santhya and Dasvarma (1998) found in south India that while one-third of symptomatic women had communicated their problem to their husbands, older and better educated women were significantly more likely than younger or less educated women to do so, suggesting disparities in female autonomy. Working women were, surprisingly, less likely to communicate their problem with their husbands, a finding attributed to their greater economic independence and ability to seek care for themselves. Apart from husbands, women were reluctant to discuss their problem with other family members, neighbours or friends (fewer than 20 per cent did so). In fact, this study finds that partner notification is a crucial step in getting treatment: 85 per cent of symptomatic women who sought treatment had notified their husbands, compared to 26 per cent who did not (Santhya and Dasvarma, 1998).

Women are also reluctant to discuss symptoms – for example, discharge, menstrual problems or prolapse – with providers unless given an opportunity, through sensitive probing by the provider. Two studies from rural Rajasthan, India found that few women with symptoms of morbidity revealed these symptoms to visiting providers until probed by the provider or interviewer (Oomman, 1996; Sharada et al., 1997). Another study in rural Maharashtra, India highlights the oblique nature of the communication; rather than convey the problem directly to the provider, women often describe their condition as 'weakness', leading the unfamiliar provider to prescribe treatment for anaemia rather than discharge (Bang and Bang, 1994).

Treatment seeking behaviours: choice of treatment and providers

Once morbidity is recognized, women opt for one or more of a range of treatments, often sequentially. These include self-denial and inaction, self-care, untrained sources of care, chemists, and finally – usually when symptoms become unbearable – allopathic health facilities (Aral and Wasserheit, 1998). The sequential nature of treatment seeking is clear from several studies.

Inaction

Inaction is reported in several studies from India. A study of young married women in rural Tamil Nadu indicates that 65 per cent of those reporting one or more gynaecological symptoms had not sought treatment (Prasad et al., 1999). Similarly, a majority of rural Rajasthani women had sought no treatment for their gynaecological problems – from 54 per cent for white discharge to 82 per cent for prolapse. Only a small percentage had sought care from allopathic providers (Oomman, 1996). A study of women in Karnataka, India found that in approximately one-sixth of all illness episodes reported, no action was taken; this figure rose to as high as 30 per cent for illnesses of a genito-urinary nature (Bhatia and Cleland, 1999).

Preferred providers and treatments

It is usually only when symptoms become severe that the woman has no choice but to address them. Even so, the first choice of treatment is rarely the allopathic health care facility. Studies from a variety of settings report that among women who sought any treatment, a continuum of actions could be discerned. Typically, women begin with self-medication at home, largely because of the opportunity it provides to treat symptoms of gynaecological morbidity in secret (see, for example, Brabin, Raleigh and Dumella, 1992; Ogden and Kyomuhendo, 1996). Among those who opt to consult a provider, there is a preference for herbalists or other unqualified practitioners rather than allopathic health care facilities.

The reluctance to use allopathic health care facilities is documented in several studies. In rural Mexico, douching with benzal, vinegar and herbal preparations ranked first among treatment options reported by women (Miranda et al., 1999).

The study of young married women in south India found that among those who had sought some treatment, 21 per cent used home remedies, 57 per cent chose unqualified private practitioners and only 9 per cent sought care from government primary health centres (Prasad et al., 1999). A study of rural Rajasthan, which sought to evaluate a reproductive tract infection intervention, observed that a total of 29 per cent of the clients of this intervention had formerly sought care from unqualified providers (Sharada et al., 1997). Studies in rural Bangladesh report that women prefer the services of traditional healers, medicine shops and the private sector to government health facilities (Hawkes, 1996; Ross et al., 1998). While 42 per cent of women sought treatment from an allopathic provider, a majority sought care from non-allopathic providers, including 31 per cent from practitioners of indigenous systems of medicine and 27 per cent from untrained providers (Hawkes, 1996). In a study of women in Uganda who experienced vaginal or ure-thral discharge, 56 per cent sought no treatment, 19 per cent sought help in the informal sector and 25 per cent from the formal sector. In cases of genital ulcerative disease, the corresponding rates were 29 per cent, 30 per cent and 42 per cent respectively, suggesting that this condition was more likely to be perceived as worthy of formal health care (Mulder, 1994). The reluctance to seek care from health centres is also observed among high-risk populations. For example, a study in Kinshasa, Zaire observes that although 87 per cent of sex workers participating in the study reported symptoms suggestive of a STI in the 12 months preceding the survey, only 32 per cent had visited an official health care facility (Piot and Laga, 1991).

Evidence suggests that the choice of health care also depends on the perceived mode of transmission. One study of health seeking in Ado-Ekiti, Nigeria reports that informal health care tends to be the treatment of choice for conditions per-ceived to be of natural causation (Erwin, 1993). Pharmaceutical outlets may also be sought, but relatively few approach a medical establishment as their first source of care. The health seeking path of an infertile woman, for example, often pro-gressed from herbal treatment by a traditional provider, to doctors at a state hospi-tal, to a combination of a spiritual healer and intermittent use of drugs procured from a pharmacy. However, women who perceived their symptoms to be sexually transmitted were more likely than others to approach a public or private sector medical establishment as the first source of care.

Sequential treatment seeking

Sequential health seeking is also evident from several studies. The cohort study of health seeking in Uganda confirms that the first course of treatment for vaginal dis-charge is herbs (oral or intravaginal). If this regimen is ineffective, traditional healers are consulted or drugs purchased from local shops. The formal health sector is approached only if all these remedies fail (Mulder, 1994). A qualitative study of women in Nigeria similarly reports that uncomfortable symptoms are first treated with home remedies, then herbal mixtures purchased in the market, followed by visits to traditional practitioners (Olukoya and Elias, 1996). Again, it is only when self-treatment is recognized to have failed that medical facilities are approached (Kaharuza et al., 1996; Olukoya and Elias, 1996). In Vietnam, a qualitative study reveals a similar sequence of treatment seeking: 'When I am not seriously ill, I buy medicine and take it at home. When I am seriously ill, I go to the commune health centre' (Gorbach et al., 1997). And in rural India, 95 per cent of women experiencing white discharge resort to home remedies on the advice of 'old experienced women' or village herbalists and traditional healers. If these treatments fail to give relief *and* if husbands are understanding, an allopathic provider, preferably private and preferably female, is consulted. And if there is still no relief, treatment is once again sought from the traditional provider (Bang and Bang, 1994).

The reluctance to seek care from allopathic facilities can result in considerable delay in treatment of gynaecological morbidity. One study of patients presenting at health centres in Kenya reports that, on average, about half of all women with a symptom (vaginal discharge, lower abdominal pain or genital ulcers) waited at least a week between the onset of symptoms and attendance at a health centre. One-fifth waited at least a month (Moses et al., 1994, reported in Rowley and Berkley, 1998). Yet there is compelling evidence that women who respond immediately to symptoms of chlamydial or gonococcal infection are less likely to experience PID and its sequelae than other women (Washington, Aral and Wolner-Hanssen, 1991).

Increasing use of allopathic treatments by traditional providers

Home remedies and treatments provided by traditional practitioners increasingly include allopathic treatments. In Nigeria, for example, although women report that they first treat uncomfortable symptoms with home remedies, these remedies include both oral and vaginal herbal preparations and other traditional medicines, as well as self-medication with antibiotics purchased over the counter and douching with various detergent agents. Traditional practitioners, moreover, tend to prescribe a combination of herbal, spiritual and allopathic treatments (Olukoya and Elias, 1996). Similarly, herbalists (all women) in Kampala, Uganda, who routinely treat women and men for symptoms of STIs, menstrual pain, infection and infertility, report that they occasionally prescribe allopathic medication as well (Wallman, 1996).

In many settings, where over-the-counter drugs are easily available, the chemist is the preferred treatment provider (Wasserheit, 1989). Studies in Ethiopia report that large proportions of women with PID gave a history of self-medication or prior antibiotic treatment (Brabin, Raleigh and Dumella, 1992). In southwest

Nigeria, the first source of treatment for STI clinic patients is chemists, patent medicine sellers and traditional providers; private hospitals and clinics are approached only when the condition deteriorates (Akinnawo and Oguntimehin, 1997). A study of lay perspectives on STIs in Lusaka, Zambia observes that local pharmacies are the preferred source of treatment for STIs. Easily available antibiotics, provided without much information or a prescription, allow 'self-care' as a predominant option for treating STIs (Msiska et al., 1997).

Compliance

Once care is sought, failure to comply with prescribed therapy regimens poses another barrier to recovery. By some accounts, non-compliance rates may exceed 65 per cent, particularly if the condition is asymptomatic (Aral and Wasserheit,1998; Washington, Aral and Wolner-Hanssen, 1991).

Barriers to treatment seeking

A range of factors inhibits women from seeking care, particularly allopathic services and those offered in official health care facilities. A fundamental barrier, as mentioned earlier, is the asymptomatic nature of many reproductive tract infections and consequent difficulty in recognizing the need for care. But even when a symptom is recognized, women must overcome a number of social, cultural and economic obstacles before care is provided.

Perceptions of severity

The widely-held perception that such symptoms as excessive discharge, menstrual disturbances or lower back and abdominal pain are 'normal' and 'women's lot' has been documented in several studies (Egypt: Khattab, 1992; India: Gittelsohn et al., 1994, Kanani, Latha and Shah, 1994, Koenig et al., 1998). These studies underscore the point that symptoms of reproductive morbidities are either not considered serious, are considered self-limiting or simply a normal consequence of marriage and childbearing, and for all these reasons not severe enough to warrant attention. Studies have also observed, however, that when multiple conditions are experienced, women are significantly more likely to consult a physician. In the Giza study, for example, women with two or more complaints were twice as likely, and women with four or more complaints four times as likely, as those with a single complaint to consult a physician (Zurayk, forthcoming).

Reluctance to undergo physical examination

Reluctance to undergo clinical examination is a significant constraint in several settings. In rural Rajasthan, for example, only a quarter of respondents with symptoms had agreed to undergo a physical examination, and the main factor underlying refusal was modesty ('shyness') (Sharada et al., 1997). This reluctance is, in many settings, a central factor leading women to prefer traditional providers and chemists.

Lack of confidentiality and stigmatization

Several studies report that the social stigma attached to STIs can result in women seeking care from alternative providers or not seeking any care (Gerbase, Rowley and Mertens, 1998). For example, an in-depth qualitative study of STI patients in a clinic in Zimbabwe reports that a leading reason for women not seeking care from clinics is that the stigma, shame and social isolation associated with STIs is particularly acute for women (Pitts, Bowman and McMaster, 1995). Case studies in Kampala, Uganda conclude that shyness, shame and fear of stigmatization are major factors inhibiting women (as well as men) from seeking timely care (Kaharuza et al., 1996). A review of reproductive tract infection interventions in Rajasthan suggests that women are reluctant to seek treatment for reproductive tract infections because of their association with 'promiscuous' behaviour and consequent fears of stigmatization (Sharada et al., 1997). Similarly, a review of available evidence cites cultural inhibitions and shame as major deterrents to health seeking for gynaecological morbidities (McDermott et al., 1993). Confidentiality, or the fear of violation of confidentiality, poses a major threat to health seeking in some settings, particularly among adolescents.

Service quality and accessibility

Poor perceived quality of care, inaccessibility of services and cost also pose barriers to health seeking for gynaecological morbidity. A review of available evidence suggests that such factors as non-availability of physicians in rural areas, communication barriers between women and male gynaecologists, and prohibitive costs can act as major obstacles to reproductive tract infection treatment seeking (McDermott et al., 1993).

A number of studies on quality of care within STI facilities – generally catering to men as well as smaller numbers of women – have highlighted the serious shortcomings that exist for such services. A study of STI facilities in rural South Africa found through employing simulated patients that only 9 per cent of the cases were correctly managed and only 48 per cent received appropriate counselling. Exit interviews conducted with actual clients revealed that 39 per cent had been required to wait more than one hour to be seen, and only 37 per cent had been consulted in privacy (Harrison et al., 1998). A study of STI patients in Zambia found high levels of dissatisfaction with treatment in such areas as privacy, adequate information to clients and general treatment by providers (Ndulo, Faxelid and Krantz, 1995). An observation study of STI facilities in Chennai, India found that while

70 per cent of clients received adequate examination and history taking, only 6 per cent were instructed on condom use and only 27 per cent were encouraged to notify their partners (Mertens et al., 1998). An observational study of a representative sample of public sector STI clinics in Jamaica also found that fewer than 60 per cent were counselled to refer their partners or to use condoms, and fewer than 30 per cent were either offered condoms or asked whether they had any questions (Bryce et al., 1994). In exit interviews among women attending STI clinics in South Africa, 63 per cent reported lack of privacy during the consultation, 55 per cent were not informed about their symptoms and/or told that infection can be asymptomatic, and 39 per cent waited longer than one hour to see the provider (Harrison et al., 1998).

Women clearly view waiting time, lack of privacy and confidentiality as major obstacles to health seeking (see, for example, Matamala, 1998). A study in Bangladesh reports that women preferred to rely on traditional healers, partly because of the paucity of trained providers and partly because traditional healers are perceived as less threatening (Ross et al., 1998). Similarly, a study in Nigeria notes that in many cases, the type of care sought reflected the practicalities of accessibility and cost rather than deeply held beliefs (Olukoya and Elias, 1996). In Zambia, shortages of drugs, lack of privacy, long queues, opposite-sex providers and cost were negatively associated with obtaining STI treatment at government health centres and hospitals (Msiska et al., 1997). Other studies have documented women's apprehension of higher-order medical services in seeking to resolve their gynaecological problems (Khattab, 1992) as well as the frequently poor and stigmatizing treatment that women receive at STI facilities (Nataraj, 1994). In Kampala, Uganda, delay in seeking care was partly attributed to inadequate services at public facilities (Kaharuza et al., 1996).

Interaction with providers is, moreover, perceived to be threatening and uncaring. In-depth interviews with clients and providers at selected health facilities in Chile documents mistreatment, expressed either verbally or through threatening attitudes. Providers themselves acknowledge that 'if a patient behaves very badly . . . we have to shout at women because they . . . don't understand our instructions and they lose control'. Providers can also be insensitive to the realities of women's lives. The Chilean study relates the case of a woman who was told she had to go without sexual relations for a week: 'My husband didn't believe me, and I didn't know how to explain it to him . . . The doctors forbid you to do something but they don't know how to put themselves in your place' (Matamala, 1998: 16 for both quotes). Providers can also be dismissive of women, providing incomplete information on the problem women are facing. Many women in rural south India complain that 'they will not tell clearly' or 'the doctor will not say anything in detail' (Santhya and Dasvarma, 1998: 14).

Treatment-related costs

Few studies have assessed the economic costs of gynaecological morbidity to individual women. The sparse available evidence confirms that inability to pay for a service is a leading deterrent to seeking care (see, for example, Zurayk, forthcoming). Yet a large proportion of expenses incurred on women's own health goes towards treatment of reproductive morbidities. One study in Karnataka, India assessed, among women with young infants, expenses incurred on their own illnesses over a 12-month period (Bhatia and Cleland, 1999). Results suggest that women incurred approximately one-third of the total health expenditure on themselves for treating diseases of the reproductive system. The Zambian study, cited earlier, reports corruption and extortion of undue fees as characterizing government STI facilities (Msika et al., 1997). In a study of Kampala, Uganda, lack of resources was the leading reason that women cited for delays in seeking care (Kaharuza et al., 1996; Wallman, 1996).

Women's autonomy and health seeking behaviour

Limited awareness of the symptoms and modes of transmission of disease, as well as limited decision-making authority, seclusion practices and limited mobility, and lack of control over resources may inhibit women's ability to seek care. For example, limited health seeking has been attributed to the practice of seclusion, or requiring permission from the husband or other family members, and the reluctance of these powerful members to permit their wives to be examined (for Nigeria, see Adekunle and Lapido, 1992; for India, see Mulgaonkar et al., 1994; Santhya and Dasvarma, 1998). In south India, women with greater levels of autonomy were more likely to seek treatment than other women, but the relationship was weak and not significant, perhaps reflecting the universal constraints faced by women in seeking treatment (Bhatia and Cleland, 1995). Autonomy among young women is particularly constrained, and this may contribute to the finding that they are more disadvantaged than older women in acquiring care (south India: Bhatia and Cleland, 1995; Nigeria: Brabin et al., 1995 where fewer than 3 per cent of symptomatic adolescent females had sought treatment).

In south India, exposure to health information emerged as a major predictor of treatment seeking behaviour (Bhatia and Cleland, 1995). However, the authors caution that the results are tentative since reverse causation cannot be ruled out, and it may be that women who experience gynaecological symptoms are more likely than others to seek out information.

A study of health seeking among 147 women in Kampala, Uganda reporting a recent morbidity observes that the majority (81) made the decision independently on what action to take, while for 34 women, the decision was made by the husband alone. While health seeking was independent of educational level, the type of care sought was clearly associated with education. Better educated women were more likely to seek care from doctors and hospitals, whereas the less educated were more likely to seek care from nurses, shops and chemists (Wallman, 1996). This study suggests that women's treatment choices reflect the types of resources available to them – those with resource constraints are more likely to seek care from personal networks, informal connections and their own health care knowledge, while those with relatively easier access to cash tend to seek care directly from formal health facilities (Bantebya-Kyomuhendo and Ogden, 1996).

The context of treatment seeking

The array of barriers – ranging from lack of awareness of symptoms, available treatments and location of appropriate health facilities, to family-level constraints inhibiting women's decision-making authority, to norms stigmatizing women with symptoms of morbidity, to health system level constraints on access, sensitive treatment and follow-up – interact to inhibit women's timely and appropriate health seeking for reproductive tract infections. The experience of a rural Indian woman who has suffered from excessive vaginal discharge for the three years since the birth of her second child is illustrative:

In the beginning I used home remedies but they did not work. I talked to my husband about my infection. He took me to the *badava* [traditional healer] but the disease was not cured. Now my husband does not listen to me. He says that I do not have any disease as I can walk, eat and work too . . . He cannot understand my problem. I cannot talk to anybody, as they will give me the evil eye, which would make the disease more severe. I talked to the health worker but she also cannot do anything as she does not have the medicine. Recently I went to the nearby dispensary. The doctor gave me tablets. It did not help, so I stopped using them. I went to the PHC [primary health centre], and there also the doctor gave me capsules. He did not check me. This medicine also did not work . . . Now it is very difficult to bear the pain. (Patel, 1994.)

Recommendations for future research priorities

The objectives of this chapter have been to shed light on what is known about the social context of gynaecological morbidity, its behavioural antecedents, the consequences of morbidity for women's lives, and women's health seeking patterns surrounding it, and suggest a set of research questions that need to be explored in subsequent studies on the behavioural context of gynaecological morbidity. What has become clear is that although a fair amount of evidence is available, it is scattered and uneven in terms of both geographic and thematic coverage. Studies assessing gynaecological morbidity have tended, by and large, to focus on prevalence, rather than the social context. Much of the evidence on determinants and consequences comes from studies on HIV/AIDS and related sexual risk behaviours.

Major gaps clearly remain. This review highlights the need for research on gynaecological morbidity to illuminate the socio-economic, behavioural and bio-medical causes and consequences of gynaecological morbidity for the quality of women's lives, and the factors underlying the importance women attach to these problems. It also highlights the need for research that explores treatment seeking behaviours, and factors that inhibit and facilitate timely and appropriate treatment. Few studies are likely to be able to address all the pathways of influence outlined in Figure 3.1. The following research questions deserve priority:

Studies need to further explore all the risk behaviours outlined as intervening factors contributing to gynaecological morbidity. We have seen, for example, that studies emerging from South Asia report that gynaecological morbidity may, to a large extent, result from iatrogenic factors, while those from sub-Saharan Africa focus more on sexually transmitted factors. Few have addressed endogenous factors. Research is needed that probes and weighs all three sets of risk factors: sexual behaviours (minimally, the circumstances at sexual debut, the extent of casual sexual relations and use of condoms); iatrogenic risks (including place of and attendance at delivery, conditions surrounding abortion, sterilization or IUD insertion, complications and, where appropriate, circumstances surrounding circumcision); and behaviours associated with endogenous factors (for example, douching, practices relating to menstruation and the ways in which menstrual flow is absorbed, the insertion of vaginal agents for sexual pleasure and previous antibiotic use). Clearly, implications for action will be quite different, depending on which risk behaviours predominate in a particular setting.

Research needs to go beyond standard sociodemographic factors to explore the social and cultural background determinants of gynaecological morbidity. Social and cultural background factors encompass several domains. For example, morbidity has been associated with misinformation and misperceptions relating to risk behaviours and practices (sexual, iatrogenic and endogenous) and the links of these to infection, and with regard to perceptions of 'normal' and 'abnormal' symptoms. Traditional cultural norms and attitudes, particularly with regard to sexual activity, as well as delivery practices, can also influence the risk environment. At the same time, gender relations and women's lack of autonomy are observed to play an important role in shaping the risk situation. Research needs to assess the ways in which women's lack of autonomy in relation to, for example, decision-making, mobility, access to resources, the threat of violence or spousal communication influences their morbidity profiles. Clearly, more research is needed to determine whether the relationship between, for example, physical and sexual violence and gynaecological morbidity is causal or whether they are co-factors, as well as the specific mechanisms involved. Finally, research needs to pay attention to the service environment, particularly women's access to and experience with reproductive health services.

This review has underscored the special vulnerability of young women to both STIs and iatrogenic infection, and has outlined a host of possible reasons. *Few studies to date, however, have focused exclusively on the situation of young women.*

Although studies have rarely explored the social consequences of gynaecological morbidity, there is scattered evidence that social consequences can be severe. Ranging from disruption of their domestic and economic activities, to sexual rejection, verbal or physical abuse, and even abandonment and divorce by their partner, morbidities can seriously undermine the quality of women's lives. Other consequences, such as concerns about infidelity and breach of trust, fear of stigmatization and recognition of their powerlessness to abandon a potentially threatening relationship can also affect women's well being. There is a need for sensitively designed studies that probe these consequences.

Finally, our review has also highlighted the paucity of studies addressing health seeking behaviours and their correlates. This lack of information is a major gap in designing programmes to provide woman-centred services. Studies need to address the host of constraints women face in accessing care. Research questions are numerous and include the following:

- One set of questions pertains to the kinds of action taken on recognition of symptoms. Was there a period when no action was taken? Was action sequential? If so, what was the sequence of responses, what treatment was obtained from each provider, for how long was the treatment taken, and what was the outcome of that treatment?
- A second set of questions relates to cost. Typically, how much did women spend on various treatments taken, including consultation, drugs, investigations and travel? To what extent did women have to rely on their husbands or other family members to cover treatment costs?
- A third set of questions relates to communication patterns with regard to symptoms. To whom were symptoms first communicated? What was the reaction? To what extent were such communications largely within versus between genders?
- A fourth set of issues relates to women's autonomy in seeking care. Who made such decisions? How much voice did the woman have? Did women have the required physical mobility or control over resources to seek care?
- A fifth area of priority concerns the private sector and reproductive health care, which for many if not most women (and men) remains the predominant source of reproductive health care. More research is needed on the quality of private sector care and the extent to which it effectively addresses or exacerbates gynaecological morbidity problems.
- Finally, research needs to establish the constraints women face in gaining access to services. Are women aware of available services? How do prevailing norms, or concerns regarding social isolation and stigmatization, inhibit health seeking

from public health facilities? How is care at health facilities perceived? How do women rate such services in terms of access to providers, provider skills, quality of care provided, confidentiality, effectiveness of treatment, cost, and so on? What was the experience of women who have received treatment at health facilities?

In conclusion, this review has highlighted the need for research that explores the sociocultural and behavioural causes and consequences of gynaecological morbidity for the quality of women's lives in various settings, and the factors that impede women from paying attention to these problems and seeking appropriate treatment. Solid research evidence on these issues can make a significant contribution toward informing the design of appropriate and acceptable reproductive health information and services.

REFERENCES

Adekunle AO, Lapido OA (1992) Reproductive tract infections in Nigeria: challenges for a fragile health infrastructure. In Germain A et al., eds. *Reproductive tract infections: global impact and priorities for women's reproductive health*, pp. 297–316. New York, Plenum Press.

Agarwala P, Malik S, Padubidri V (1990) A study of psychiatric morbidity in a gynaecology outpatient clinic. *Indian journal of psychiatry*, 32: 57–63.

Akinnawo EO, Oguntimehin F (1997) Health-seeking behaviour of STD patients in an urban area of southwest Nigeria: an exploratory study. *Health transition review*, 7(Suppl.): 307–313.

Aral, SO (1992) Sexual behaviour as a risk factor for sexually transmitted disease. In: Germain A et al., eds. *Reproductive tract infections: global impact and priorities for women's reproductive health*, pp. 185–198. New York, Plenum Press.

Aral SO, Wasserheit JN (1998) Social and behavioural correlates of pelvic inflammatory disease. *Sexually transmitted diseases*, 25(7): 378–385.

Arrowsmith S, Hamlin EC, Wall LL (1996) Obstructed labour injury complex: obstetric fistula formation and the multifaceted morbidity of maternal birth trauma in the developing world. *CME review article*, 51(9): 568–574.

Bang RA, Bang AT (1994) Women's perceptions of white vaginal discharge: ethnographic data from rural Maharashtra. In: Gittelsohn J et al., eds. *Listening to women talk about their health: issues and evidence from India*, pp.79–94. New Delhi, Har-Anand Publications.

Bang RA, Bang AT, Baitule M et al. (1989) High prevalence of gynaecological diseases in rural Indian women. *Lancet*, 1(8629): 85–88.

Bantebya–Kyomuhendo G, Ogden J (1996) Six women. In: Wallman S, ed. *Kampala women getting by: wellbeing in the time of AIDS*, pp.189–205. East African Studies Series. London, James Currey Ltd.

Bergstrom S (1992) Reproductive failure as a health priority in the third world: a review. *East African medical journal*, 69(4): 174–180.

Bhatia JC, Cleland J. (1995) Self-reported symptoms of gynaecological morbidity and their treatment in south India. *Studies in family planning*, 26(4): 203–216.

Bhatia JC, Cleland J (1999) Health seeking behaviour of women and costs incurred: an analysis of prospective data. In: Pachauri S, Subramanian S, eds. *Implementing a reproductive health agenda in India: the beginning*, pp. 207–232. New Delhi, The Population Council.

Bhatia JC, Cleland J, Bhagavan L, Rao NSN (1997) Gynaecological morbidity in south India. *Studies in family planning*, **28**(2): 95–103.

Brabin L (1996) Providing accessible health care for adolescents with sexually transmitted disease. *Acta Tropica*, **62**: 209–216.

Brabin L, Gogate A, Gogate S et al. (1998) Reproductive tract infections, gynaecological morbidity and HIV seroprevalence among women in Mumbai, India. *Bulletin of the World Health Organization*, **76**(3): 277–287.

Brabin L, Kemp J, Obunge OK et al. (1995) Reproductive tract infections and abortion among adolescent girls in rural Nigeria. *Lancet*, **345**: 300–304.

Brabin L, Raleigh VS, Dumella S (1992) Pelvic inflammatory disease: a clinical syndrome with social causes. *Annals of tropical medicine and parasitology*, **86**(Suppl. 1): 1–9.

Brown JE, Ayowa OB, Brown RC (1993) Dry and tight: sexual practices and potential AIDS risk in Zaire. *Social science and medicine*, **37**: 989–994.

Bryce J, Vernon A, Brathwaite AR et al. (1994) Quality of sexually transmitted disease services in Jamaica: evaluation of a clinic-based approach. *Bulletin of the World Health Organization*, **72**(2): 239–247.

Bulut A, Filippi V, Marshall T et al. (1997) Contraceptive choice and reproductive morbidity in Istanbul. *Studies in family planning*, **28**(1): 35–43.

Byrne P (1984) Psychiatric morbidity in a gynaecology clinic: an epidemiological survey. *Journal of psychiatry*, **144**: 28–34.

Cain M (1986) The consequences of reproductive failure: dependence, mobility, and mortality among the elderly of rural South Asia. *Population studies*, **40**(3): 375–388.

Carael M (1997) Urban–rural differentials in HIV/STDs and sexual behaviour. In: Herdt G, ed. *Sexual cultures and migration in the era of AIDS: anthropological and demographic perspectives*, pp. 107–126. Oxford, Oxford University Press.

Carael M, Cleland J, Deheneffe C et al. (1995) Sexual behaviour in developing countries: implications for HIV control. *AIDS*, **9**: 1171–1175.

Chaturvedi S, Chandra P, Isaac MK et al. (1993) Somatization misattributed to non-pathological vaginal discharge. *Journal of psychosomatic research*, **17**: 575–579.

Coker AL, Richter DL (1998) Violence against women in Sierra Leone: frequency and correlates of intimate partner violence and forced sexual intercourse. *African journal of reproductive health*, **2**(1): 61–72.

Dallabetta GA, Miotti PG, Chiphangwi JD et al. (1995) Traditional vaginal agents: use and association with HIV infection in Malawian women. *AIDS*, **9**: 293–297.

de Zoysa I, Sweat MD, Denison JA (1996) Faithful yet fearful: reducing HIV transmission in stable relationships. *AIDS*, **10** (Suppl. A): S197–S203.

Dirie MA (n.d.) Female circumcision in Somalia: medical and social implications. (Unpublished paper.)

El-Zanaty F, Hussein EM, Shawky GA et al. (1996) *Egypt demographic and health survey, 1995*. Cairo and Calverton, Maryland, Demographic and Health Surveys.

Elias C (1996) Introduction and overview. In: *Reproductive tract infection: lessons learned from the field: where do we go from here?* New York, The Population Council.

Elias C, Leonard A, Thompson J (1993) A puzzle of will: responding to reproductive tract infections in the context of family planning programmes. Paper presented at the Africa Operations Research and Technical Assistance Project Conference, Nairobi, October.

Erwin, JO (1993) Reproductive tract infections among women in Ado-Ekiti, Nigeria: symptoms recognition, perceived causes and treatment choices. *Health transition review*, **3**(Suppl.): 136–149.

EVALUATION Project (1997) *Uttar Pradesh: male reproductive health survey, 1995–1996.* Chapel Hill, Carolina Population Center.

Faundes A, Tanaka AC (1992) Reproductive tract infections in Brazil: solutions in a difficult economic climate. In: Germain A et al., eds. *Reproductive tract infections: global impact and priorities for women's reproductive health*, pp. 253–273. New York, Plenum Press.

Foxman B, Aral SO, Holmes KK (1998) Interrelationships among douching practices, risky sexual practices, and history of self-reported sexually transmitted diseases in an urban population. *Sexually transmitted diseases*, **25**(2): 90–99.

Ganatra BR, Hirve SS, Walawalkar S et al. (2000) Induced abortions in a rural community in Western Maharashtra: prevalence and patterns. (Unpublished paper.)

George A, Jaiswal S (1995) Understanding sexuality: an ethnographic study of poor women in Bombay, India. *Women and AIDS/research program report Series, No. 12.* Washington, DC, International Center for Research on Women.

Gerbase AC, Rowley JT, Mertens TE (1998) Global epidemiology of sexually transmitted diseases. *Lancet*, **351**: S1112–S1114.

Gittelsohn J, Bentley ME, Pelto PJ et al., eds. (1994) *Listening to women talk about their health: issues and evidence from India.* New Delhi, Har-Anand Publications.

Glantz NM, Halperin DC (1996) Studying domestic violence: perceptions of women in Chiapas, Mexico. *Reproductive health matters*, **7**: 122–128.

Gogate A, Brabin L, Nicholas S et al. (1998) Risk factors for laparoscopically confirmed pelvic inflammatory disease: findings from Mumbai (Bombay), India. *Sexually transmitted infection*, **74**: 426–432.

Gorbach PM, Hoa DTK, Eng E et al. (1997) The meaning of RTI in Vietnam – a qualitative study of illness representation: collaboration or self-regulation? *Health education and behaviour*, **24**(6): 773–785.

Graham W, Ronsmans C, Filippi V et al. (1995) Asking questions about women's reproductive health in community-based surveys: guidelines on scope and content. London, London School of Hygiene and Tropical Medicine, Maternal and Child Epidemiology Unit.

Gupta GR, Weiss E, Whelan D (1996) Women and AIDS: building a new HIV prevention strategy. In: Mann JM, Tarantola DJM, eds. *AIDS in the world II: global dimensions, social roots and responses. The Global AIDS Policy Coalition*, pp. 215–229. New York, Oxford University Press.

Harrison A, Wilkinson D, Lurie M (1998) Improving the quality of sexually transmitted disease case management in rural South Africa. *AIDS*, **12**: 2329–2335.

Hawkes S (1996) A study of the prevalence of reproductive tract infections in rural Bangladesh. (Unpublished paper.)

Hawkes S, Morison L, Foster S (1999) Reproductive tract infections in women in low-income, low-prevalence situations: assessment of syndromic management in Matlab, Bangladesh. *Lancet*, **354**: 1776–1781.

Heise L, Pitanguay J, Germain A (1994) *Violence against women: the hidden health burden*. World Bank Discussion Paper No. 255. Washington, DC, The World Bank.

Inhorn M (1996) *Infertility and patriarchy: the cultural politics of gender and family life in Egypt*. Philadelphia, University of Pennsylvania Press.

International Institute for Population Sciences (IIPS) (1998) *India, National Family Health Survey 1988–1999: Woman's Questionnaire (NFHS)*. Mumbai, IIPS.

Isarabhakdi P (1995) The determinants of sexual behaviour that influence the risk of pregnancy and disease among rural Thai young adults. (Unpublished final report to the UNDP/UNFPA/WHO/World Bank Special Programme of Research, Development and Research Training in Human Reproduction, World Health Organization, Geneva.)

Joesoef MR, Sumampouw H, Linnan M et al. (1996) Douching and sexually transmitted diseases in pregnant women in Surabaya, Indonesia. *American journal of obstetrics and gynecology*, **174**(1): 115–119.

Kaharuza F et al. (1996) Private disease. In: Wallman S, ed. *Kampala women getting by: wellbeing in the time of AIDS*, pp. 166–188. East African Studies Series. London, James Currey Ltd.

Kanani S, Latha K, Shah M (1994) Application of qualitative methodologies to investigate perceptions of women and health practitioners regarding women's health disorders in Baroda slums. In: Gittelsohn J et al., eds. *Listening to women talk about their health: issues and evidence from India*, pp. 116–130. New Delhi, Har-Anand Publications.

Kaufman J, Liqin Y, Tongyin W et al. (1996) A survey of RTI prevalence, risk factors and field-based diagnosis methods among 2,020 rural Chinese women in Yunnan province. (Unpublished paper.)

Keshavarz H, Duffy SW, Sotodeh-Maram E et al. (1997) Factors related to cervicitis in Qashghaee nomadic women of southern Iran. *Revue d'Epidemiologie et de la Sante Publique*, **45**: 279–285.

Khattab H (1992) *The silent endurance: social creation of women's reproductive health in rural Egypt*. Amman, UNICEF; Cairo, The Population Council, Regional Office for West Asia and North Africa.

Khattab H, Zurayk Z, Kamal OI et al. (1997) An interview questionnaire on reproductive morbidity: the experience of the Giza morbidity study. *The policy series in reproductive health*. Policy Series in Reproductive Health, No. 4. Cairo, The Population Council Regional Office for West Asia and North Africa.

Kleinman A (1980) *Patients and healers in the context of culture*. Berkeley, University of California Press.

Koenig M, Jejeebhoy S, Singh S et al. (1998) Investigating gynaecological morbidity in India: not just another KAP survey. *Reproductive health matters*, **6**(11): 84–97.

La Ruche G, Nogbou, Messou, Ali-Napo L et al. (1999) Vaginal douching: association with lower genital tract infections in African pregnant women. *Sexually transmitted diseases*, **26**(4): 191–196.

Lahai-Momoh JC, Ross MW (1997) HIV/AIDS prevention-related social skills and knowledge among adolescents in Sierra Leone, West Africa. *African journal of reproductive health*, **1**(1): 37–44.

Macro International (1999) *Demographic and health surveys: Model A – Women's Questionnaire*. Version 6.3 (March 12). Calverton, Maryland, Macro International.

Maggwa ABN, Ngugi EN (1992) Reproductive tract infections in Kenya: insights for action from research. In: Germain A et al., eds. *Reproductive tract infections: global impact and priorities for women's reproductive health*, pp. 275–295. New York, Plenum Press.

Matamala MI (1998) Gender-related indicators for the evaluation of quality of care in reproductive health services. *Reproductive health matters*, **6**(11): 10–21.

Mathai R, Ross MW, Hira S (1997) Concomitants of HIV/STD risk behaviours and intention to engage in risk behaviours in adolescents in India. *AIDS CARE*, **9**(5): 563–575.

Mbizvo MT, Mashu A, Chipato T (1996) Trends in HIV–1 and HIV–2 prevalence and risk factors in pregnant women in Harare, Zimbabwe. *Central African journal of medicine*, **42**(1): 14–21.

McDermott J, Bangser M, Ngugi E et al. (1993) Infection: social and medical realities. In: Koblinsky M, Timyan J, Gay J, eds. *The health of women: a global perspective*, pp. 91–103. Boulder, Westview Press.

Mertens TE, Smith GD, Kantharaj K et al. (1998) Observations of sexually transmitted disease consultations in India. *Public health*, **112**: 123–128.

Miranda J, Azocar F, Komaromy M et al. 1998. Unmet mental health needs of women in public-sector gynaecologic clinics. *American journal of obstetrics and gynaecology*, **178**(2): 212–217.

Miranda MEC, Gurvich NG, Ryan G et al. (1999) Understanding reproductive tract infections from women's perspectives: a study in urban and rural Mexico. Presented at the meeting on Factors Affecting the Safe Provision of IUDs in Resource-poor Settings, Washington, DC.

Moses S, Ngugi EN, Bradley JE et al. (1994) Health care-seeking behaviour related to the transmission of sexually transmitted diseased in Kenya. *American journal of public health*, **84**: 1947–1951.

Msiska R, Nangawe E, Mulenga D et al. (1997) Understanding lay perspectives: care options for STD treatment in Lusaka, Zambia. *Health policy and planning*, **12**(3): 248–252.

Mulder DW (1994) Disease perception and health-seeking behaviour for sexually transmitted diseases. In: Network of AIDS Researchers of Eastern and Southern Africa, Nairobi, Kenya (NARESA) ed. *Prevention and management of sexually transmitted diseases in eastern and southern Africa: current approaches and future directions*, pp. 83–89. NARESA Monograph No. 3. Nairobi, NARESA.

Mulgaonkar, VB, Parikh IG, Taskar VR et al. (1994) Perceptions of Bombay slum women regarding refusal to participate in a gynaecological health programme. In: Gittelsohn J et al., eds. *Listening to women talk about their health: issues and evidence from India*, pp. 145–167. New Delhi, Har-Anand Publications.

Mundigo AI, Indriso C, eds. (1999) *Abortion in the developing world*. New Delhi, Vistaar Publications.

Murphy M (1981) Social consequences of vesico-vaginal fistula in northern Nigeria. *Journal of biosocial science*, **13**: 139–150.

Nataraj S (1994) The magnitude of neglect: women and sexually transmitted diseases in India.

In: Mirsky J et al., eds. *Private decisions, public debate: women, reproduction and population*, pp. 7–20. London, Panos Publications Ltd.

Ndulo J, Faxelid E, Krantz I (1995) Quality of care in sexually transmitted diseases in Zambia: patients' perspective. *East African medical journal*, **72**(10): 641–644.

Newton W, Keith LG (1985) Role of sexual behaviour in the development of pelvic inflammatory disease. *Journal of reproductive medicine*, February, **30**(2): 82–88.

Njovana E, Watts C (1996) Gender violence in Zimbabwe: a need for collaborative action. *Reproductive health matters*, **7**(May): 46–54.

Ogden J, Bantebya–Kyomuhendo G (1996) Home treatment. In: Wallman S, ed. *Kampala women getting by: wellbeing in the time of AIDS*. East African Studies Series. London, James Currey Ltd.

Okumu CV, Kamu PK, Rogo K (1993) The prevalence and socio-demographic correlates of sexually transmitted diseases in pregnancy in Nairobi, Kenya. In: Medical Women's International Association, Kenya Medical Women's Association, ed. *The health of women and safe motherhood: presentations at the first regional congress of the Medical Women's International Association, Near East and Africa Region*. Nairobi, Medical Women's Association.

Olukoya AA, Elias C (1996) Perceptions of reproductive tract morbidity among Nigerian women and men. *Reproductive health matters*, **7**(May): 56–65.

Oomman N (1996) *Poverty and pathology: comparing rural Rajasthani women's ethnomedical models with biomedical models of reproductive morbidity: implications for women's health in India*. PhD dissertation thesis, Johns Hopkins University, Baltimore, Maryland.

Orubuloye IO, Oguntimehin F, Sadiq T (1997) Women's role in reproductive health decision making and vulnerability to STD and HIV/AIDS in Ekiti, Nigeria. *Health transition review* **7**(Suppl.): 329–336.

Patel BC, Barge S, Kolhe R et al. (1994) Listening to women talk about their reproductive health problems in the urban slums and rural areas of Baroda. In: Gittelsohn J et al., eds. *Listening to women talk about their health: issues and evidence from India*, pp.131–144. New Delhi, Har-Anand Publications.

Patel P (1994) Illness beliefs and health seeking behaviour of the Bhil women of Panchamahal district, Gujarat State. In: Gittelsohn J et al., eds. *Listening to women talk about their health: issues and evidence from India*, pp. 55–66. New Delhi, Har-Anand Publications.

Patel V, Oomman N (1999) Mental health matters too: gynaecological symptoms and depression in South Asia. *Reproductive health matters*, **7**(November): 30–39.

Patten J, Susanti I (1998) Reproductive health in Bali, Indonesia: findings from a needs assessment survey among rural women. *Venereology*, **11**(1): L11–L18.

Phan thi Lien, Elias C, Uhrig J et al. (1999) The prevalence of reproductive tract infections at the MCH/FP Centre in Hue, Vietnam: a cross-sectional descriptive study (draft 6). Bangkok, The Population Council.

Piot P, Laga M (1991) Current approaches to sexually transmitted disease control in developing countries. In: Wasserheit J, Aral SO, Holmes KK et al., eds. *Research issues in human behaviour and STD in the AIDS era*, pp. 281–295. Washington, DC, American Society for Microbiology.

Piot P, Rowley J (1992) Economic impact of reproductive tract infections and resources for their control. In: Germain A et al., eds. *Reproductive tract infections: global impact and priorities for women's reproductive health*, pp. 227–249. New York, Plenum Press.

Pitts M, Bowman M, McMaster J (1995) Reactions to repeated STD infections: psychosocial aspects and gender issues in Zimbabwe. *Social science and medicine*, **40**(9): 1299–1304.

Plichta SB, Abraham C (1996) Violence and gynaecologic health in women <50 years old. *American journal of obstetrics and gynaecology*, **174**(3): 903–907.

Prasad JH, George V, Lalitha MK et al. (1999) Prevalence of reproductive tract infection among adolescents in a rural community in Tamil Nadu. Vellore, Christian Medical College. (Unpublished draft.)

Ramasubban RB, Singh BR (2001) Ashaktapana (weakness) and reproductive health in a slum population in Mumbai, India. In: Obermeyer CM, ed. *Cultural perspectives on reproductive health*. Oxford, Clarendon Press.

Roddy RE (1993) Predisposing factors for pelvic inflammatory disease. Identifying and educating women at risk may reduce the incidence of PID. *Journal of the American Academy of Physician Assistants*, **6**(1): 42–47.

Ross JL, Laston SL, Nahar K et al. (1998) Women's health priorities: cultural perspectives on illness in rural Bangladesh. *Health*, **2**(1): 91–110.

Ross MW, Caudle C, Taylor J (1991) Relationship of AIDS education and knowledge to AIDS-related social skills in adolescents. *Journal of school health*, **61**(8): 351–354.

Rowley J, Berkley S (1998) Sexually transmitted diseases. In: Murray, CJL, Lopez AD, eds. *Health dimensions of sex and reproduction*, pp. 19–110. Cambridge, Massachusetts, Harvard University Press.

Rugpao S (1995) Sexual behaviour in adolescent factory workers. (Unpublished final report to the UNDP/UNFPA/WHO/World Bank Special Programme of Research, Development and Research Training in Human Reproduction, World Health Organization, Geneva.)

Santhya KG, Dasvarma GL (1998) Spousal communication on reproductive illness: a case study of rural women in southern India. Paper presented at the IUSSP Seminar on Gender Inequalities in Reproductive Health, Brazil, November.

Schei B (1990) Psycho-social factors in pelvic pain: a controlled study of women living in physically abusive relationships. *Acta Obstetricia and Gynecologica Scandinavica*, **69**(1): 67–71.

Schei B (1991) Physically abusive spouse – a risk factor of pelvic inflammatory disease. *Scandinavian journal of primary health care*, **9**: 41–45.

Schei B, Bakketeig LS (1989) Gynaecological impact of sexual and physical abuse by spouse: a study of a random sample of Norwegian women. *British journal of obstetrics and gynaecology*, **96**(12): 1379–1383.

Serbanescu F, Morris L (1998) *Young adult reproductive health survey Romania, 1996: final report*. Atlanta, Centers for Disease Control and Prevention.

SEWA-Rural (1994) Gynaecological aspects of women's health: a cross-sectional study. Jhagadia (Gujarat, SEWA-Rural). (Unpublished paper.)

Sharada AL, Bhandari R, Dutta K et al. (1997) RTI intervention in Bundi district: a process evaluation. (Unpublished report for UNFPA, India, November.)

Srinivasa DK, Narayan KA, Oumachigui A et al. (1997) Prevalence of maternal morbidity and health seeking behavior in a south Indian community. Pondicherry, Jawaharlal Institute of Postgraduate Medical Education and Research. (Unpublished paper.)

Stevenson MM, Radcliffe KW (1995) Preventing pelvic infection after abortion. *International journal of STD and AIDS*, **6**: 305–312.

Tangchonlatip K (1997) Husbands' and wives' attitudes towards husbands' use of prostitutes in Thailand. (Unpublished final report to the UNDP/UNFPA/WHO/World Bank Special Programme of Research, Development and Research Training in Human Reproduction, World Health Organization, Geneva.)

Unisa S (1999) Childlessness in Andhra Pradesh, India: treatment-seeking and consequences. *Reproductive health matters*, **7**(13): 54–64.

van der Straten A, King R, Grinstead O et al. (1995) Couple communication, sexual coercion and HIV risk reduction in Kigali, Rwanda. *AIDS*, **9**: 935–944.

Venier JL, Ross MW, Akande A (1998) HIV/AIDS-related social anxieties in adolescents in three African countries. *Social science and medicine*, **46**(3): 313–320.

Visaria, L (1997) Gynaecological morbidity in rural Gujarat: some preliminary findings. Gujarat Institute of Development Research. (Unpublished paper.)

Wallman S (1996) *Kampala women getting by: wellbeing in the time of AIDS*. East African Studies Series. London, James Currey Ltd.

Ward H, Mertens TE, Thomas C (1997) Health seeking behaviour and the control of sexually transmitted disease. *Health policy and planning*, **12**(1): 19–28.

Washington AE, Aral SO, Wolner-Hanssen P et al. (1991) Assessing risk for pelvic inflammatory disease and its sequelae. *Journal of the American Medical Association*, **266**(18): 2581–2586.

Wasserheit JN (1989) The significance and scope of reproductive tract infections among Third World women. *International journal of gynaecology and obstetrics*, **13**(Suppl.): 145–168.

Wasserheit JN, Holmes KK (1992) Reproductive tract infections: challenges for international health policy, programs and research. In: Germain A et al., eds. *Reproductive tract infections: global impact and priorities for women's reproductive health*, pp. 227–249. New York, Plenum Press.

Wasserheit JN, Harris JR, Chakraborty J et al. (1989) Reproductive tract infections in a family planning population in rural Bangladesh. *Studies in family planning*, **20**(2): 69–80.

Wellings K (1996) Sexual behaviour in young people. *Ballieres clinical obstetrics and gynaecology*, **10**(1): 139–160.

Wingood GM, DiClemente RJ (1998) Gender-related correlates and predictors of consistent condom use among young adult African-American women: a prospective analysis. *International journal of STD and AIDS*, **9**(3): 139–145.

Wolner–Hanssen P, Eschenbach D, Paavonen J et al. (1990) Association between vaginal douching and acute pelvic inflammatory disease. *Journal of the American Medical Association*, 263: 1936–1941.

World Health Organization (1990) *Guidelines for qualitative research on partner relations and knowledge, attitudes, beliefs and practices*. Geneva, World Health Organization Global Programme on AIDS.

World Health Organization (1995) *A rapid assessment of health seeking behaviour in relation to sexually transmitted disease*. SEF/PRS/STD. Geneva, World Health Organization Global Programme on AIDS.

World Health Organization (1998) Family planning and sexual behaviour in the era of HIV/AIDS/STDs: Questionnaires. Geneva, UNDP/UNFPA/WHO/World Bank Special Programme of Research, Development and Research Training in Human Reproduction.

Yarber WL, Parrillo AV (1992) Adolescents and sexually transmitted diseases. *Journal of school health*, **62**(7): 331–338.

Younis N, Khattab H, Zurayk H et al. 1993. A community study of gynaecological and related morbidities in rural Egypt. *Studies in family planning*, **24**(3): 175–186.

Zurayk H. (forthcoming) Measurement of reproductive morbidity: the usefulness of perceived/reported morbidity on reproductive tract infections. In Campbell O, Mundigo A, eds. *Innovative approaches to the assessment of reproductive health*.

4

Reproductive health: men's roles and men's rights

Sarah Hawkes[1] and Graham Hart[2]

[1] London School of Hygiene and Tropical Medicine, London, UK; [2] Medical Research Council, Glasgow, UK

Introduction: why men?

Recent years have seen several shifts in the emphasis and direction of reproductive health programmes. There has been a paradigm shift away from narrow concerns on demographic targets (through a concentration on population control and the delivery of family planning services) towards a more client-centred individual approach which is, in theory at least, both holistic and responsive to an individual's needs and well-being (Pachauri, 1999). This shift has arisen from separate directions that have combined to challenge the largely demographic imperative of lowering population growth rates towards a broader refocusing on human welfare and individual choice, and the public health goal of reducing reproductive and gynaecological morbidity (Collumbien and Hawkes, 2000). Proponents of the wider conceptual framework have defined reproductive health to include both 'family planning and sexual health care' (United Nations, 1994). Operationalizing this definition at a programme level implies provision of 'the widest range of services without any form of coercion'. However, most of the policy and programme initiatives arising from this paradigm shift have so far been directed at women.

Much of this focus on women is largely historical. From the development of modern methods of contraception to the delivery of family planning programmes and the monitoring of outcomes via fertility surveys, women have been the central focus (Becker, 1996). Only recently has there been a recognition that a broadening of the reproductive health agenda away from fertility control to incorporate components such as management of sexually transmitted infections (STIs) or effective behaviour change communication, will necessitate the inclusion of men into previously predominantly female domains.

Until now, however, there has been little interest directed at the *rights* of men. Most concern is still focused on men's *roles* and *responsibilities* in relation to the health of their female partners. For men themselves, there have so far been relatively few service outcomes from this broader reproductive health agenda. Men tend to be seen as important only in respect to their female partner's health and use of services. Much of the lack of interest and subsequent service provision for the reproductive and sexual health needs of men has arisen from the starting point that women suffer by far the greater burden of reproductive ill health. An analysis of the burden of reproductive disease highlights the predominance of morbidity (and consequent risk of mortality) experienced by women compared to men (World Bank, 1993). The annual global disease burden of pregnancy alone (looking at adverse outcomes such as haemorrhage, sepsis and eclampsia) is estimated to be almost 30 million disability-adjusted life years lost. Similarly, cancers of the reproductive system occur far more frequently in women. In the case of STIs such as HIV and syphilis, however, the number of cases in men outnumbers that reported in women.

The prevention and control of STIs have increasingly become a priority. Among the historically discernible influences resulting in this change, three stand out. First, women's health advocates and other interest groups voiced dissatisfaction with the vertical contraceptive delivery systems, which overlooked other issues in reproductive health (Collumbien and Hawkes, 2000; Sen, Germain and Chen, 1994). Secondly, the growing HIV pandemic raised awareness of other STIs, especially in the acknowledged interrelationship of the two epidemics (see, for example, Wasserheit, 1992). Finally, the influential 1993 *World Development Report* enumerated the burden of ill health caused by STIs, including HIV/AIDS (World Bank, 1993).

Given the gender distribution of morbidity and mortality resulting from STIs, there is a necessity to incorporate men as potential participants, partners and 'consumers' of expanded reproductive health services, which now include the control of these infections. Policy makers, programme planners, researchers and health advocates alike recognize that men's reproductive health and their sexual behaviour, along with their gender roles, have direct effects not only on their own risk of morbidity, but also directly influence women's health outcomes. The 1994 International Conference on Population and Development (ICPD) in Cairo explicitly sanctioned signatory countries to develop reproductive and sexual health programmes that are comprehensive in scope and coverage, and are accessible by *both* men and women. The ICPD Programme of Action states that all countries should strive to develop 'innovative programmes . . . to make information, counselling and services for reproductive health accessible to . . . adult men' (United Nations, 1994: 45). Moreover, the ICPD declaration targets men for STI control strategies. Countries are advised to 'encourage and enable men to take responsibility for their sexual and reproductive behaviour . . . and to accept the major responsibility for the prevention of sexually transmitted diseases' (United Nations, 1994: 30).

Attempts to incorporate men into programmes and interventions to improve the reproductive health status of both themselves and their female partners reveal a relative paucity of details in the intervention literature. Instead we find that interest in men has focused mainly on the knowledge and use of male methods of contraception (for example, Hulton and Falkingham, 1996; Ringheim, 1995), approaches to increase support for the partner's use of contraception through joint decision-making (Bankole and Singh, 1998; Johansson et al., 1998; Karra, Stark and Wolf, 1997; Lasee and Becker, 1997; Mahmood and Ringheim, 1997) and preventing the spread of STIs by promoting more 'responsible' male sexual behaviour. In both the ICPD document and the published literature more generally, relatively little attention is given to men's own reproductive and sexual health concerns.

Basu (1996) points to the overwhelming imbalance towards women's rights and men's responsibilities: a near-exclusive demand for female reproductive health since gender issues remain at the forefront of concern. The concept of gender has often been used to refer specifically to women's status, rather than to the social relations between women and men that have resulted in gender inequalities, not least in the area of health (Hunt and Annandale, 1999). In relation to sexual and reproductive health, unless men are included in the simple but often overlooked social and epidemiological equation, interventions are going to continue along a path that not only excludes the needs of men, but also fails to address the contextual constraints of women. There is a need to ensure that the so-far women-centred focus of programmes post-Cairo does not result in a potential discounting of the needs of poor and disadvantaged men in terms of health, equality and empowerment.

Key observers in the reproductive health field have questioned the wisdom of including men in programmes. They worry that men will come to dominate the arena of reproductive health, not only as policy makers, programme managers, scientists and researchers, but also as consumers of reproductive health services (see, for example, Berer, 1996). Concern is voiced that allowing men to enter into previously female domains (for example, family planning clinics now transformed into comprehensive reproductive health care centres), may discourage women from continuing to access such services (for a review, see Wegner et al., 1998).

We believe that whilst it is necessary to incorporate men into reproductive health programmes as 'partners', a framework which views men only as 'responsible partners', with the burden of accountability for women's reproductive ill health laid firmly at their feet, may act to ignore the complex interplay between health outcomes and other socio-economic risk factors, not just gender. We highlight in this chapter how a continued women-only focus in reproductive health care research and service provision may act to miss the root causes of many of the reproductive health problems suffered by women. Whilst the role of male partners is explored in the contribution to women's reproductive ill health, this chapter goes beyond this to examine what is known about the reproductive and sexual ill health of men themselves, and how incorporating men into programmes for STIs/reproductive tract infection control in their own right, not just as partners of women, also may act to reduce the burden of disease for women. This chapter considers why researchers, health care providers and programme and policy makers should take into account the reproductive and sexual health needs of men as well as women; how programmes and surveys can be designed that acknowledge and are responsive to men's sexual health needs and concerns; and how by doing so, the outcome is likely to be beneficial not only to the men accessing services, but also to the health of women as well.

> • Summary point
> Men have rights as well as responsibilities in sexual and reproductive health care. Programmes and interventions aimed at women alone cannot succeed in reducing the global burden of ill health due to STIs. The reproductive health and sexual behaviour of men affect not only their own risk of morbidity but also directly influence women's health outcomes. Men also exert an indirect influence on women's health through social and gender relations. Programmes that respond to men's sexual and reproductive health concerns are likely to benefit both men and women.

Who are men?

In undertaking research among men, it is important to recognize from the outset that men, like women, are not a homogeneous group with the same needs and concerns globally. Men are characterized not only by their sex and gender, but also by their age, ethnicity, sexuality, income, educational status, occupation, geographical location, their position within a family, access to information and their ability to put such information to use. These social and demographic factors must be taken into account when researchers wish to look beyond the prevalence of sexual ill health in men and seek to discover its determinants. Moreover, men's sexual and reproductive health needs are not static but are likely to change over the course of a lifetime.

A survey carried out in India has shown that men with higher levels of education, higher economic status, and those living in urban areas have a better knowledge of reproductive health matters, seek treatment more frequently and are more likely to protect themselves against STIs than do other men (Singh, Bloom and Tsui, 1998). Younger men exhibit lower levels of understanding about fertility and the female menstrual cycle compared to older men (Drennan, 1998). Young men in their late teens in a working-class area of Glasgow, UK, who were at various stages of sexual engagement with young women, held very different views as to the nature of sexual relationships, and were highly variable in their adoption of safer sexual practices, even though they were knowledgeable about HIV risk factors. Thus there was significant variation among these young men even though they were recruited because they shared similar age, class and neighbourhood characteristics (Wight, 1993). These studies highlight the importance of thoroughly assessing the social, cultural, economic and demographic characteristics of men when designing surveys and interventions. The issues to be addressed will clearly differ according to a number of characteristics defining the men in a target group.

> • Summary point
> Men are not a homogeneous group. Survey methods and intervention designs must recognize and accommodate the disparate and changing needs and characteristics of men in the target population.

Empirical evidence on men's reproductive and sexual health

Historically, the sexual health of men in low- and middle-income countries has received very little attention, both from the research community and from public sector health care planners and providers. Similarly, in high-income countries, the sexual and reproductive health of men has, until relatively recently, remained hidden from academic, medical or policy scrutiny (Pfeffer, 1985). The HIV epidemic has changed this somewhat, with many interventions aimed specifically at informing men about safer sexual practices. When men have been included in reproductive health surveys and programmes, they have featured mainly as influences upon women's fertility. Whilst there is now an increasing emphasis on exploring the fertility requirements of couples rather than just women (Becker, 1996), relatively few surveys have been undertaken that concentrate on determining men's other sexual and reproductive health concerns and needs.

Many studies that have included men as participants have focused on family planning, and more specifically, on how men determine the fertility choices of their wives. Demographic and health surveys carried out in the 10-year period 1987–97 have shown that many men know, and approve of, a variety of family planning methods (Drennan, 1998). Combined data from Demographic and Health Surveys (DHS) in 21 countries show that a majority of men in most surveys can name at least one method of contraception – in 15 of the 21 countries included in one analysis, more than 90 per cent of men could name a contraceptive method (Drennan, 1998). The level of men's approval for family planning is generally determined by a number of factors, including country of residence, socio-economic and educational status. Male methods of contraception (condoms and vasectomy) are generally the least used of all contraceptive methods, although this varies greatly between countries. Use of condoms as a couple's major method of family planning varies from less than one per cent (in much of sub-Saharan Africa) to over 40 per cent (in Japan). Similarly, vasectomy rates range from 0 per cent in a large number of countries to over 10 per cent in some East Asian societies.

Beyond knowledge of, and attitudes towards, contraceptive methods, however, men in general have been found to have very little knowledge of basic reproduction (Singh, Bloom and Tsui, 1998), often misinterpret the signs of possible infection in the reproductive tract (Olukoya and Elias, 1996), and are unaware of the danger signs their partners may exhibit during potentially complicated pregnancies or labour (EVALUATION Project, 1997).

> • **Summary point**
> There is little published data on the extent of men's reproductive and sexual ill health, their knowledge of the issues of reproductive health and consequences of ill health, or an understanding of their sexuality. Most studies to date have focused on men's roles in family planning decision-making.

Sexually transmitted infections in men

Surveys undertaken in both lower and higher income countries have shown a high prevalence of psychosexual concerns among men. From a public health point of view, however, men suffering from STIs are a high priority. This is the result of a number of known sequelae of untreated or mistreated STI in men:
- Chronic pain, strictures and infertility.
- Increased risk of acquiring or transmitting HIV.
- Transmission of STIs to female partners in whom chronic complications and adverse sequelae are more common.

From what do men suffer?

The most common presenting symptoms in men infected with STIs fall into four main categories: urethral discharge; genital ulcer disease; scrotal swelling; and inguinal bubo. In addition, men may complain of pain passing urine – a sign either of a STI or, less commonly, of a non-STI in the urogenital system. Whilst men, like women, may suffer from a wide variety of STIs (over 25 common infections), the main pathogens causing symptoms in the reproductive tracts of men are listed below. These are categorized according to four recognizable syndromes. A syndrome is defined as a set of symptoms and/or signs that an individual suffers from and may present within health care settings. Such an approach is consistent with WHO recommendations for STI management (WHO 1991, 1994):

- Urethral discharge: *Chlamydia trachomatis, Neisseria gonorrhoeae.*
- Scrotal swelling: *C. trachomatis, N. gonorrhoeae.*
- Genital ulcer disease: *Treponema pallidum* (syphilis), *Haemophilus ducreyi* (chancroid), herpes simplex virus.
- Inguinal bubo: *C. trachomatis* (lymphogranuloma venereum).

Other common sexually transmitted infections include genital warts (caused by the human papilloma virus – HPV), HIV and the hepatitis B virus (found more commonly in men who report same-sex behaviour in developed countries, but linked mainly to maternal–fetal routes of transmission in much of the developing world).

Prevalence of sexually transmitted infections among men

Whilst there are many published reports of STI prevalence among men in specific settings (for instance, sexually-transmitted disease (STD) clinic attendees, blood donors and men in the workplace), community-based surveys of STI prevalence in men have been undertaken in a much smaller number of situations. Table 4.1 outlines the results from eight community- and population-based studies.

Asymptomatic carriage of sexually transmitted infections among men

Previously thought to be predominantly a feature of infections among women, there is now increasing evidence to suggest that a large percentage of men infected with the STI gonorrhoea and/or chlamydia exhibit no symptoms at all. Surveys carried out among rural populations in Uganda and Tanzania have shown that over half of men infected with gonorrhoea were asymptomatic, and among those infected with *C. trachomatis*, between 80 and 90 per cent did not report any symptoms (Grosskurth et al., 1996; Paxton et al., 1998). Overall, reliance upon reported symptoms would have missed over 80 per cent of men with either gonorrhoea or chlamydia in the Ugandan survey carried out by Paxton et al. (1998). The implications of asymptomatic carriage for morbidity survey design are clear: assessing self-reports of the presence of current symptoms will result in an underestimate of STI prevalence. In order to calculate sexually transmitted infection prevalence with greater accuracy, it is necessary to undertake more sensitive measurements of infection status. This will usually be through laboratory-based diagnosis of the presence of infection (see Chapter 10).

Table 4.1. Community-based surveys of sexually transmitted infection prevalence among men

Site of study	Year	Men in survey	Number	HIV (%)	Syphilis (%)	Gonorrhoea (%)	Chlamydia (%)	Others (%)
Tanzania (Grosskurth et al., 1995, 1996; Mosha et al., 1993)	1990–92	Rural community; stratified random population-based survey, plus laboratory examination for men with symptoms	5857 men in survey, 1664 with symptoms or a positive urine test	3.7	8.1	8.8	2.7	
Zimbabwe (Gomo et al., 1997)	1991	Rural community living on sugar estates	601			14.0		
Tanzania (Klouman et al., 1997)	1991–92	Rural community – total village population	517	0.7	1.2 (active)	0.4	9.6	Genital warts 0.9
Ethiopia (Fontanet et al., 1998)	1994	Cluster sampling from 0 to 49-year-olds in the capital, Addis Ababa	1463	6.0				
South Africa (Colvin et al., 1998)	1995	Cross-sectional survey of adults in 110 homesteads	259	10.5	8.8 (active)	4.5	6.1	
Bangladesh (Hawkes, 1998)	1995–96	Rural community, random selection of men aged 15–50 years from demographic survey lists	969	0	0.5 (active)		0.5	
Uganda (Paxton et al., 1998)	1995	Rural community, aged 15–59 years; community clustering	5140			0.9	2.1	
Bangladesh (Sabin et al., submitted)	1996	Urban slum dwellers aged 15–50 years; cluster household sampling	540	0	8	1	1	

• Summary point

Men suffer from a wide variety of STIs. Many of the more serious sexually transmitted infections infect men without causing any symptoms. Population-based surveys relying only upon self-reported morbidity will miss the majority of infected men. Objective measures requiring laboratory validation are needed for sexually transmitted infection prevalence estimates.

The predictive value of sexually transmitted infections symptoms in men: consequences for management

Surveys of self-reported morbidity are commonly undertaken to enable health planners to assess the likely needs of a community with respect to the use of health services. However, self-reports of health status are notoriously difficult to interpret and compare across surveys (Ross and Vaughan, 1986). This is partially because there is a lack of standardization in survey methods and definition (see Chapter 8 for a more detailed discussion). In women, symptoms of vaginal discharge, for example, may be due either to the STI or to non-sexually transmitted endogenous infections. This makes both the sensitivity and specificity of the WHO-recommended syndromic diagnostic and treatment algorithms variable in women. In contrast to the situation among women, however, when men do have symptoms these are more likely to be due to a STI than to other causes.

For example, Alary et al. (1998) working in Benin showed that among men attending clinics specifically for relief of symptoms suggestive of a STI (urethral discharge or pain passing urine), the use of simple algorithms for patient management was both sensitive to (over 85 per cent in this case; therefore, few false negatives) and predictive of (over 65 per cent; relatively few false positives) the STIs causing the symptoms (*N. gonorrhoeae* or *C. trachomatis*). In contrast, the same researchers found that the algorithms for managing women seeking care for symptoms of vaginal discharge were equally sensitive (85 per cent) but were poor predictors of infection (predictive value of only 11 per cent). In part this was because the women in the study had a much lower prevalence of STIs compared to the men (7.8 per cent compared to 44.8 per cent). Poor predictive value results in over- or ineffective treatment. This carries both financial and social implications for the women receiving an erroneous diagnosis of a STI, obvious financial implications for any STI control programme as well as the risk of promoting antimicrobial resistance. Researchers in Indonesia evaluated the recommended algorithms for treating men with urethral discharge presenting at a sexually transmitted disease (STD) clinic. The clinical algorithm was found to be highly sensitive among men (100 per cent; no false negatives) and had a low rate of overdiagnosis. Cost calculations using this simple algorithm approach compared very favourably with the high cost of using microbiological diagnosis (Djajakusumah et al., 1998).

These results, showing the high efficacy of simple management protocols among symptomatic men, are in contrast to many studies detailing a relatively poor performance using the clinical algorithms to treat STIs among symptomatic women complaining of vaginal discharge (see for example, Dallabetta, Gerbase and Holmes, 1998). In resource-poor settings where microbiological diagnosis is either unavailable or prohibitively expensive for widespread use, there is every reason to recommend the use of the syndromic approach to diagnose and treat symptomatic men.

Treatment algorithms aim not only for microbiological cure, but also cover aspects of counselling, prevention and partner management. It has been argued that treating symptomatic men may increase the number of asymptomatic but infected women who enter the treatment framework (Hawkes, 1998). This, of course, relies upon men informing their female sexual partners that they need treatment. In many societies it may be more acceptable for a man to initiate STI treatment than for a woman to try to persuade her male partner that he should seek care. Thus, targeting men for STI service provision, which includes partner notification strategies, may potentially result in more couples receiving appropriate care than if women are the sole focus of programme activities.

> • **Summary point**
> It is clinically easier and more effective to treat STI symptoms in men than in women. The predictive value of these symptoms in men is high: they are more likely to be due to a STI than to anything else. The picture in women is more problematic as endogenous, non-STIs are more common. Management of men with STI should always include treatment options for their sexual partners as well.

What are the consequences of untreated sexually transmitted infections in men?

Infertility

Untreated or mistreated STIs have the potential to result in inflammation, scarring and occlusion of normally open tubes. It is widely known that reproductive tract infections that reach the upper reproductive tract of women can result in chronic and serious complications; the forementioned pathological processes may lead, via pelvic inflammatory disease (PID), to tubal blockage and resultant infertility. Infertility can also affect men who suffer from acute bilateral epididymitis –

inflammation of both epididymes (a convoluted tube comprising the first portion of the excretory duct of the testis). The most common cause in sexually active young men is either gonorrhoea or chlamydia. Whilst this complication is less common in men than women, in areas of high STI prevalence and poor treatment possibilities or outcomes, epididymitis is the leading cause of male infertility (Berger, 1999).

Risk of HIV transmission

The presence of an untreated symptomatic STI is now known to act as a cofactor in the risk of HIV acquisition and transmission (Grosskurth et al., 1995). Moreover, HIV-positive men with STI shed more virus than HIV-positive men without a STI (Cohen et al., 1997). Many countries are now incorporating STI control programmes as an integral part of their HIV control strategies.

Transmission to women

STIs, including HIV, are more easily transmitted from men to women than women to men (Jones and Wasserheit, 1991). Indeed, women are twice as likely to become infected by a variety of sexually transmitted pathogens as men (Harlap, Kost and Forrest, 1991) and the efficiency of male-to-female transmission of HIV is approximately four times higher than female-to-male transmission (Aral, 1993). Moreover, apart from the increased biological risk of transmission, women may be at greater risk of acquiring STIs from men owing to social or cultural norms of behaviour that preclude women the ability to refuse sexual intercourse with their partners or to insist upon the use of barrier methods of protection. Once a woman is infected with a STI, we have seen in the foregoing that the treatment options available to her are limited by the high rate of asymptomatic carriage of the infecting organisms, and the lack of sensitivity and specificity of the syndromic diagnostic and treatment interventions used in resource-poor settings. Moreover, once a woman is infected with a STI, she has a higher chance that infection will result in an acute or chronic complication (such as PID, chronic pain, infertility, cervical cancer or transmission to an unborn child) than the equivalent infections in men (Cates and Brunham, 1999; Stamm et al., 1984).

> • **Summary point**
> Untreated STIs in men can lead to male infertility, acquisition and transmission of HIV, and STI transmission to female sexual partners, who may subsequently pass the infection to their unborn children. Not only is male-to-female STI transmission more efficient biologically, social and cultural factors often inhibit women's ability to protect themselves from infection.

Where do men go for treatment?

Although it has been suggested that policies to provide clinical services for men may, as a consequence, reach asymptomatic but infected women through partner notification strategies, such interventions are only likely to succeed if men initially seek care from providers who are trained to give appropriate and effective care. Such care would include not just determining the appropriate antibiotics to use for symptomatic men, but would also involve training health workers in other aspects of STI management, such as counselling, condom promotion and treatment for partners.

Concerns around the provision of services for men often centre on how to integrate men's services into the existing health care system; for example, how to bring men into the family planning system or the primary health care system (especially if the latter is predominantly a site of maternal and child health services) (Wegner et al., 1998). It is clear, however, that men already do seek care for their sexual health concerns, and it may be a better starting point to try to determine where and why they seek such care. In this way, programme managers, for example, can determine which health providers need to be included in training programmes, and the needs and incentives governing these providers.

Surveys carried out among men in both rural and urban areas of Bangladesh found that most men with symptoms do seek care, and that the vast majority (95 per cent) do so in the multifaceted private sector (Hawkes, 1998; Sabin et al., submitted). Given that the public sector primary health care services are mainly concerned with issues of maternal and child health, it is perhaps not surprising that men are forced to go to private providers with their sexual health problems. In contrast, a study among men in rural Tanzania found that most men with symptoms suggestive of a STI sought care in the 'official' health sector (Newell et al., 1993). In designing an appropriate response to such a finding, policy makers and programme managers have to take into account whether men can be persuaded to go to services traditionally seen as being a female domain; whether the public sector can afford to now start seeing men as well; and the costs and possibilities for training private providers in appropriate and effective care strategies compared to training public sector workers to treat more men.

> • **Summary point**
> Men with reproductive and sexual health concerns, including STI symptoms, often seek care. Understanding reasons for choice of provider may help in the design of appropriate interventions, such as provider training programmes.

What are men concerned about?

Given the number and variety of reproductive health surveys undertaken among women to determine the prevalence and associated risk factors of gynaecological morbidity and their associated reproductive health needs, we have seen in the foregoing that very little is known about the sexual and reproductive health needs of men. However, if we are aiming to establish appropriate programmes, interventions and services which see men as full participants, we must begin to understand men's own thoughts, feelings and concerns around the issue of sexual health. Whilst it is undoubtedly a step in the right direction to start encouraging men to access family planning services, this is unlikely to be a sufficient incentive for their full involvement in the reproductive health agenda. Men, like women, require holistic and comprehensive sexual health services that are responsive to their needs. To ascertain which services will be appropriate, it is vital to determine the sexual health needs and concerns of the men in the community being served.

Data from population-based studies carried out in Orissa, India and rural Bangladesh illustrate some men's perceptions of their sexual health problems: over 1000 men in two recent surveys indicated that their major sexual health concerns were related to psychosexual disorders (Collumbien and Hawkes, 2000). Worries about semen loss were predominant in Orissa, whereas in Bangladesh men were more concerned with a wider variety of problems of a psychosexual nature; concerns about semen loss and 'nocturnal emissions' were volunteered by over 15 per cent of the men questioned in Bangladesh. Other commonly reported problems concerned sexual performance: premature ejaculation and inability to maintain an erection. Such concerns were mirrored in concomitant clinic attendance figures for newly established male sexual health clinics in rural Bangladesh. Over 40 per cent of attendees reported psychosexual dysfunction as their main reason for coming to the clinic (Hawkes, 1998).

The prevalence of reported psychosexual anxieties among men in these two studies is not dissimilar to that from other published reports. Analyses of large numbers of studies carried out in both Europe and the United States among community- and clinic-based samples found a surprisingly consistent percentage of men who self-report psychosexual concerns of premature ejaculation (35–38 per cent), male erectile dysfunction (4–9 per cent) and inhibited male orgasm (4–10 per cent) (Nathan et al., 1986; Spector and Carey, 1990).

Thus, in designing both survey instruments to study men's sexual health, and in thinking about the range of possible interventions suitable for improving men's sexual health, both researchers and programme planners need to consider the full range of concerns voiced by men. Whilst the international community of policy makers, health advocates and programme planners may be concerned with, and focused upon, the problems of STIs, men themselves may have a wider set of concerns. If men are to be encouraged to access services, services must reflect and respond to men's stated concerns.

> • **Summary point**
> Whilst researchers, policy makers and programme managers may be concerned about one area of men's sexual health – STIs – men themselves may have other worries and sexual health concerns. Appropriate and responsive interventions must take into account the concerns of the recipient community.

The role of sexuality

Throughout the world, there is often a fixed notion of men's sexuality. Categories of sexual behaviour are sometimes seen as immutable and somewhat rigid: 'heterosexual' (straight), 'homosexual' (gay) or 'bisexual'. However, it is clear that there is fluidity and temporal variation in men's sexual behaviour and sexual identities. Studies indicate that, amongst ostensibly homosexual men, there are reportedly high levels of heterosexual experiences, with up to 10 per cent of men recruited to investigate homosexual behaviour reporting sex with female partners in the previous year (Davies et al., 1993; Fitzpatrick et al., 1989). Studies of the same-sex behaviour of 'heterosexual' men are difficult to find, and it is often not clear whether reports of homosexual behaviour are by men whose primary sexual experience is heterosexual. Nevertheless, in one of the few surveys of a representative sample of men and women carried out in the UK – the National Survey of Sexual Lifestyles (NATSAL) – it was found that 6.1 per cent of men reported some lifetime homosexual experience (Johnson et al., 1994).

In some regions, notably Central and South America, in countries such as Mexico (Liguouri, Block and Aggleton, 1996), the Dominican Republic (de Moya and Garcia, 1996) and Peru (Caceres, Reingold and Watts, 1996), bisexual behaviour among men is accepted much more readily than in other parts of the world, particularly among those who are the insertive partners in anal intercourse. Indeed, in many of these countries, the majority of cases of HIV infection occurring in women early in the HIV/AIDS epidemic were a consequence of secondary transmission of the infection from male partners who had contracted the infection through homosexual sex (Mann, Tarantola and Netter, 1992). It is also apparent that in many countries male sex workers who receive payment for sex from other men do not primarily identify as gay, and may be married or have regular female partners (see Aggleton, 1999). Transgender males are also prevalent in many cultures (*hijras* in India and Pakistan, *katoeys* in Thailand and Laos, and *waria* in Indonesia), many of whom are sex workers providing anal and oral sex to men who do not self-identify as homosexual or bisexual (Beyrer, 1998).

While the pattern of HIV transmission in developed countries is often dichoto-
mized into homosexual versus heterosexual, there is evidence that in resource-poor
countries partner-mixing patterns may be more complex. A study of Royal Thai
Army conscripts in northern Thailand (who are recruited from the population of
young Thai men by a lottery system and are therefore likely to be representative),
found that those who had male or transvestite (*katoey*) sex partners were more
likely to be married, have girlfriends and visit female sex workers than men who
had sexual intercourse only with female partners (Beyrer et al., 1996). These men
who have sex with men had more female lifetime sex partners and were more likely
to be infected with HIV than men who reported sexual intercourse with only female
partners.

The evidence from developed countries also indicates that men who have sex
with men are more likely to acquire a STI. More than half the men in the UK
NATSAL study who had five or more homosexual partners in the last 5 years
reported attendance at an STD clinic, compared to only one in seven of the men
reporting five or more heterosexual partners. A recent study of homosexual men in
Scotland (Hart et al., 1999a) found that respondents were 4.5 times more likely to
report ever having a lifetime experience of a sexually transmitted infection than
heterosexual men who reported STD clinic attendance in the NATSAL study (36
per cent vs. 8 per cent), and 12 times more likely to report a STI in the last year (11
per cent vs. 0.9 per cent).

The data suggesting that men's sexuality often lies on a continuum between strict
heterosexuality and strict homosexuality, taken together with the higher STI
prevalence rates among men who have sex with men, have several implications for
both research and service provision. The first is that provision of sexual and reproductive services for men, as well as research on the sexual behaviour of men which
do not take into account the range of expression of men's sexuality in different cultures, are likely to exclude those behaviours with the greatest potential for disease
transmission. Comprehensive service provision, including health promotion, will
be compromised unless there is open discussion of sexual behaviour, including
same-sex experiences. Infections of the anus and rectum are often asymptomatic;
thus an accurate history as well as a thorough physical examination are essential.
Non-judgemental attitudes are required of health care workers with regard to the
reported sexual behaviour of patients, as proscriptive attitudes are likely to result
in delayed treatment seeking or even the avoidance of services altogether. The
implications for research point to the need for qualitative studies to gain a comprehensive understanding of the local cultural categories and language of sexuality and
sexual relations before embarking upon surveys of the sexual behaviour of men.

Furthermore, these findings have implications for the dynamics of STI transmission to women. The high prevalence of reported STI in homosexual and bisexual
men indicates the potential for transmission of STI, including HIV, to female part-

ners. Women have a significant risk of acquiring the infections contracted by their male partners, whether through heterosexual or homosexual sex, jeopardizing their own sexual and reproductive health and the health of their unborn children. Efforts to reduce these risks require an understanding of the often complex patterns of sexual behaviour of their male partners.

> • Summary point
> An understanding of men's reproductive and sexual health needs must take into account their sexuality as well as their sexual behaviour. Providers and researchers who assume exclusive heterosexuality or exclusive homosexuality in their male patients and respondents may be missing those behaviours that have the greatest potential for STI transmission.

How do men's actions influence women's health?

Exposing women to infection

A direct relationship has been observed between men's actions and health outcomes among women. Studies of STI risk factors among married women have shown a consistently strong association between a woman's risk of having a STI and the reported sexual behaviour of her husband rather than the woman herself (Hunter et al., 1994; Moses et al., 1994; Thomas et al., 1996). Gangakhedkar et al. (1997) found that women with no history of commercial sex work attending STD clinics in Pune, India had an HIV prevalence rate of over 13 per cent, and prevalence rates of cervicitis, vaginitis and genital ulcer disease that surpassed those of female sex workers attending the clinics. The only significant reported risk for these women was sex with their husbands. Results from Africa show a similar type of relationship. Duncan et al. (1994) found a higher than expected rate of STIs among monogamous women married to their first and only sexual partner.

There are social, economic and cultural reasons why married men are more likely to contract primary STIs compared to their wives. Men may be more likely to be involved in sexual networks that include more than one partner; they are generally more mobile and more often involved in inter- or intra-country patterns of migration pursuing employment opportunities; and finally, men are more likely to be the purchasers of commercial sex (see Greene and Biddlecom, 1997 for a review). In societies where sanctions against non-marital sex are less harsh for men than for women, and women are subjected to tight social and cultural control, their non-commercial non-marital sexual relations may be less common than in other societies. Furthermore, labour migration and the predominantly male demographic phenomenon of urbanization in developing countries may increase both the opportunity and demand for commercial sexual relations. Finally, in many societies, social norms and expectations exist that view men's non-monogamous sexual attitudes and lifestyles benevolently or even positively.

These sociocultural parameters are compounded by the biological transmission risk of STI between men and women. Men generally report higher rates of sexual risk behaviour compared to women, and if infected with a sexually transmissible pathogen, they are more likely to infect their subsequent female partners during unprotected sex.

Women's inability to negotiate safer sex

As seen in the foregoing, gender relations, sociocultural roles, social norms and men's economic position may act to encourage men's at-risk sexual lifestyles, and place them at a higher initial risk of contracting STIs. However, for many women, even if they are aware of their partner's sexual behaviours, there are many barriers preventing the negotiation of safer sexual relationships (Greene and Biddlecom, 1997). The risk or threat of domestic violence, or loss of economic support, may act to dissuade women from even starting to discuss protective measures with their sexual partners. Violence against women is reported not just by women, but admitted to by men themselves (see, for example, Martin et al., 1999b; Schafer, Caetano and Clark, 1998).

In Uttar Pradesh, India a study found that men who engaged in extramarital sex and those with current STI symptoms were more likely to have sexually coerced their wives through the use of force (Martin et al., 1999a). Unplanned pregnancies were also more common among wives of physically or sexually abusive men. There is a clear need for further research to elucidate the cultural, socio-economic and psychosocial determinants of these interrelated male behaviours. In this setting, risky sexual behaviour, STI, and physical and sexual abuse were found to be associated and are likely to require a comprehensive and holistic intervention focused on men.

Given the conditions of violence, coercion and economic dependency that many women face, asking a male sexual partner to use condoms or refusing sex when they are concerned that a man is infected with a STI is often not possible. Such is the case even when women believe or know that their partners are infected with HIV (Blanc et al., cited in Drennan, 1998). A study of reasons for resistance to condom use among higher-risk women (women who injected drugs or whose partners were drug users) in New York City, USA found that decision-making around condom use is bound with a mixture of social, economic and cultural factors (Worth, 1989). Decisions on the use of condoms are made on a per relationship basis; even when women perceive their partners to be infected with HIV, they do not insist on condom use as it carries too many short-term costs (possible disruption of a relationship through violence or loss of economic support) compared to the perceived long-term benefit of avoiding a STI.

Comparable results have been found in studies carried out in a variety of African countries. A study in Zaire (Kamenga et al., reported in Becker, 1996) found that among HIV serodiscordant couples, condom use was significantly higher among male HIV-negative female HIV-positive couples, compared to male HIV-positive female HIV-negative couples. Similar results are reported by Becker (1996) from studies in Uganda and Rwanda. These results highlight the relative powerlessness of women in negotiating condom use, even in the face of a known HIV risk.

Although men more often control sexual decision-making, a further study from Rwanda (van der Straten et al., 1995) found that strategies to increase couple communication over the 2 years of the study resulted in an increase in reported condom use by the couple. This was especially true for HIV-serodiscordant couples. This wide-ranging and intensive study was somewhat limited by its predominant focus on women. However, the authors conclude that 'before attempting to improve women's negotiating skills, their male partners should be brought to the negotiating table to make them collaborators rather than opponents in the safer-sex process' (van der Straten et al., 1995: 42).

Men's control over health seeking

The influence men exert on the reproductive health of their female partners is not limited to the direct effects of STI exposure. Men are often the decision-makers on the care-seeking behaviour of household members. While the most serious sequelae of reproductive tract infections in women could be prevented with timely and effective treatment, in regions where women lack key resources and autonomy, the permission of male relatives is often required to gain access to medical care for symptoms or routine health examinations for asymptomatic infection.

The predominance of male decision-making is found in diverse areas of reproductive health: contraceptive use (Cook and Maine, 1987), desired family size (although Greene and Biddlecom (1997) review this area substantially and find that surveys start with the hypothesis that men act as barriers to women's contraceptive use, they report finding no studies that examine the possibility that men block women who want to have more children), as well as the ability of women to seek health care. A community-based study in Gujarat, India found that half the women in this rural population who reported symptoms suggestive of a reproductive tract infection and agreed to come to a health camp for diagnosis and treatment subsequently failed to attend for clinical services. One of the main reasons provided by the women for this poor turnout was that the men and elders in their families either did not give permission or were not available to grant permission. A study in Bolivia found that men act as gatekeepers to health care for their wives. Husbands were making care-seeking decisions as this was seen to fit in with the 'authority' of their 'traditional' role (Kaune, 1997).

In other areas of female reproductive health care seeking, the characteristics of the male partner have been found to have an impact on the health outcomes of the women. For example, a case-control study of maternal deaths in rural Maharashtra, India found that women whose husbands were more educated had a lower risk of mortality from matched pregnancy complications compared to women with illiterate husbands, after controlling for other socio-economic factors (Ganatra, Coyaji and Rao, 1998). The education of the woman herself was found to have no effect on her survival, reflecting the peripheral decision-making role women play, especially when ill. In this study as in many others, variables such as distance from an appropriate health facility were found to be predictive of the woman's survival (see, for example, Ronsmans et al., 1997). Whilst gender relations are an important component of the variety of barriers to reproductive health care for women, physical, cultural, technical, economic and other social factors often play the most critical roles.

Men's ability to influence women's health outcomes are perhaps not difficult to analyse in terms of the interplay between social and economic power and gender differentials. Men are generally the economically stronger figure in many households, and their control of the family's 'pursestrings' may have a direct influence on the type of health care services that women and girls in the family can legitimately seek and purchase. However, as the literature reviewed in the foregoing has shown (see, for example, Olukoya and Elias, 1996; Singh, Bloom and Tsui, 1998), men's reluctance may arise more out of lack of knowledge than a position of wilful neglect. The appropriate interventions, in many cases, would be to work not only toward the longer-term goal of socio-economic equality for women and men, including at the household level, but also to achieve shorter-term aims, such as educating both girls and boys on sexual and reproductive health, and implementing information, education and communication (IEC) campaigns directed at men. Such strategies may enable men more fully to understand their own reproductive and sexual health needs as well as the concerns and needs of their female partners.

> • **Summary point**
> Men are generally the decision-makers on a range of issues that have a direct impact on women's health. Examples include whether or not to use condoms or practise other risk reduction measures, and acting as 'gatekeepers' to women's access to appropriate health care. Understanding the sociocultural, economic or educational determinants underlying men's decisions will promote the development of effective interventions with health benefits for their female partners as well as the men themselves.

Conclusions

This chapter has illustrated how a resurgence of interest in the control of STIs has resulted in greater interest in the sexual health of men. For the most part, this interest is focused on strategies to 'encourage and enable men to take responsibility for their sexual and reproductive behaviour and their social and family roles' (United Nations, 1994). Whilst men are deemed to have 'responsibility', women are said to have 'rights' with regard to making choices about reproductive health and accessing appropriate and effective services. It has been argued, however, that in the case of STIs, services and interventions can only succeed in their aim of managing infected persons and preventing transmission if they are equally accessible to both men and women. Whilst provision of services and interventions against STIs in men should not be at the expense of those for women, it is often clinically easier and more effective to diagnose and treat men with STI compared to women in resource-poor settings. Moreover, it may even prove to be an effective strategy in controlling the spread of STIs, and hence reducing the disproportionate burden of their complications suffered by women.

If we go beyond the assumption of the 'responsibility' of men for sexual and reproductive behaviour, and affirm that access to sexual and reproductive health services is a human right that should be available to both men and women, then it is possible to begin to think about how these services should be designed to be attractive to men and provide comprehensive health care for men. In this regard, it is important to recognize the concerns and needs of men themselves. Surveys carried out among men have historically focused on their reproductive concerns as they relate to their female partners. Few resources have been allocated to research to assess men's own sexual and reproductive health needs although, as we have seen, methods for doing this have been available for some time, and are being constantly developed and refined in response to new and challenging health threats. The time has now come to determine the sexual and reproductive health needs of men if they are to participate fully as healthy and responsible partners in improving sexual and reproductive health for all.

REFERENCES

Aggleton P (1999) *Men who sell sex*. London, UCL Press.
Alary M, Baganizi A, Guedeme A, et al. (1998) Evaluation of clinical algorithms for the diagnosis of gonococcal and chlamydial infections among men with urethral discharge or dysuria and women with vaginal discharge in Benin. *Sexually transmitted infections*, **74**(Suppl. 1): S44–S49.
Aral S (1993) Heterosexual transmission of HIV: the role of other sexually transmitted infections

and behavior in its epidemiology, prevention and control. *Annual review of public health*, **14**: 451–467.

Bankole A, Singh S (1998) Couples' fertility and contraceptive decision-making in developing countries: hearing the man's voice. *International family planning perspectives*, **24**(1): 15–23.

Basu AM (1996) The International Conference on Population and Development, Cairo, 1994. Is its Plan of Action important, desirable and feasible? ICPD: what about men's rights and women's responsibilities? *Health transition review*, **6**: 225–227.

Becker S (1996) Couples and reproductive health: a review of couple studies. *Studies in family planning*, **27**(6): 291–306.

Berer M (1996) Men. *Reproductive health matters*, **7**: 7–10.

Berger RE (1999) Acute epididymitis. In: Holmes K et al., eds. *Sexually transmitted diseases*, pp. 847–858. New York, McGraw Hill Publications.

Beyrer C (1998) *War in the blood*. London, Zed Books Ltd.

Beyrer C, Kunawararak P, Celentano DD et al. (1996) The epidemiology of HIV and syphilis among male commercial sex workers in northern Thailand [letter]. *AIDS*, **10**(1): 113.

Caceres CF, Reingold A, Watts D (1996) Male bisexuality in Peru and the prevention of AIDS. In: Aggleton P (ed.) *Bisexualities and AIDS*. London: Taylor and Francis.

Cates W, Brunham RC (1999) Sexually transmitted diseases and infertility. In: Holmes K et al., eds. *Sexually transmitted diseases*, pp. 1079–1088. New York, McGraw Hill Publications.

Cohen MS, Hoffman IF, Royce RA et al. (1997) Reduction of concentration of HIV-1 in semen after treatment of urethritis: implications for prevention of sexual transmission of HIV-1. AIDSCAP Malawi Research Group. *Lancet*, **349**(9069): 1868–1873.

Collumbien M, Hawkes S (2000) Missing men's message: does the reproductive health approach respond to men's sexual health needs? *Culture, health and sexuality*, **2**(2): 135–150.

Colvin M, Abdool Karim SS, Connolly C et al. (1998) HIV infection and asymptomatic sexually transmitted infections in a rural South African community. *International journal of STD and AIDS*, **9**: 548–550.

Cook RJ, Maine D (1987) Spousal veto over family planning services. *American journal of public health*, **77**(3): 339–344.

Dallabetta GA, Gerbase AC, Holmes KK (1998) Problems, solutions and challenges in syndromic management of sexually transmitted diseases. *Sexually transmitted infections*, **74**(Suppl. 1): S1–S11.

Davies PM, Hickson FCI, Weatherburn P et al. (1993) *Sex, gay men and AIDS*. Basingstoke, Falmer.

de Moya EA, Garcia R (1996) AIDS and the enigma of bisexuality in the Dominican Republic. In: Aggleton P, ed. *Bisexualities and AIDS*, pp. 121–135. London, Taylor and Francis.

Djajakusumah T, Sudigdoadi S, Keersmaekers K et al. (1998) Evaluation of syndromic patient management algorithm for urethral discharge. *Sexually transmitted infections*, **74**(Suppl. 1): S29–S33.

Drennan M (1998) Reproductive health: new perspectives on men's participation. *Population reports*, Series J, No. 46. Baltimore, Johns' Hopkins University School of Public Health, Population Information Program.

Duncan ME, Tibaux G, Pelzer A et al. (1994) A socioeconomic, clinical and serological study in an African city of prostitutes and women still married to their first husband. *Social science and medicine*, **39**(3): 323–333.

EVALUATION Project (1997) Uttar Pradesh Male Reproductive Health Survey 1995–1996. Evaluation Project, North Carolina.

Fitzpatrick R, Hart G, Boulton M et al. (1989) Heterosexual sexual behaviour in a sample of homosexually active men. *Genitourinary medicine*, **65**: 259–262.

Fontanet AL, Messele T, Dejene A et al. (1998) Age- and sex-specific HIV-1 prevalence in the urban community setting of Addis Ababa, Ethiopia. *AIDS*, **12**: 315–322.

Gangakhedkar RR, Bentley ME, Divekar AD et al. (1997) Spread of HIV infection in married monogamous women in India. *Journal of the American Medical Association*, **278**(23): 2090–2092.

Ganatra BR, Coyaji KJ, Rao VN (1998) Too far, too little, too late: a community-based case-control study of maternal mortality in rural west Maharashtra, India. *Bulletin of the World Health Organization*, **76**(6): 591–598.

Gomo E, Ndamba J, Nhandara C et al. (1997) Prevalence of gonorrhoea and knowledge of sexually transmitted infections in a farming community in Zimbabwe. *Central African journal of medicine*, **43**(7): 192–195.

Greene ME, Biddlecom AE (1997) *Absent and problematic men: demographic accounts of male reproductive roles.* Population Council Working Paper no. 103. New York, Population Council.

Grosskurth H, Mayaud P, Mosha F et al. (1996) Asymptomatic gonorrhoea and chlamydial infection in rural Tanzanian men. *British medical journal*, **312**: 277–280.

Grosskurth H, Mosha F, Todd J et al. (1995) Impact of improved treatment of sexually transmitted diseases on HIV infection in rural Tanzania: randomised control trial. *Lancet*, **346**: 530–536.

Harlap S, Kost K, Forrest J (1991) *Preventing pregnancy, protecting health: a new look at birth control choices in the United States.* New York, Alan Guttmacher Institute.

Hart GJ, Flowers P, Der GJ et al. (1999a) Gay men's HIV-related sexual risk behaviour in Scotland. *Sexually transmitted infections*, **75**: 242–246.

Hart GJ, Pool R, Green G et al. (1999b) Women's attitudes to condoms and female controlled means of protection against HIV and STDs in south-western Uganda. *AIDS Care*, **11**: 687–698.

Hawkes S (1998) Why include men? Establishing sexual health clinics for men in rural Bangladesh. *Health policy and planning*, **13**(2): 121-130.

Hulton L, Falkingham J (1996) Male contraceptive knowledge and practice: what do we know? *Reproductive health matters*, **7**: 90–99.

Hunt K, Annandale E (1999) Relocating gender and morbidity: examining men's and women's health in contemporary Western societies. *Social science and medicine*, **48**: 1–5.

Hunter DJ, Maggwa BN, Mati JK et al. (1994) Sexual behaviour, STDs, male circumcision and risk of HIV infection among women in Nairobi, Kenya. *AIDS*, **8**(1): 93–99.

Johansson A, Nguyen TN, Tran QH et al. (1998) Husbands' involvement in abortion in Vietnam. *Studies in family planning*, **29**(4): 400–413.

Johnson A, Wadsworth J, Wellings K et al. (1994) *Sexual attitudes and lifestyles.* Oxford, Blackwell.

Jones RB, Wasserheit JN (1991) Introduction to the biology and natural history of sexually transmitted diseases. In: Wasserheit JN et al., eds. *Research issues in human behaviour and sexually* transmitted diseases in the AIDS era, pp. 11–137. Washington, DC, American Society for Microbiology.

Karra MV, Stark NN, Wolf J (1997) Male involvement in family planning: a case study spanning five generations of a south Indian family. *Studies in family planning*, **28**(1): 24–34.

Kaune V (1997) Auto-diagnosis of community problems: the involvement of men in facilitating access to health care for women. (Unpublished report, cited in Popline http://www.jhuccp.org/popline/popline Document No. PIP 140010.)

Klouman E, Masenga EJ, Klepp KI et al. (1997) HIV and reproductive tract infections in a total village population in rural Kilimanjaro, Tanzania: women at increased risk. *Journal of acquired immune deficiency syndromes and human retrovirology*, **14**(2): 163–168.

Lasee A, Becker S (1997) Husband–wife communication about family planning and contraceptive use in Kenya. *International family planning perspectives*, **23**(1): 15–20.

Liguori AL, Block MG, Aggleton P (1996) Bisexuality and AIDS in Mexico. In: Aggleton P, ed. *Bisexualities and AIDS*, pp. 76–98. London, Taylor and Francis.

Mahmood N, Ringheim K (1997) Knowledge, approval and communication about family planning as correlates of desired fertility among spouses in Pakistan. *International family planning perspectives*, **23**(2): 122–129.

Mann J, Tarantola DJM, Netter TW (1992) *AIDS in the world*. Cambridge, MA, Harvard University Press.

Martin SL, Kilgallen B, Tsui AO et al. (1999a) Sexual behaviors and reproductive health outcomes: associations with wife abuse in India. *Journal of the American Medical Association*, **282**(20): 1967–1972.

Martin SL, Tsui AO, Maitra K et al. (1999b) Domestic violence in northern India. *American journal of epidemiology*, **150**(4): 417–426.

Moses S, Muia E, Bradley JE et al. (1994) Sexual behaviour in Kenya: implications for STD transmission and control. *Social science and medicine*, **39**: 1649–1656.

Mosha F, Nicoll A, Barongo L et al. (1993) A population-based study of syphilis and sexually transmitted disease syndromes in north-western Tanzania – 1. Prevalence and incidence. *Genitourinary medicine*, **69**: 415–420.

Nathan DM, Singer DE, Godine JE et al. (1986) Non-insulin-dependent diabetes in older patients: complications and risk factors. *American journal of medicine*, **81**(5): 837–42.

Newell J, Senkoro K, Mosha F et al. (1993) A population-based study of syphilis and sexually transmitted disease syndromes in north-western Tanzania – 2. Risk factors and health seeking behaviour. *Genitourinary medicine*, **69**: 421–426.

Olukoya AA, Elias C (1996) Perceptions of reproductive tract morbidity among Nigerian women and men. *Reproductive health matters*, 7:56–63.

Pachauri S (1999) Moving towards reproductive health: issues and evidence. In: Pachauri S, ed. *Implementing a reproductive health agenda in India: the beginning*, pp. xiii–xvii New Delhi, Population Council.

Paxton LA, Sewankambo N, Gray R et al. (1998) Asymptomatic non-ulcerative genital tract infections in a rural Ugandan population. *Sexually transmitted infections*, **74**: 421–425.

Pfeffer N (1985) The hidden pathology of the male reproductive system. In: Homans H, ed. *The sexual politics of reproduction*, pp. 30–44. Aldershot, Gower Press.

Ringheim K (1995) Evidence for the acceptability of an injectable hormonal method for men. *International family planning perspectives*, 21(2): 75–80.

Ronsmans C, Vanneste AM, Chakraborty J et al. (1997) Decline in maternal mortality in Matlab, Bangladesh: a cautionary tale. *Lancet*, 350: 1810–1814.

Ross DA, Vaughan JP (1986) Health interview surveys in developing countries: a methodological review. *Studies in family planning*, 17(2): 78–94.

Sabin K, Rahman M, Hawkes S et al. (submitted) Prevalence of STIs in Dhaka slum communities. *Sexually transmitted infections*.

Schafer J, Caetano R, Clark CL (1998) Rates of intimate partner violence in the United States. *American journal of public health*, 9: 47–56.

Sen G, Germain A, Chen LC (1994) Reconsidering population policies: ethics, development, and strategies for change. In: Sen G et al., eds. *Population policies reconsidered: health, empowerment, and rights*, pp. 3–11. Cambridge, MA, Harvard University Press.

Singh KK, Bloom SS, Tsui AO (1998) Husbands' reproductive health knowledge, attitudes and behaviour in Uttar Pradesh, India. *Studies in family planning*, 29(4): 388–399.

Spector IP, Carey MP (1990) Incidence and prevalence of the sexual dysfunctions: a critical review of the empirical literature. *Archives of sexual behaviour*, 19(4): 389–408.

Stamm WE, Guinan ME, Johnson C et al. (1984) Effect of treatment regimens for *Neisseria gonorrhoeae* on simultaneous infection with *Chlamydia trachomatis*. *New England journal of medicine*, 310: 545–549.

Thomas T, Choudhri S, Kariuki S et al. (1996) Identifying cervical infection among pregnant women in Nairobi, Kenya: limitations of risk assessment and symptom-based approaches. *Genitourinary medicine*, 72: 334–338.

United Nations (1994) Programme of Action of the UN International Conference on Population and Development. New York, United Nations.

van der Straten A, King R, Grinstead O et al. (1995) Couple communication, sexual coercion and HIV risk reduction in Kigali, Rwanda. *AIDS*, 9: 935–944.

Wasserheit JN (1992) Epidemiological synergy. Interrelationships between human immunodeficiency virus infection and other sexually transmitted diseases. *Sexually transmitted diseases*, 19(2): 61–77.

Wegner MN, Landry E, Wilkinson D et al. (1998) Men as partners in reproductive health: from issues to action. *International family planning perspectives*, 24(1): 38–42.

Wight D (1993) Constraints or cognition? Young men and safer heterosexual sex. In: Aggleton P et al., eds. *AIDS: facing the second decade*, pp. 41–60. London, Falmer.

World Bank (1993) *World development report: investing in health*. New York, Oxford University Press.

World Health Organization (1991) Management of patients with sexually transmitted diseases. Report of a WHO steering group. *WHO technical report series 810*. Geneva, World Health Organization.

World Health Organization (1994) *Management of sexually transmitted diseases*. WHO/GPA/TEM/94.1. Geneva, World Health Organization.

Worth D (1989) Sexual decision-making and AIDS: why condom promotion among vulnerable women is likely to fail. *Studies in family planning*, 20(6): 297–307.

5

Study design for the measurement of gynaecological morbidity

Huda Zurayk

American University of Beirut, Beirut, Lebanon

This chapter addresses design issues in the measurement of gynaecological morbidity. Recognizing that gynaecological morbidity is a complex phenomenon, the possible study designs are reviewed and their shortcomings and strengths are highlighted. Finally, I shall focus on community-based studies as they provide a holistic view of gynaecological morbidity from various perspectives.

In considering designs for the measurement of gynaecological morbidity, three questions need to be asked: Why are we concerned with measuring gynaecological morbidity (or, what is our aim)?; Who is our target population?; What concepts are we trying to measure?

The aims of measuring gynaecological morbidity are, in my view, to establish the prevalence of morbidity conditions, and to understand perspectives, behaviours and experiences, as well as determinants, for the purpose of guiding policies and programmes aimed at reducing reproductive morbidity. Interventions can then be designed, on the basis of such studies, to reduce the burden of gynaecological morbidity. Accurate measurement of morbidity is required, in turn, to evaluate these interventions.

In focusing on women's reproductive health, and specifically on the component of gynaecological morbidity, the target population is not only women in the reproductive ages. Adolescents in preparation for healthy sexuality and reproduction, and women past reproduction still sexually active or not and experiencing the consequences of reproduction, are part of the target population. In addition, women's reproductive health cannot be separated from men's health and behaviours, particularly in terms of such concerns as sexually transmitted infection (STI), contraception and psychological well-being, all relevant to the concept of reproductive morbidity.

In attempting to answer the crucial question of what concepts represent our concern with gynaecological morbidity, a more complex issue needs to be faced. It is believed that several measurement concepts need to be used to represent gynaecological morbidity, defined to refer to the occurrence of states of ill health associated with the reproductive system. A holistic meaning for gynaecological morbidity includes the concept of disease conditions, which could be asymptomatic, or symptomatic with the individual aware or unaware of the symptoms. It also includes the concept of illness, where the individual has a perception of a problem according to a framework of health that could be close to or different from the biomedical model.

Starting with this broad meaning of gynaecological morbidity, three measurement concepts are proposed, which, taken together, can produce greater understanding of the magnitude of gynaecological 'ill health' in a population. The relevance and significance of these measurement concepts became clear during the Giza morbidity study in 1989–91, undertaken in a small community in rural Egypt by the Regional Reproductive Health Working Group (Khattab, 1992; Khattab, Younis and Zurayk, 1999; Younis et al., 1993; Zurayk et al., 1993). The aim of the study was to assess the magnitude and context of gynaecological and related morbidity in two villages in rural Giza. We were an interdisciplinary team of medical, social science and statistical specialists.

The three measurement concepts representing this interdisciplinary perspective are:
- Occurrence of a disease condition.
- Occurrence of symptoms of a disease condition.
- Perception of a state of ill health.

In considering study designs for the measurement of reproductive morbidity, it is important to be aware at the outset of the meanings incorporated in the outcome of 'ill health', and of the resulting three measurement concepts that can represent its complexity. It is also essential to adopt a wide framework that goes beyond the measurement of outcome to include concern for individual experience, associated behaviours and the underlying social context. In this way, an analytical perspective can generate a rich body of information to support the development of realistic and effective multifaceted policy actions to improve health.

Nevertheless, I shall organize the review of relevant designs for gynaecological morbidity around the three 'outcome' measurement concepts mentioned in the foregoing, while giving due consideration to the wider framework of representation. The extent to which a study design meets the criteria of validity and reliability, as well as feasibility and affordable cost will be considered. When the term survey is used, it is assumed that proper statistical techniques are utilized in defining the relevant population frame, determining the appropriate sample size and adopting the proper selection mechanism. Many surveys and other designs for measuring gynaecological morbidity do not necessarily stand alone but are part of larger studies with wider aims. For example, both the Demographic and Health

Surveys (DHS) and the Pan Arab Project for Child Development (PAPCHILD) include modules for measuring symptoms of maternal and gynaecological morbidity, although both are primarily concerned with childhood illnesses. Such larger studies include components of morbidities that can be interdependent and viewed relative to one another.

Designs for the measurement of occurrence of disease conditions

The concept of 'occurrence of a disease condition' is often referred to as 'observed morbidity', implying that the presence of the disease condition is being assessed by a trained observer, most often a physician, using clinical or diagnostic examinations (Murray and Chen, 1992). Designs that aim to measure occurrence of disease conditions will be divided into population-based and facility-based approaches.

Population-based designs
Medical examination survey

The medical examination survey involves measuring the occurrence of gynaecological morbidity conditions through medical assessments, by clinical and/or laboratory examinations carried out on a sample from the target population. The Giza morbidity study (Khattab, Younis and Zurayk, 1999) included a medical examination survey as one of its components. It is useful to this survey as an illustration, explaining first its sampling strategy.

The Giza morbidity study defined the eligible population as all ever-married women in two Giza villages. These villages were selected because they represented the networking and dynamics of a rural society, the poor socio-economic environment of the residents and their relative proximity to Cairo, which simplified logistics. Moreover, because of the previous experience of one of the researchers in the area, entry to the village was available to the research team. Considerations of possible levels of prevalence of morbidity conditions under study, particularly reproductive tract infections, were used to statistically lead to a sample size by providing the sampling error that would be tolerated with 95 per cent confidence. Prevalence of reproductive tract infections was estimated at 0.10, and the sampling error was fixed at 0.02, calculating thus the sample size at

$$[(1.96)^2 \times (0.10) \times (0.90)]/(0.02)^2 = 875$$

As the study progressed, the analysis of data from the first 250 completed cases revealed a higher prevalence of gynaecological morbidity than expected, particularly for reproductive tract infections. In view of the complexity of the data collection process and the cost of laboratory testing, it was decided to restrict the sample size to 500 women.

For the actual selection of women, age quotas were determined so that the age distribution of the sample would be similar to the population pattern of these villages indicated in the most recent Egyptian census results. A map was drawn for each village where streets, alleys and housing blocks were identified. A random sample of streets and alleys was selected in one village and a random sample of housing blocks in the other. Households were visited sequentially in the selected areas. Eligible women were invited to join the study and were told about all the phases involved.

Initially, some women refused to participate despite efforts by the research team to involve them and the community in study preparations. Following intensive efforts by the field workers to suit the convenience of the women, the response improved. As the study progressed, most women who had refused to participate sought out the field team to join the study. The total response rate at the end of the study was an impressive 92 per cent (see Khattab, Chapter 7).

The medical examination was conducted at the village health centre. Field workers accompanied women to the centres following the second interview with them according to a schedule of preset appointments. The physicians in charge of each health centre were trained to undertake the clinical examination in a standard way under the constant supervision of one of the study obstetrician-gynaecologists. Table 5.1 shows the range of gynaecological and related conditions covered by the clinical tests and/or laboratory examinations. Some laboratory tests were undertaken at the village health centre by a specially trained laboratory technician, while the more complex tests were undertaken at a specialized laboratory in Cairo. Table 5.2 shows the prevalence of conditions detected (for details, see Khattab, Younis and Zurayk, 1999; Younis et al., 1993).

The medical examination survey has the potential of offering a valid representation of the occurrence of disease conditions, yet validity depends on the feasibility and affordability of using 'gold standard' diagnostic tests. Some gynaecological and related disease conditions are diagnosed by clinical examination alone, such as genital prolapse. Other conditions need simple diagnostic tests, such as blood pressure reading to detect hypertension and the measurement of haemoglobin for anaemia. Clinical examination and simple diagnostic tests can be easily incorporated in a medical examination survey. The reliability of measurement then depends on the competence of the observer, which can be maximized through standardization and training.

Other conditions, such as the occurrence of reproductive tract infections, are more difficult to establish in a field situation. Reproductive tract infection can be identified by a clinical examination for signs of discharge and its characteristics of amount, colour, consistency and accompanying itching. Reproductive tract infection can be measured by 'surrogate' tests that can be carried out in a field laboratory,

Table 5.1. Measurement of gynaecological and related morbidity

Morbidity conditions	Interview questionnaire (symptoms)	Clinical examination	Laboratory test
Gynaecological morbidity			
Reproductive tract infections			
Lower			
Vaginitis	✗		✗
Cervicitis	✗	✗	
Upper (pelvic inflammatory disease)	✗	✗	
Cervical ectopy (erosion)		✗	
Cervical cell changes			✗
Genital prolapse	✗	✗	
Menstrual problems	✗		
Problems with intercourse	✗		
Infertility	✗		
Related morbidity			
Urinary tract infections	✗		✗
Anaemia			✗
Obesity		✗	
High blood pressure		✗	
Syphilis			✗

such as potassium hydroxide odour and Ph-levels for bacterial vaginosis. Other reproductive tract infection conditions need more sophisticated laboratory diagnosis, such as Syva Miers Track for *Chlamydia trachomatis*.

Validity for an expanded medical examination survey depends on the existence of 'gold standard' tests, and on the feasibility and affordability of implementing these tests in a field situation. Interesting questions arise when such tests are neither feasible nor affordable. For instance, does the clinical assessment of reproductive tract infections adequately represent the actual occurrence of the condition? Studies have shown that agreement is likely to be poor between clinical and laboratory diagnoses (Bulut et al., 1995; Kaufman et al., 1999; Zurayk et al., 1995). Do surrogate tests that can be undertaken in a field situation link well to the 'gold standard' laboratory tests? This question is important to explore as biomedical science continues to work on less costly diagnostic tests that can be applied in a field situation, particularly for reproductive tract infection diagnosis (Berkely, 1994; Bayer, Stryker and Smith, 1995).

Table 5.2. Prevalence of gynaecological and related morbidity conditions

Condition	Percentage
Reproductive tract infections	51
Vaginitis[a]	44
Bacterial vaginosis	22
Trichonomas	18
Candida	11
Cervicitis[b]	10
Pelvic inflammatory disease[b]	2
Cervical ectopy[b]	22
Cervical cell changes[a]	11
Genital prolapse[b]	56
Urinary tract infection[a]	14
Syphilis[a]	1
Anaemia (Hg $<$ 12 g/dl)[a]	63
High blood pressure (diastolic $>$90)[b]	18
Obesity (weight/height^2 $>$25)[b]	43
Number of women	*n* 502

Notes:
[a] Laboratory test.
[b] Clinical examination.

Most applications of a medical examination survey, including the Giza morbidity study, have required respondents to visit a clinic, to which they are either brought or asked to come on their own. This required visit has been a significant contributory factor to the non-response associated with medical examination surveys. With the simplification of medical tests, the household can increasingly be used as a site for gathering medical data. This has been shown to work in some studies; for example, the collection of self-administered swabs from women at their homes (Gray and Wawer, 1996) and a physician visiting households and conducting an actual gynaecological examination at home (Al-Qutob, Mawajdeh and Massad, 2001). In such studies, efforts should be made to ensure the reliability of measurements under conditions in the home.

Reliability of measurement in a medical examination survey depends on the technical competence of the observers and on the availability of supplies, instruments and equipment, as well as the proper environment. In the Giza morbidity study, the physician at each of the two health centres was given the responsibility of conducting the medical examination for the sample of women. Both physicians were female and were general practitioners who had been practising at the health centres for some time. To raise their level of competence, they were given specially designed training at a University Medical Centre and hands-on training at the health centres. The medical examination to assess the occurrence of gynaecological and related disease conditions was standardized, and special forms prepared for recording the results. The physicians were constantly supervised by one of the study obstetrician-gynaecologists. The same procedure was followed for the laboratory technicians. To improve reliability, some upgrading of the physical facilities was also undertaken in order to ensure cleanliness, privacy, proper lighting and the availability of required medical supplies, instruments and equipment.

Medical examination surveys are costly undertakings. Grants supported the medical assessment of 509 women in the Giza morbidity study, and were used to upgrade the facilities, train and supervise the health centre staff, pay for the extra services they were providing and cover the costs of the laboratory tests. Women in the sample who came for the medical examination were given token presents of soap and biscuits. Field workers, who were also supported by grants, invested a lot of time working with women to ensure that they came for the medical examination, which led to a response rate of 92 per cent. All these elements of cost must be taken into account when planning a medical examination survey.

The important role that community engagement plays in ensuring the collaboration of women in coming to the medical examination is to be noted. A low response rate and a self-selected sample of women with complaints can lead to biased estimates of the level of gynaecological morbidity in a community (Koenig et al., 1998). It is, therefore, important to guard against the possibility of a low response rate to the medical examination at the initial stage of the design as well as what may be a natural situation for women of accepting to undertake the medical examination only when suspecting a problem. The potential for women's collaboration in the study should be established from the very beginning, and an investment of the field worker's time be made only if positive potential is indicated, to maximize response. If it is judged from the outset, as has happened in studies of conservative communities, that the response rate to the medical examination is likely to be low, then designs other than the medical examination survey must be adopted to explore the level and nature of gynaecological morbidity (see Koenig and Shepherd, in this volume).

In conclusion, when considering the medical examination survey as a design for the assessment of gynaecological morbidity in the community, the potential for satisfaction of three basic criteria must be properly assessed at the outset:

- Validity of measurement: Are 'gold standard' diagnostic tests affordable and feasible?

- Reliability of measurement: Can the competence of medical observers and the availability of supplies, instruments and equipment, as well as the proper environment for medical examination, be assured?
- Sample coverage: Are women likely to respond to the medical examination thus avoiding bias introduced by non-response and self-selection?

The questionnaire survey

Questionnaire surveys can be used to measure the occurrence of disease conditions by including questions on whether the individual has a particular disease condition, or whether the individual has been diagnosed with a particular disease condition on a recent visit to a health facility. One positive feature of a questionnaire survey is that it is usually feasible and much less costly to implement than a medical examination survey. However, the validity of measuring the occurrence of disease conditions based on reported morbidity depends on the extent to which a population is exposed to biomedical information as well as on the extent to which medical services are accessible and used.

Reliability is also a concern for questionnaire surveys. In measuring disease occurrence by a question on diagnosis at a recent visit to a health facility, the response is highly dependent on memory and the extent to which the physician communicated clear information on the diagnosis. The performance of questions relying on memory can be improved by using short reference periods, such as the previous two weeks.

In Peru, a follow-up survey was undertaken in 1994 on a subsample of 1370 women initially interviewed in the 1991–92 Peru DHS. Among the questions asked were six questions that attempted to 'assess reproductive morbidity experienced by the women during the period January 1, 1991 to the date of interview in 1994' (admittedly too long a recall period). These included questions on general health, hospitalization and the reason for hospitalization, visits to a medical facility for one's own health, information provided by the health professional, and the resolution of the problem. Some information elements in these questions were used to develop estimates of reproductive morbidity in Peru (Jain et al., 1996).

The validity of these estimates could not be tested. However, given differential and mostly low health information and accessibility of health services in Peru, the validity of the estimates provided by the study is questionable. Moreover, the long recall period is likely to have affected the reliability of the responses. Nevertheless, questionnaire surveys like the one used in Peru could be a useful tool for asking direct questions on the occurrence of gynaecological disease conditions in the recent past in more medicalized settings.

Facility-based designs

Record review

All or a sample of the medical records in a health facility (or facilities) serving a particular population, or data extracted from such records by a statistical system, can be reviewed to determine the prevalence of visits for gynaecological conditions in that population. The validity of estimates of occurrence of disease conditions arising from such a review depends on the representativeness of visits in terms of the actual burden of disease in the population as well as on the type of examinations and diagnostic tests used at the facility. The quality and completeness of records determine reliability, and even feasibility.

In many developing countries, facility-based record reviews (or data systems) are not a feasible design for learning about the occurrence of gynaecological disease conditions for three main reasons: health facilities are not uniformly accessible across population groups; women in particular may not be aware of the need to present to the health services for symptoms of gynaecological conditions; and the quality of records at health facilities may be low, which discredits their use as sources of information.

In developed countries, however, facility-based record reviews (or data systems) provide very useful information on the occurrence of gynaecological disease conditions. For example, a study was recently undertaken in the United States to assess rates of visits to emergency departments for gynaecological disease conditions among reproductive age women. Data were used from the National Hospital Care Survey for 1992–94, which is an annual national probability sample of visits to emergency and outpatient departments of non-federal short-stay hospitals. Approximately 1.4 million gynaecological visits were made annually, for an average of 24.3 visits per 1000 women. The main complaint was reproductive tract infections, which are largely preventable. Younger women as compared to older women, and black women as compared to white, were more likely to visit emergency departments. The study demonstrated that the emergency department is a significant source of care for gynaecological conditions in the US, raising serious questions, particularly for young and black women, about access to and acceptability of more appropriate reproductive health care services (Curtis et al., 1998).

Survey of visits

A random sample of facilities are selected and all, or a sample of visits, are observed for a particular time period to determine the prevalence of gynaecological conditions. This facility-based design avoids using records and adopts the direct observation of encounters. Observation of patient–provider encounters must be carefully planned to avoid a biased performance by the provider, or lack of privacy for the woman, and also to ensure proper recording of relevant elements of the encounter. As such, these observations are not only useful to determine the type and frequency of gynaecological problems being seen at the facility, but also to assess the quality of care being given by the providers. However, deriving population estimates of the occurrence of gynaecological disease conditions from these observations leads to biased estimators because they are based on visitors to facilities. Validity is further dependent on the type of examinations and diagnostic tests used. Other possible approaches are to interview health providers at these facilities to determine their usual load of gynaecological conditions, or to interview women at exit to find out about diagnoses given for their complaints. Such procedures rely on memory and on the actual exchange of information during visits, and are less reliable than actual observation of visits.

A particularly used variant of this visit-based design is to invite visitors to a health centre for non-gynaecological complaints to undertake a gynaecological examination during their visit. While we sound the usual caution about women's reticence to undertake a clinical examination, it may be more probable that women agree when already in the health centre than when they are invited from their home to visit the health centre for a medical examination. Nevertheless, the criteria of validity and reliability of medical measurement, and the representativeness of visitors at the health facility, must be assessed.

Inviting visitors to undertake a gynaecological examination has been used in family planning clinics in developing countries in order to assess the prevalence of gynaecological disease conditions among women seeking family planning services. For example, such a study was conducted in one of the Family Planning Association of Kenya clinics in Nairobi. Randomly selected women (520) attending the clinic between May and December 1994 were invited to participate in a study of reproductive tract infections and cervical dysplasia. A general physical examination, including a pelvic assessment, was undertaken by the physician in charge and selected laboratory tests were conducted. The results showed that 20 per cent of the women had reproductive tract infection pathogens, with trichomoniasis accounting for nearly half the cases. Also, HIV-1 testing was positive in 10 per cent of the sample and pelvic inflammatory disease was clinically diagnosed among 4 per cent. The study concluded that the high level of STI prevalence was consistent with other recent studies of family planning clinics in Nairobi, and recommended that the scope of reproductive health services be broadened beyond family planning and maternity care to include care for reproductive tract infections (Temmerman et al., 1998).

Designs for the measurement of occurrence of symptoms of disease conditions

From the foregoing it can be seen that eliciting information on the occurrence of disease conditions is difficult. Medical examination surveys are costly and not always feasible. Seeking information through health facilities does not yield valid estimates in developing countries as visitors to health facilities are not usually representative of the general population. Moreover, record keeping at health facilities is often incomplete or inaccurate. As indicated earlier, questionnaire surveys sometimes have been used as a feasible alternative to determine disease occurrence by asking individuals to report whether they have a particular disease condition. This self-reported morbidity is equally problematic in developing countries.

More frequently, however, questionnaire surveys have focused not on the direct measurement of occurrence of disease conditions but on whether an individual experiences a known symptom of a particular condition. Rather than ask a woman whether she is suffering from a reproductive tract infection such as vaginitis, the questionnaire asks about symptoms of reproductive tract infection, including discharge and its characteristics of colour, consistency, odour and itching, which are all within the woman's realm of experience. Although this measure is called self-reported or perceived morbidity (Murray and Chen, 1992), it in fact reflects reporting of symptoms that the biomedical system identifies with a particular disease condition. An individual may or may not be aware of the significance of these symptoms, and thus using terms like self-reported morbidity or perceived morbidity for self-reports of predetermined symptoms is actually misleading (Zurayk and Kabakian, 1996). Moreover, some disease conditions like chlamydia do not usually manifest themselves through symptoms.

Questionnaire surveys have been asking individuals about symptoms of disease conditions because these questions can easily be asked of large samples (see, for instance, Bhatia and Cleland, 1995; Khattab, Khalil and Younis, 1996). The literature has generally shown that reporting of symptoms does not correspond well with the occurrence of disease (Kaufman et al., 1999; Zurayk et al., 1995). In the Giza morbidity study, women were asked to report symptoms of gynaecological and related morbidity before being taken to the village health centre for medical assessment. The results show that reporting the symptom of discharge, even when taking into account its salient characteristics such as amount, colour and consistency, was not associated with the laboratory diagnosis of reproductive tract infection. Similarly, reporting of symptoms of prolapse, taken to be a 'feeling of heaviness below' and/or 'protrusion of genital organs', was not associated with the clinical diagnosis of prolapse upon examination (Zurayk et al., 1995).

Table 5.3. Symptoms of gynaecological and related morbidities

Condition/symptom	Percentage who reported symptoms
Reproductive tract infection	
Discharge present	77
Discharge 'not her nature'	13
Lower abdominal pain	18
Menstrual problems	44
Problems with intercourse	41
Genital prolapse	
Heaviness below and/or protrusion of organs	31
Infertility	
Delay in conception	48
Urinary tract infection	
At least one of seven symptoms	59
Number of women	*n* 509

It is now recognized that the value of asking about symptoms of disease conditions in questionnaire surveys does not lie in their ability to measure prevalence of disease. Questionnaire surveys can provide valuable policy-relevant information by asking detailed questions on symptoms. Of particular relevance are investigations of behaviours associated with reports of symptoms, or reports of disease conditions, in terms of home remedies or of seeking care from health services. Table 5.3 highlights the percentage of women in the Giza morbidity study reporting selected symptoms of gynaecological and related morbidity conditions, and reveals a high level of reporting. Table 5.4 shows, for women who reported each symptom, the proportion consulting a physician or 'others' for these symptoms. An interesting pattern emerges whereby women consult most often for complaints related to infertility and least often for complaints related to sexual intercourse, which throws light on women's priorities with a view to their social context.

It is also possible to pursue, in questionnaire surveys, issues of compliance with treatment prescribed and quality of health care provided for those using services for reported symptoms. For those experiencing symptoms but not using health services, it is important to investigate awareness of the seriousness of these symptoms and reasons for non-use. Such questions provide a wealth of information of relevance to a reproductive health policy concerned with improving the accessibility and quality of reproductive health services. In the end, it is symptoms that reflect the potential for visiting health services. The magnitude of experience of

Table 5.4. Consultation for medical symptoms

Symptom	n	Percentage who consulted	
		physician	others[a]
Reproductive tract infection			
Discharge (not her nature)	68	32	7
Lower abdominal pain	89	27	6
Menstrual problems	162	28	15
Intercourse related complaints	192	14	4
Genital prolapse			
Heaviness below and/or protrusion of organs	158	30	6
Infertility			
Delay in conception during reproductive cycle	243	54	56
Urinary tract infection			
At least one of seven symptoms	301	27	5

Note: [a] Others include: daya, family, neighbours, friends.

symptoms, particularly the severity of this experience, is thus relevant for health services planning.

The Giza morbidity study has shown that although reporting of symptoms did not serve as a valid measure of occurrence of disease conditions, they correlated well with the observation of signs, indicating the reliability of measurements, such as the presence of discharge. Thus a report by a woman of discharge correlated well with whether a physician observed discharge on clinical examination (Zurayk et al., 1995). Considerable effort was spent in the planning stage for the questionnaire to make sure that the questions were phrased using appropriate terminology. Field workers were also instructed on interviewing techniques, and on the importance of ensuring that they visit at a time convenient to the women. These are important considerations for gathering reliable information, well worth the investment involved in training field workers and in the extended time duration of the survey (Khattab, Khalil and Younis, 1996).

Perception of ill health

Perception of ill health incorporates an individual's awareness of an abnormality, whether or not it is medically defined. It is important to understand this concept since it can explain women's perspectives on gynaecological ill health and can help to improve how the health system serves women, particularly in terms of the quality of communication between health providers and their clients. Qualitative methodologies, such as in-depth interviews and participant observation, are best suited to investigate women's perceptions of health and ill health. Such methodologies can solicit information on how women define and experience gynaecological ill health, what are its perceived causes and consequences, and the care given or sought while contextualizing this information within a larger socio-economic and health services environment.

Questionnaires can also collect information on perceptions of ill health but with much less depth of description. In the Giza morbidity study, 77 per cent of women reported on a structured interview questionnaire that discharge was present, many of them providing descriptions of medically suspicious characteristics when asked to elaborate on the symptoms. However, only 13 per cent responded negatively to the question in the interview schedule on whether this discharge was 'of her nature'. The finding that most women considered the discharge, even if accompanied by medically suspicious characteristics, to be 'their nature', demonstrates the extent to which women are distant from the biomedical framework in understanding ill health.

The qualitative data collected in the Giza morbidity study elaborated further on women's perceptions and the social context of their health situation. Case studies of women who were diagnosed with serious gynaecological disease conditions, and referred for further medical investigation and care, were especially revealing. Through in-depth recording of the experience of these women, the case studies showed the lack of attention women gave to symptoms and the many social and economic constraints they had to overcome in seeking medical care for the few symptoms that worried them, such as bleeding. These case studies also revealed the lack of sensitivity of health providers to women's perspectives, their needs and the social conditions of their lives (Khattab, 1992).

Such direct experience of the social context of women's health and ill health provided by the Giza morbidity study encouraged the regional Reproductive Health Working Group to conduct further work in this area. The Group has initiated and brought together studies of the Middle East that explore women's perceptions of ill health, its consequences and perceived treatment options, as well as perceptions of the body and sexuality. These valuable studies reveal significant common patterns, and will be used as training materials to sensitize health providers to women's world and their health perceptions (see Ghannam and Sholkamy, 2002).

Similar studies have been carried out in India (Mulgaonkar et al., 1994) and are especially relevant for policy in the developing world. All these studies use qualitative methodologies on small samples. They are not costly except for the time required for the principal investigator to gather and analyse large bodies of data. They are valuable on their own, but also very revealing when included as separate components of a study design using other methodologies of measurement, such as medical examination surveys and/or questionnaire surveys.

Community-based studies

After focusing on the three measurement concepts for gynaecological morbidity and the designs that could best be used to represent each concept, community-based studies are considered the most valuable method to learn about gynaecological morbidity in a community because such studies offer the opportunity of synthesizing all these designs. Community-based studies are studies like the Giza morbidity study, conducted on small, contained geographical communities, which involve the simultaneous consideration of the three measurement concepts and give due attention to the social context of ill health. Community-based studies are expensive, and hence not always feasible, and in these cases, clinic-based designs are a reasonable alternative, bearing in mind that samples studied may not be representative of women at large.

A community-based study thus defined uses a multitude of data collection methods. It undertakes a medical examination survey on a sample of women from the community using, to the extent possible, valid, reliable and feasible medical assessment techniques. It uses a questionnaire survey at various stages of the study. The questionnaire survey can be used in the initial stages to collect socio-economic and demographic information, and general information on health status, experience with childbearing, contraceptive behaviour as well as information relevant to the status of women, family dynamics and support. The questionnaire survey can also be used to investigate the occurrence and experience of symptoms of disease conditions, perceptions of causes and consequences, associated behaviours, particularly in terms of making use of health services, compliance with prescribed treatments and satisfaction with quality of care. After the results of the medical examination survey are available, the questionnaire survey can be used to elicit information from those diagnosed with disease conditions on their experience and awareness of these conditions. Finally, the community-based study uses qualitative methodologies continuously throughout the study to initiate a smooth entry into the community and to explore women's perceptions, experiences and the social context of their health and ill health.

The community-based study allows the application of these methods to men as well as to women. It can also target key informants and key groups in the community, such as health providers. Through this wide framework, it can provide a rich understanding of the health situation in a community.

Because of its complexity, however, the community-based study requires several conditions:

• The study team should be multidisciplinary, and include anthropologists, biostatisticians and demographers. Physicians in relevant disciplines, particularly obstetrics–gynaecology, laboratory sciences and public health, should be part of the team. While it is not always feasible to assemble such a team, at the very least what is required are individuals with expertise in social science, medicine and quantitative methods, with others serving as consultants on the team. These researchers must be respectful of each others' disciplines and able to work together in a collaborative manner.

- The team should begin work together in an initial period of conceptualization and planning so that a comprehensive study framework is designed and a rapport developed with the community before the initiation of data collection.
- The community should be carefully selected in terms of variability of relevant population characteristics, potential for response from women, particularly to the medical examination, availability of adequate health facilities, and relative closeness to a specialized laboratory.
- The community should be involved from the very beginning in the planning of the study, and time should be invested to ensure that the community collaborates and benefits. It is particularly important to plan for treatment of those revealed by medical diagnosis to be suffering from gynaecological morbidity.
- Standardized definitions and instruments of data collection should be used with a view to replication in other communities yielding comparable measures.
- Analysis strategies should allow for the synthesis of results from various data sources, giving due attention to the outcome of ill health as well as to the wider framework of experience, behaviours and the social context of ill health.

By necessity, such a complicated design needs to be applied to a small-size community, which raises the significant question of representation. We argue that a community-based study is useful in providing a rich body of data that cannot be provided by larger studies that are structured and limited in the information they can gather.

Community-based studies are costly and time-intensive, and rely on community support and women's response. They are cost-effective in the benefit they add, through the depth of information they produce, to the process of developing realistic interventions and policy formulations to improve women's reproductive health in different communities and social groups. However, in situations where support and response from the community are judged (or determined through pilot surveys) not to be forthcoming, or where funds are not available to cover the many components of a community-based study, it may be more appropriate to rely on other designs, such as questionnaire surveys or facility-based surveys. Despite some of the limitations of these designs that have been discussed, they are more feasible and easier to undertake. They provide useful information on gynaecological morbidity among specific groups while yielding a less rich and comprehensive profile of illness in a community.

REFERENCES

Al-Qutob R, Mawajdeh S, Massad D (2001) Can a home-based pelvic examination be used in assessing reproductive morbidity in population-based studies? A Jordanian experience. *Journal of Advanced nursing*, **33**(5): 603–612.

Bayer R, Stryker J, Smith MD (1995) Testing for HIV infection at home. *New England journal of medicine*, **332**(19): 1296–1299.

Berkely S (1994) Diagnostic tests for sexually transmitted diseases: a challenge. *Lancet*, **343**:685–686.

Bhatia JC, Cleland J (1995) Self-reported symptoms of gynaecological morbidity and their treatment in south India. *Studies in family planning*, **26**(4): 203–216.

Bulut A, Yolsal N, Filippi V et al. (1995) In search of truth: comparing alternative sources of information on reproductive tract infection. *Reproductive health matters*, **6**: 31–39.

Curtis KM, Hillis SD, Kieke BA et al. (1998) Visits to emergency departments for gynaecologic disorders in the United States, 1992–1994. *Obstetrics and gynaecology*, **91**(6): 1007–1012.

Ghannam F, Sholkamy H (Eds) (2002) The social construction of well-being in the Middle East: studies of perceptions and strategies. Cairo, The American University in Cairo Press. (Forthcoming.)

Gray RH, Wawer MJ (1996) Clinical/laboratory methods for the diagnosis of reproductive morbidity in population-based studies. Paper presented at the Seminar on Innovative Approaches to the Assessment of Reproductive Health organized by the IUSSP Committee on Reproductive Health and the Population Institute, University of the Philippines, Manila, 24–27 September.

Jain AK, Stein K, Arends-Kuenning M et al. (1996) *Measuring reproductive morbidity with a sample survey in Peru*. Program Division Working Paper, No. 9. New York, The Population Council.

Kaufman J, Liqin Y, Tongyin W et al. (1999) A study on field-based methods for diagnosing reproductive tract infections in rural Yunnan province, China. *Studies in family planning*, **30**(2): 112–119.

Khattab H (1992) *The silent endurance: social conditions of women's reproductive health in rural Egypt*. Cairo, The Population Council and UNICEF-Amman.

Khattab H, Khalil K, Younis N (1996) Socio-medical dimensions of women's utilization of reproductive health services in Giza, Egypt. Paper presented at the Arab Regional Population Conference in Cairo organized by the IUSSP, Cairo, 8–12 December.

Khattab H, Younis N, Zurayk H (1999) *Women, reproduction and health in rural Egypt*. Cairo, The American University in Cairo Press.

Koenig M, Jejeebhoy S, Singh S et al. (1998) Investigating gynaecological morbidity in India: not just another KAP survey. *Reproductive health matters*, **6**(11): 84–97.

Murray CJL, Chen LC (1992) Understanding morbidity change. *Population and development review*, **18**(3): 481–503.

Mulgaonkar VB, Parikh IG, Taskar VR et al. (1994) Perceptions of Bombay slum women regarding refusal to participate in a gynaecological health programme. In: Gittelsohn J et al., eds. *Listening to women talk about their health*, pp. 145–167. New Delhi, Har-Anand Publications.

Temmerman M, Kidula N, Tyndall M et al. (1998) The supermarket for women's reproductive health: the burden of genital infections in a family planning clinic in Nairobi, Kenya. *Sexually transmitted infections*, **74** (3): 202–204.

Younis N, Khattab H, Zurayk H et al. (1993) A community study of gynaecological and related morbidities in rural Egypt. *Studies in family planning*, **24**(3): 175–186.

Zurayk H, Khattab H, Younis N et al. (1995) Comparing women's reports with medical diagnoses of reproductive morbidity conditions in rural Egypt. *Studies in family planning*, **26**(1): 14–21.

Zurayk H, Kabakian T (1996) Measurement of reproductive morbidity: the usefulness of perceived/reported morbidity on reproductive tract infections. Paper presented at the Seminar on Innovative Approaches to the Assessment of Reproductive Health organized by the IUSSP Committee on Reproductive Health and the Population Institute, University of Philippines, Manila, 24–27 September.

Zurayk H, Khattab H, Younis et al. (1993) Concepts and measures of reproductive morbidity. *Health transition review*, **3**(1): 17–40.

6

Alternatives to community-based study designs for research on women's gynaecological morbidity

Michael Koenig and Mary Shepherd

Johns Hopkins University, Baltimore, USA

Since 1990, the issue of women's gynaecological morbidity has received increasing attention and priority from health policy makers and programme managers in many developing countries. Although recognized by women's health advocates as an important public health and gender issue more than a decade ago (Dixon-Mueller and Wasserheit, 1991), findings from carefully designed, community-based research studies have played a critical role in drawing wider attention to the issue of gynaecological morbidity in developing countries. Published studies in India, Egypt, Nigeria, Tanzania, Uganda and China have effectively highlighted the magnitude and scope of sexually transmitted infections (STIs) (Mosha et al., 1993; Wawer et al., 1998), and of gynaecological morbidity more broadly (Bang et al., 1989; Bhatia et al., 1997; Brabin et al., 1995; Kaufman et al., 1999; Younis et al., 1993), among women in developing countries.

Community-based gynaecological morbidity studies have served as important tools for epidemiological surveillance, health services planning, and in particular, for policy advocacy. While the experience since the 1990s has illustrated the importance of such studies, it has also served to highlight the numerous logistical and methodological challenges of undertaking prevalence studies at the community level; and that in many settings or contexts, true community-based studies may prove unfeasible (Koenig et al., 1998).

Community-based studies of gynaecological morbidity prevalence frequently face three interrelated sets of constraints. One set of constraints are heavy logistical demands, including the need for efficient systems for the transportation of specimens, timely access to sophisticated laboratory facilities and the availability of highly trained clinicians amenable to travelling to and working in community settings. These challenges rise significantly the more rural and remote the study areas are.[1] A

---

[1] See Khanna (1997) for a description of the multiple hurdles they confronted during their study in rural India, and Kaufman et al. (1999) for a similar description.

second and related set of constraints are the costs of such studies. While many research costs are fixed (e.g. laboratory tests), the expenses associated with research rise significantly the further one extends into more remote rural areas.

A third and clearly central constraint confronting community-based studies of gynaecological morbidity in many settings is their overall feasibility, specifically with regard to the willingness of communities/ respondents to participate in such studies. Given the personal and often culturally sensitive nature of much of the information obtained in respondent surveys, and the highly intrusive nature of clinical examinations or in some cultures drawing blood for laboratory analysis, there may be an understandable reluctance on the part of many women to participate in such studies. A subsequent chapter describes the extensive preparatory efforts undertaken by three prominent community-based studies to engage the community and enlist respondent participation in the study (see Chapter 7). Despite such efforts, high rates of respondent non-participation and sample loss may still be inevitable in many settings. While many of the previous studies cited have achieved impressive rates of respondent participation, many others – often unpublished and mainly from India where numerous community-based studies have been attempted – have failed to attain at least a requisite sample response rate, defined by Elias and colleagues (see Chapter 8) as 75 per cent of sampled women (Table 6.1). Higher levels of sample attrition are associated with a greater likelihood of self-selection among participating respondents, and a lower likelihood that study findings can be generalized to the larger community (Koenig et al., 1998). The difficulties in eliciting respondent participation appear to be most pronounced in settings such as rural India – characterized by women's low status and a highly conservative cultural environment, and where women seeking care for gynaecological problems represent the exception rather than the rule.[2]

As Zurayk discusses in Chapter 5, community-based studies are now widely recognized as the 'gold standard' for establishing the prevalence and patterns of gynaecological morbidity. Due to the various reasons outlined earlier, however (cost, feasibility and most importantly, anticipated levels of respondent participation), true community-based surveys are likely to prove impractical in many settings. Moreover, depending upon the research objectives of the investigator, population-based approaches may not be the most appropriate or optimal study design. Our objective here is to outline and assess alternatives to community-based designs for research on gynaecological morbidity. Four alternative approaches to conventional community-based designs are considered: community-based studies of client populations; clinic-based studies of clients seeking routine reproductive

---

[2] Some important exceptions to this rule do exist, most notably the study in Iran on cervicitis (Keshavarz et al., 1997). The authors do not provide information on how the study achieved a respondent compliance rate of 100 per cent.

Table 6.1. Participation rates for clinical components of community-based gynaecological morbidity studies

Setting	Authors	Study population[a]	Participation level (%)[b]
Egypt – rural	Younis et al. (1993)	509 ever married women	91
Turkey – urban	Bulut et al. (1997)	867 female contraceptive users	80
Nigeria – rural	Brabin et al. (1995)	439 married and unmarried women aged 10–19 years and 520 aged 20–39 years	93 & 88
Tanzania – urban and rural	Mosha et al. (1993)	4173 married and unmarried men and women aged 15–54 years	81[c]
Tanzania – rural	Grosskurth et al. (1995)	12537 married and unmarried men and women aged 15–54 years	85[c]
Uganda – rural	Wawer et al. (1998)	12827 married and unmarried men and women aged 15–59 years	91[c]
China – rural	Kaufman et al. (1999)	2020 women aged 15–49 years	85–90
India – urban	Latha et al. (1997)	Urban slum women in Mumbai and Baroda, Gujarat	65 & 72
India – rural	Bhatia et al. (1997)	417 women <35 years	88
	Bang et al. (1989)	1104 married and unmarried women	59
	Latha et al. (1997)	Rural women in Gujarat and West Bengal	35 & 45
	Visaria (1997)	324 married women	29
	Khanna (1997)	94 married women	20
	Oomman (1996)	51 married women	19

Notes:

[a] Currently married women, unless otherwise specified.

[b] Denominator is women eligible for participation in the clinical component.

[c] Blood samples only.

health services; non-medical facility-based studies; and clinic-based studies of clients seeking gynaecological services.

Community-based studies of client populations

A variant on conventional community-based study designs is the study at the community level of special populations of users of services. The rationale for this design is to investigate the gynaecological health of a particular type of client – most notably, contraceptive users. A prominent example of this is the study by Wasserheit et al. (1989) in rural Bangladesh. The study was conducted in 1985 in the Matlab intervention area of the International Centre for Diarrhoeal Disease Research. In the intervention area, one-half (40 out of 80) of female community health workers were randomly chosen, and instructed to interview all women within each of their catchment areas who were currently using modern contraception (intrauterine contraceptive devices (IUDs), oral contraception, injectables and tubectomy) regarding symptoms of gynaecological morbidity.[3] A systematic sample of 20 per cent of non-users of contraception was also interviewed as a comparison group. All women reporting symptoms consistent with reproductive tract infections were referred to community health centres for clinical examination by female nurse mid-wives and/or obtaining specimens for laboratory testing. Of the women surveyed, 22 per cent reported symptoms suggestive of a reproductive tract infection. Of these symptomatic women, 24 per cent refused to participate in the subsequent clinical component. Of the 472 symptomatic women who did undergo an examination, almost 7 in 10 had clinical or laboratory evidence of a reproductive tract infection. The study also found that relative to non-contraceptors, IUD and tubectomy acceptors were substantially more likely to have a self-reported or diagnosed reproductive tract infection. Although characterized by several methodological limitations,[4] this study none the less represents an important early attempt to assess the prevalence of reproductive tract infections among an important population subgroup.

A more recent study by Bulut et al. (1997) in Istanbul, Turkey also focused upon contraceptive users as its primary study population. The sampling universe was all women of reproductive age who had ever used a method of contraception and who resided in the catchment area surrounding a mother and child health–family planning clinic in an urban area of Istanbul. Women were initially interviewed in their residence regarding sociodemographic information, contraceptive histories and

---

[3] This task was facilitated by the existence of up-to-date computerized record-keeping books maintained by each community health worker.

[4] These include sampling based upon women's self-reports of morbidity, which have been shown to have a poor level of correspondence with laboratory/clinic assessments, exclusion of the large group of asymptomatic women with infections, and potential reporting bias by contraceptive users who indicated gynaecological morbidity.

past and current reproductive morbidities. All non-pregnant, interviewed women were requested to come to the health centre for a detailed assessment of reproductive morbidity, which included a questionnaire, clinical examination and laboratory tests; 20 per cent of these women declined to participate in the clinical phase of the study. The significant findings that emerged from this study included the low correspondence between perceived and diagnosed gynaecological morbidity, and the apparent association between IUD use and reported menstrual disorders.

Clinic-based studies of clients seeking routine reproductive health services

A second more common approach has been investigation of reproductive tract infection/STI prevalence based upon clients seeking routine reproductive health services, typically family planning or antenatal care clients. Clinic-based study populations have been commonly used over the past three decades to assess the prevalence of STIs (Wasserheit, 1989). Table 6.2 summarizes several of the main studies that used clinic-based designs to assess the prevalence of reproductive tract infection/STI.

One of the earliest examples was a study by Hopcraft and colleagues (1973), which investigated the prevalence of selected STIs among women attending family planning clinics in Nairobi, Kenya. The study included laboratory testing for gonorrhoea, candidiasis and trichomoniasis of randomly selected samples of 100 married and 100 unmarried new or continuing family planning clients. The study found that overall, 54 per cent of these clients had one or more of these infections, most commonly candidiasis (28 per cent), followed by trichomoniasis (26 per cent) and gonorrhoea (18 per cent). A comparison of the sociodemographic profile of this family planning client population with a random sample of clients attending health centres indicated that the study sample was drawn from a population of higher socio-economic status, not unexpected given the likelihood that acceptors of family planning represented innovators at that time. Additional studies of family planning clients reported moderately high rates of reproductive tract infections in a study in Nairobi, Kenya (Temmerman et al., 1998) and extremely high rates of STIs among clinic attenders in Addis Ababa, Ethiopia (Duncan et al., 1997), although the latter group appeared to be a particularly self-selected, high risk population.

The study by Char and Vaidya (2000) of female sterilization clients in rural Maharashtra, India represents a contrasting clinic-based study design. In this study, the investigators recruited the first 20 women who came for a sterilization procedure at a weekly primary health clinic to participate in their study of gynaecological morbidity. The study took place on 31 clinic days over a 15-month study period during 1997–98.[5] It resulted in 511 women completing the questionnaire, clinical

---

[5] Given the low volume of clients in the summer months, data collection was suspended for part of the observation period.

Table 6.2. Summary of clinic-based studies of clients seeking routine reproductive health services

Author	Setting	Study period	Study population	Main findings
Hopcraft et al. (1973)	Nairobi, Kenya	NA	100 married and 100 unmarried new or continuing family planning clients	54% with at least one infection – 28% with candidiasis, 26% with trichomoniasis; 18% culture-positive for gonorrhoea
Temmerman et al. (1998)	Nairobi, Kenya	1994	520 randomly selected women attending a family planning clinic	8% reported symptoms of genital tract infection; 20% had an infection detected, most prevalently trichomoniasis (10%) and chlamydia (4%)
Duncan et al. (1997)	Addis Ababa, Ethiopia	NA	542 family planning clinic attenders	66% gonorrhoea; 64% chlamydia; 54% pelvic inflammatory disease (PID)
Char and Vaidya (2000)	Rural Maharashtra, India	1997–98	511 married women attending a sterilization clinic	39% with self-reported and 29% with clinically diagnosed gynaecological morbidity; 21% with infection detected; 7% with syphilis and 7% with bacterial vaginosis
Mayaud et al. (1995)	Rural Tanzania	1992–93	1149 consecutive women attending 12 antenatal clinics	RTI symptoms reported by 66% of women; 49% with laboratory-confirmed infection, most commonly trichomoniasis (27%)
Wessel et al. (1998)	Cape Verde	1993	350 women attending an antenatal clinic	41% of women were found to have lab-confirmed infection; 31% with bacterial vaginosis

Note: NA, not ascertained; RTI, reproductive tract infection.

and laboratory procedures (a compliance rate of 96 per cent). Preliminary study findings indicate significant levels of gynaecological morbidity among this client population: 39 per cent of women based upon self-reports, 29 per cent of women based upon clinical diagnosis and 21 per cent with laboratory-confirmed infections.[6] The results of this study make a compelling case for the integration of reproductive tract infection/STI services – screening, counselling and treatment – into existing family planning services.

The testing of antenatal clinic attenders has been the backbone of HIV/AIDS surveillance efforts since early in the epidemic (Zaba, Boerma and White, 2000). A good example of the investigation of the prevalence of reproductive tract infection/STI through antenatal clinic attendees is the study by Mayaud et al. (1995) in rural Tanzania. At each of 12 selected clinic sites, the study enrolled 100 consecutive attendees for antenatal care over a 2-week period. Each participant was administered a questionnaire on obstetric and gynaecological history and current symptoms, and received a gynaecological examination together with cervical and vaginal specimen swabs. Only 8 out of the 1149 women enrolled in the study refused to participate in the examination.[7] Laboratory results of the remaining 964 women confirmed that 39 per cent had evidence of one or more STIs, with almost half having one or more reproductive tract infections.

A second example of this approach is a study of 350 pregnant women attending an antenatal clinic in the capital of Cape Verde, West Africa (Wessel et al., 1998). The study enrolled the first 8–12 first or second trimester prenatal clinic attendees each day who consented to participate in the study (out of approximately 20 daily attendees), over a 3-month period. The study found an overall high rate of genital infections for the three conditions tested for: 41 per cent of study women were found to be infected with one or more infections, with bacterial vaginosis by far the most prevalent (31 per cent), followed by chlamydia (13 per cent) and gonorrhoea (5 per cent). Given the very high rate of registration for antenatal care in the catchment area (94 per cent), the authors posited that their study population was likely to be representative of the broader population of pregnant women, although an unspecified selected number of women declined to participate in the study, primarily because they were reluctant to undergo a pelvic examination.

Non-medical facility-based studies

A third approach to assessing the prevalence of gynaecological morbidity is through the examination of populations attending non-medical facilities, most notably mil-

---

[6] This figure includes lifetime exposure to syphilis through TPHA (*Treponema pallidum* haemagglutination) testing.

[7] An additional 16 per cent of specimens cultured were unusable because of contamination.

itary recruits (Catterson and Zadoo, 1993; Gaydos et al., 1998), workplace-based populations (Borgdorff et al., 1995; Ray et al., 1998; Ryder et al., 1990; Sahlu et al., 1998) and school-based populations (Baganizi et al., 1997; Cohen et al., 1999; Reitmeijer et al., 1997). Given the requirement in such settings of minimally invasive testing procedures, this approach has thus far been used primarily to test for HIV infection from blood samples, and to a lesser extent, for chlamydia and gonorrhoea screening from urine samples. As less invasive laboratory tests for other reproductive tract infections become available at a reasonable cost, this study design is likely to become increasingly common as a means to study gynaecological morbidity.

A good example of this approach is the study of Gaydos et al. (1998) of chlamydial infection among female Army recruits at a South Carolina recruitment facility. All women recruits who presented on Sundays during the calendar years 1996 and 1997 were invited to participate in the study, which consisted of the completion of a social and behavioural questionnaire and provision of a urine sample for analysis. The study used DNA-amplification assays to detect the presence of chlamydial infection. The study reported an overall prevalence rate of 9.2 per cent, with prevalence declining sharply with increasing age, and identified a number of specific sociodemographic and behavioural risk factors that were predictive of the risk of infection. Even with this non-intrusive specimen collection approach, it is noteworthy that 20 per cent of the recruits declined to participate in the study.[8] As shown in Table 6.3 similar results were reported in an earlier study of 476 largely sexually active, active duty Army females in Hawaii reporting for their annual Pap smear test: 8.2 per cent with chlamydia, and under 1.0 per cent with gonorrhoea (Catterson and Zadoo, 1993). Other inquiries have been carried out among male military recruits in northern Thailand to assess HIV/AIDS prevalence and incidence (Celentano et al., 1998; Nelson et al., 1993).

There are clear and readily apparent differences between studies of military recruits and those drawn from the broader population. Military recruit populations tend on the whole to be much younger, largely unmarried, and generally drawn from lower socio-economic and educational attainment backgrounds. Given that the armed forces are also overwhelmingly male in developing countries, this approach will also be primarily applicable to studies of men rather than women. Even in settings where women comprise a significant proportion of the military, given the likelihood that they are unmarried, the inclusion of a gynaecological examination component for women is likely to prove problematic in many developing countries. Such study populations seem particularly well suited to rapid

---

[8] Anonymous questionnaires completed by a sample of those who refused to participate indicated that they were less sexually active than volunteers, less likely to have a history of chlamydia or other STIs, and more likely to have consistently used condoms, hence they were less motivated to be screened for chlamydia in this study.

Table 6.3. Summary of studies of military recruit populations

Author	Setting	Study period	Study population	Main findings
Gaydos et al. (1998)	South Carolina, US	1996–97	13 204 army female recruits	9% prevalence of chlamydia
Catterson and Zadoo (1993)	Hawaii, US	1989–91	476 consecutive active duty army females presenting for routine pap smears	8% prevalence of chlamydia
Nelson et al. (1993)	Northern Thailand	1991	2417 young male army conscripts	12% HIV seropositive

laboratory-based assessment techniques, rather than detailed studies that include clinical examinations and detailed surveys. Nevertheless, for the study of the prevalence of specific infections among a young, frequently sexually active population, this design merits consideration.

Clinic-based studies of clients for gynaecological morbidity services

A fourth potential study design consists of clinic-based studies of clients seeking treatment for gynaecological morbidity. The objective of establishing the prevalence of morbidity is clearly inappropriate with such samples, given their self-selected nature. Study designs consisting of clients attending clinics for gynaecological care none the less have an underexploited potential for investigation of the underlying biomedical and social determinants of morbidity, as well as the social and economic consequences of such morbidity.

The recent study of pelvic inflammatory disease (PID) among hospital/clinic attenders in Mumbai, India represents perhaps the best example of this approach to date (Brabin et al., 1998; Gogate et al., 1998). Cases and controls were drawn from women attending one of three health centres in three urban hospitals/ health centres over the 1993–95 period. Cases were defined as women presenting at the clinics with either symptoms of pelvic inflammatory disease (PID) or with a history of infertility not attributable to the male partner; controls consisted of fertile women with no indication of gynaecological morbidity who were seeking tubal ligation. In addition to a social and clinical questionnaire, study participants – both cases and controls – underwent gynaecological and laparoscopic examinations, and a laboratory assessment. The final study sample consisted of 446 cases and 2433 controls, with evidently very low rates of study participation refusal. A key finding from this study was the very low prevalence of STI in all three study populations, and the unlikelihood that sexual transmission played a significant role in suspected PID cases. Subsequent analysis of risk factors for confirmed PID identified the possible roles of obstetric complications and invasive surgical procedures such as D&C (dilatation and curettage) and laparoscopy in elevating the risk of PID for this population (Gogate et al., 1998).

Strengths and limitations of clinic-based study designs

Clinic-based studies of gynaecological morbidity are characterized by both distinct disadvantages and advantages over community-based studies. The main limitation of studies derived from clinic populations is the issue of potential sample selection bias, which potentially limits the extent to which findings from such studies can be generalized to the broader population. The direction of potential selection bias in influencing levels of gynaecological morbidity is not always readily apparent, as clinic-based samples may be self-selected for either higher risk or lower risk of gynaecological morbidity relative to the general population.[9] Concern over sample selectivity is likely to be especially pronounced in settings where utilization rates for services such as antenatal care or contraception remain very low. An important component of any clinic-based study should therefore be a comparison of the socio-demographic and behavioural profile of participants and that of the general population or selected controls, in an effort to assess the potential magnitude and direction of possible sample bias.

A second potential limitation of clinic-based studies relates to ethical concerns and the potential for infringement upon clients' rights. One generic concern relates to the potential violation of client confidentiality and the right to privacy in studies based upon follow-up visits to clients at their home, especially if they had sought the service in secrecy, as is frequently the case with contraception (Castle et al., 1999). It is also possible that study participants may view their participation in such studies as mandatory and a precondition for receiving the service for which they have come to the clinic, no matter how carefully worded the study consent forms are. This is also a serious concern when the study population may not be participating on a voluntary basis, as in the case of military recruits.

Study designs derived from clinic-based populations are also characterized by distinct advantages over community-based studies, most notably their greater feasibility and the increased likelihood of respondent compliance with the clinical and laboratory components. Sample loss due to refusal tends to be very low in clinic-based studies. With few exceptions refusal rates were under 10 per cent in the studies listed in Table 6.2. It is noteworthy, however, that the studies of family planning acceptors in Turkey and Bangladesh, which returned to the community to interview clients, were characterized by significant levels of respondent refusal to participate – between one-fifth and one-quarter of study participants (Bulut et al., 1997; Wasserheit et al., 1989).

A second important advantage of clinic-based studies derives from the potentially direct link between research findings and subsequent programmatic changes. In contrast to broader population-based studies, clinic-based study designs focus on a well-defined target population which is already in direct contact with the service programme, and usually involve services whose infrastructure is well-established and which have achieved wide coverage levels (e.g. family planning, antenatal care). The findings from such studies are also likely to suggest interventions that have the potential to improve the quality of existing service programmes (e.g. screening and

---

[9] In underdeveloped settings, family planning or antenatal clients are likely to be characterized by higher socio-economic status, and by a greater tendency to address their health needs, including their reproductive health concerns. In more developed settings where private sector care is well established, public sector clinic attenders may be drawn predominantly from lower socio-economic populations. Moreover, family planning clients are by definition sexually active, and thus potentially more exposed to the risks of STIs.

treatment of reproductive tract infections among family planning acceptors) and thus have a greater likelihood of being adopted by programme managers.

Discussion

Our objective in this chapter has been to provide an overview of alternatives to community-based study designs for research on gynaecological morbidity, and to assess their relative strengths and limitations. At the core, the choice between community-based designs and alternative approaches revolves around trade-offs between concerns over potential sample representativeness versus respondent compliance and study costs. Table 6.4 presents a comparison of the relative strengths and limitations of the five main study designs described in this chapter.

In community-based studies, sample representativeness has generally been assumed to be high, although we note that few such studies have actually been based upon systematic, random sampling approaches.[10] Levels of respondent compliance have, in contrast, ranged from very low to very high, and the costs of such endeavours tend to be extremely high. In contrast, in the alternative study designs considered, sample representativeness tends to be moderately high, given the likelihood of selectivity among clinic attenders. Compliance levels, on the other hand, tend to be high in such studies, given their often direct link to service provision. Although little hard data exist, it is plausible to assume that the costs of clinic-based studies will be lower relative to community-based designs, given the reduced logistical demands and community mobilization efforts required. It is of interest to note that although all the noted study designs have the potential for yielding insight into the determinants and consequences of confirmed gynaecological morbidity, studies of gynaecological morbidity clients represent a particularly valuable, albeit underutilized, approach for this objective.

Community-based study designs continue to have an important role to play in documenting the prevalence and patterns of gynaecological morbidity within the broader community. The significance and impact of such studies is likely to be especially pronounced in settings where no such information exists, and where there is an absence of consensus on how widespread such morbidity is within the general population of women. The experience of the last decade in settings such as India and Egypt has demonstrated the power of community-based prevalence studies to play a catalyzing role in elevating gynaecological morbidity within national public health agendas. In settings where such community-based studies have not been undertaken, there remains a discernible tendency to dismiss findings

---

[10] Most successful community-based studies to date have used a sampling approach of universal coverage within a limited number of communities, usually one or two (Bang et al., 1989; Brabin et al., 1995; Younis et al., 1993). The exceptions include the study by Bhatia et al. (1997) in south India and Kaufman et al. (1999) in China.

Table 6.4. Comparison of alternate study designs for research on gynaecological morbidity

Study design	Compliance levels	Cost	Potential for estimation of prevalence	Potential for research on determinants/consequences
Community-based	Low to high	High	High	Moderate to high
Military recruits	High	Moderate	Moderate	Low to moderate
Community-based studies of client populations	Moderate to high	Moderate to high	Moderate	Moderate
Clinic-based studies of clients for other services	High	Moderate	Moderate	Moderate
Clinic-based studies of gynaecological morbidity clients	High	Moderate	Not appropriate	High

from clinic-based samples as self-selected and non-representative of the broader population. A testimony to this is the very large number of clinic-based studies of STIs that have been carried out over the last two decades – primarily in Africa – which have had at best only modest policy and programmatic impact. (See Wasserheit (1989) for a useful summary of earlier studies.) The feasibility of community-based data collection approaches will undoubtedly be further enhanced in the near future with the availability of low-cost, self-administered methods of sample collection (see Meehan et al., Chapter 10, for a discussion), which could be expected to reduce the often severe problems of respondent compliance and attendant concerns over sample selectivity.

The alternative research designs outlined represent practical alternatives to population-based surveys of gynaecological morbidity. The rationale for such alternatives is likely to be particularly strong in settings where: community-based approaches have proven unfeasible given strong community opposition and cultural conservatism concerning gynaecological examinations; community-based prevalence studies have already been undertaken and where a broad-based consensus exists concerning the public health importance of gynaecological morbidity, raising questions about the need for repeat community-based prevalence studies; or a focus on gynaecological morbidity prevalence is not the primary research issue of interest. Many of the alternative study designs described are still in the early stages of application, and much remains to be learned about both the strengths and limitations of these approaches. Regardless of the specific study design, there will continue to be a need to include in all such studies an assessment of the degree to which such special study populations are representative of the broader population from which they are drawn. This caveat aside, the range of study designs outlined can provide researchers with an expanded array of options for researching and understanding the determinants, prevalence and consequences of gynaecological morbidity for women in developing and developed countries.

REFERENCES

Baganizi E, Saah A, Bulterys M et al. (1997) Prevalence and incidence rates of HIV-1 infection in Rwandan students [letter]. *AIDS*, **11**(5): 686–687.

Bang RA, Bang AT, Baitule M et al. (1989) High prevalence of gynaecological diseases in rural Indian women. *Lancet*, **1**(8629): 85–88.

Bhatia JC, Cleland J, Bhagavan L et al. (1997) Levels and determinants of gynaecological morbidity in south India. *Studies in family planning*, **28**(2): 95–103.

Borgdorff MW, Barongo LR, Klokke AH et al. (1995) HIV-1 incidence and HIV-1 associated mortality in a cohort of urban factory workers in Tanzania. *Genitourinary medicine*, **71**(4): 212–215.

Brabin L, Kemp J, Obunge OK et al. (1995) Reproductive tract infections and abortion among adolescent girls in rural Nigeria. *Lancet*, **345**(8945): 300–304.

Brabin L, Gogate A, Gogate S et al. (1998) Reproductive tract infections, gynaecological morbidity and HIV seroprevalence among women in Mumbai, India. *Bulletin of the World Health Organisation*, **76**(3): 277–287.

Bulut A, Filippi V, Marshall T et al. (1997) Contraceptive choice and reproductive morbidity in Istanbul. *Studies in family planning*, **28**(1): 35–43.

Castle S, Konate MK, Ulin PR et al. (1999) A qualitative study of clandestine contraceptive use in urban Mali. *Studies in family planning*, **30**(3): 231– 248.

Catterson ML, Zadoo V (1993) Prevalence of asymptomatic chlamydial cervical infection in active duty Army females. *Military medicine*, **158**(9): 618–619.

Celentano DD, Nelson KE, Lyles CM et al. (1998) Decreasing incidence of HIV and sexually transmitted diseases in young Thai men: evidence for success of the HIV/AIDS control and prevention program. *AIDS*, **12**(5): F29–36.

Char A, Vaidya S (2000) Gynaecological morbidity among women seeking sterilization services in rural Maharashtra. Paper presented at the meeting; Reproductive Health in India: Evidence and Issues, Pune, India, 28 February–March 2000. (Unpublished paper.) Available on http://virtual.jhuccp.org/vl

Cohen DA, Nsuami M, Martin DH et al. (1999) Repeated school-based screening for sexually transmitted diseases: a feasible strategy for reaching adolescents. *Pediatrics*, **104**(6):1281–1285.

Dixon-Mueller R, Wasserheit J (1991) *The culture of silence: reproductive tract infections among women in the third world.* New York, International Women's Health Coalition.

Duncan ME, Tibaux G, Kloos H et al. (1997) STDs in women attending family planning clinics: a case study in Addis Ababa. *Social science and medicine*, **44**(4): 441–454.

Gaydos CA, Howell MR, Pare B et al. (1998) *Chlamydia trachomatis* infections in female military recruits. *The New England journal of medicine*, **339**(11): 739– 744.

Gogate A, Brabin L, Nicholas S et al. (1998). Risk factors for laparoscopically confirmed pelvic inflammatory disease: findings from Mumbai (Bombay), India. *Sexually transmitted infections*, **74**(6): 426–432.

Grosskurth H, Mosha F, Todd J et al. (1995) A community trial of the impact of improved sexually transmitted disease treatment on the HIV epidemic in rural Tanzania: 2. Baseline survey results. *AIDS*, **9**(8): 927–934.

Hopcraft M, Verhagen AR, Ngigi S et al. (1973) Genital infections in developing countries: experience in a family planning clinic. *Bulletin of the World Health Organization*, **48**(5): 581–586.

Kaufman J, Han L, Wang T et al. (1999) A study of field-based methods for diagnosing reproductive tract infections in rural Yunnan Province, China. *Studies in family planning*, **30**(2): 112–119.

Keshavarz H, Duffy SW, Sotodeh-Maram E et al. (1997) Factors related to cervicitis in Qashghaee nomadic women of southern Iran. *Revue d'epidemiologie et de sante publique*, **45**: 279–285.

Khanna R (1997) Dilemmas and conflicts in clinical research on women's reproductive health. *Reproductive health matters*, **9**: 168–173.

Koenig M, Jejeebhoy S, Singh S et al. (1998) Investigating women's gynaecological morbidity in India: not just another KAP survey. *Reproductive health matters*, **6**(11): 84–97.

Latha K, Kanani SJ, Maitra N et al. (1997) Prevalence of clinically detectable gynaecological morbidity in India: results of four community based studies. *Journal of family welfare*, **43**(4): 8–16.

Mayaud P, Grosskurth H, Changalucha J et al. (1995) Risk assessment and other screening options for gonorrhoea and chlamydial infections in women attending rural Tanzanian antenatal clinics. *Bulletin of the World Health Organization*, **73**(5): 621–630.

Mosha F, Nicoll A, Barongo L et al. (1993) A population-based study of syphilis and sexually transmitted disease syndromes in north-western Tanzania. 1. Prevalence and incidence. *Genitourinary medicine*, **69**: 415–420.

Nelson KE, Celentano DD, Suprasert S et al. (1993) Risk factors for HIV infection among young adult men in northern Thailand. *Journal of the American Medical Association*, **270**(8): 955–960.

Oomman N (1996) *Poverty and pathology: comparing rural Rajasthani women's ethnomedical models with biomedical models of reproductive morbidity: implications for women's health in India*. Ph.D. dissertation. Johns Hopkins University, Baltimore, Maryland.

Ray S, Latif A, Machekano R et al. (1998) Sexual behaviour and risk assessment of HIV seroconvertors among urban male factory workers in Zimbabwe. *Social science and medicine*, **47**(10): 1431–1443.

Rietmeijer CA, Yamaguchi KJ, Ortiz CG et al. (1997) Feasibility and yield of screening urine for *Chlamydia trachomatis* by polymerase chain reaction among high-risk male youth in field-based and other nonclinic settings. A new strategy for sexually transmitted disease control. *Sexually transmitted diseases*, **24**(7): 429–435.

Ryder RW, Ndilu M, Hassig SE et al. (1990). Heterosexual transmission of HIV-1 among employees and their spouses at two large businesses in Zaire. *AIDS*, **4**(8): 725–732.

Sahlu T, Fontanet A, Rinke de Wit T et al. (1998) Identification of a site for a cohort study on natural history of HIV infection in Ethiopia. *Journal of Acquired Immune Deficiency Syndromes and human retrovirology*, **17**(2): 149–155.

Temmerman M, Kidula N, Tyndall M et al. (1998) The supermarket for women's reproductive health: the burden of genital infections in a family planning clinic in Nairobi, Kenya. *Sexually transmitted infection*, **74**: 202–204.

Visaria L (1997) Gynaecological morbidity in rural Gujarat: some preliminary findings. Gujarat Institute of Development Research. (Unpublished paper.)

Wasserheit JN (1989) The significance and scope of reproductive tract infections among Third World women. *Supplement 3, International journal of gynaecology and obstetrics*, **13**: 145–168.

Wasserheit JN, Harris JR, Chakraborty J et al. (1989) Reproductive tract infections in a family planning population in rural Bangladesh. *Studies in family planning*, **20**(2): 69–80.

Wawer MJ, Gray RH, Sewankambo NK et al. (1998) A randomized, community trial of intensive sexually transmitted disease control for AIDS prevention, Rakai, Uganda. *AIDS*, **12**(10): 1211–1225.

Wessel HF, Herrmann B, Dupret A et al. (1998) Genital infections among antenatal care attendees in Cape Verde. *African journal of reproductive health*, **2**(1): 32–40.

Younis N, Khattab H, Zurayk H et al. (1993) A community study of gynaecological and related morbidities in rural Egypt. *Studies in family planning*, **24**(3): 175–186.

Zaba B, Boerma T, White R (2000) Monitoring the AIDS epidemic using HIV prevalence data among young women attending antenatal clinics: prospects and problems. *AIDS*, **14**(11): 1633–1645.

7

Community interaction in studies of gynaecological morbidity: experiences in Egypt, India and Uganda

Shireen Jejeebhoy,[1] Michael Koenig[2] and Christopher Elias[3]

[1] The Population Council, New Delhi, India; [2] Johns Hopkins University, Baltimore, USA; [3] PATH, Seattle, USA

A common element in virtually all investigations of women's gynaecological morbidity is the high level of interaction and rapport between investigators and the communities studied, irrespective of whether the study is conducted by a research group or a NGO. In this chapter we present lessons learned from the experiences of three studies in building community rapport and maximizing participation levels. Two of these were pioneer studies of women's gynaecological morbidity, conducted in the late 1980s in rural Egypt (Younis et al., 1993) and India (Bang et al., 1989). The third is a more recent and ongoing study of HIV and sexually transmitted infections (STIs), based in rural Rakai district, Uganda (Wawer et al., 1999).

The objectives of each of the three studies were largely similar: to assess levels of reproductive morbidity and, in the case of Rakai, STIs in community settings. Project sites were two villages each in Egypt and India, containing a total population of 16 500 and 4000, respectively, and an entire district in Uganda comprising a population of 384 000. Populations were largely poor and female literacy rates were uniformly low. Each of these studies have included a survey focusing on self-reported symptoms, risk behaviours and background characteristics, as well as clinical examination (Egypt and India) and/or laboratory testing. While the Ugandan study required a minimum of pelvic examinations, they were a central component of both the Egypt and India studies.

Collectively, these studies underscore that the essential steps of any community-based study of gynaecological morbidity include efforts to put together a strong research team, and meld the strengths of a variety of social, biomedical and epidemiological skills and disciplines; gain community rapport and motivate women to participate in the study, particularly to undergo a clinical examination and/or laboratory testing; and arrange to provide appropriate treatment and follow-up to those reporting or diagnosed with a morbidity. The manner in which the studies addressed these fundamental issues is strikingly similar, and is described in full in the case studies accompanying this summary. The purpose of this overview is to highlight the main insights gleaned from each study in three different contexts.

Composition of the research team

The composition of the research team is clearly shaped by study objectives. While the Rakai project is essentially a community-based, randomized trial to assess the effect of mass treatment of STIs on HIV transmission, the objective of the study in India was to assess prevalence of gynaecological morbidity. The study in Egypt, in contrast, also included a strong social and behavioural focus, including exploration of women's experiences of gynaecological ill health, their perceptions of its aetiology and actions taken. It is no surprise therefore that while principal investigator teams of both the Rakai and the Indian studies were largely medical, the Egypt study included a more multidisciplinary team.

Given the orientation of this volume towards understanding illness and disease correlates, consequences and health seeking behaviour, the experience of the Egypt study in putting together a multidisciplinary research team is especially pertinent. The principal investigators in this study represented different disciplines – the biomedical (including gynaecology and other specializations), and the social sciences (including an anthropologist and a bio-statistician). The case study also recommends, in light of the close connections between gynaecological and mental health, the inclusion of a psychologist on the research team. However, simply assembling a multidisciplinary team is not sufficient. The case study argues for close interaction between investigators, and mutual respect for and interest in each other's disciplines. It argues that the team should have a good collective understanding of both the nature of the problem and the sociocultural context in which the study is conducted. Given that researchers are increasingly interested in the social and behavioural determinants and consequences of gynaecological morbidity, as well as its prevalence, such an interdisciplinary team is an essential component of studies.

At the same time, each of the three studies demonstrated that the larger research team must contain a variety of skills. Each study included a team of field workers, as far as possible female, who represented the effective link between the research team and the community and were responsible for building rapport with study participants. In the Egyptian and Indian studies, this team was also responsible for fielding the survey; in Uganda, a separate team undertook the survey. In the Ugandan project, for example, health educators and counsellors, particularly females, appraised the community of the proposed activities; counsellors in addition provided pre- and post-test counselling and informed participants of their laboratory test results, and acted as the main interface between the community and research team. In the Egyptian and Indian projects, this team of field workers was the vital link in the chain, bearing the responsibility of building and maintaining rapport with the community, assisting study participants in a variety of ways (ranging from accompanying them to the project clinic, to distributing medication to those deemed to need any) and monitoring compliance. The cooperation and participation of local health providers in the Egyptian and Indian studies also succeeded in minimizing the distance between the research team and the community. Traditional providers were enlisted in the Indian study, including traditional birth attendants and village volunteers.

The importance of training for each of these teams is clearly evident. Where a multidisciplinary team of principal investigators exists, extensive cross-training is required. Moreover, the wide inter-clinician disparities in diagnosis observed in other studies (Koenig et al., 1998) can only be minimized through extensive training. Training is equally indispensable among those charged with building rapport, fielding surveys, conducting laboratory tests, and managing and analyzing data.

Gaining the support of women and the community

Close interaction with the community is an important determinant of the successful completion of studies investigating reproductive tract infections and gynaecological morbidity. A common element in all three studies was the high level of interaction and rapport between the investigators and the communities studied. Careful and exhaustive preparatory efforts and engagement with the communities were essential prerequisites in gaining the cooperation and active support of study communities. Several steps have been outlined.

Study site selection

Study sites need to be carefully selected. Sites should not be remote and inaccessible, and their population should fall within the size recommended for the study. Clinic facilities or potential sites should be available, and community leaders should be interested and willing to become involved in the study. For example, in the Indian study, community leaders committed to assistance for providing appropriate clinic facilities and mobilizing women to participate in the study.

Government involvement

The involvement and commitment of central and local government was found to be an essential first step in gaining community acceptance in the Ugandan project. Similarly, the Egyptian study was not initiated until government approval was obtained. Government support was observed to be central in gaining entry into communities, and in ensuring the credibility of the research team and their agenda.

Community mobilization

Intensive community mobilization efforts were a feature of all three studies. Once entry into the community is made, the research team must educate and inform communities of the objectives of the research, how the study will be conducted, and how it will benefit the community. This phase is potentially time-consuming but it is an ethical precondition for research. In the Egyptian study, this phase of rapport-building was undertaken for a full year before activities were initiated. The studies report discussions with a range of community-level gatekeepers: formal and informal leaders; NGOs; and representatives of women's groups. Through a snowball process, key local leaders representing special hard-to-reach or potentially resistant groups were also approached. The Egypt study elicited, for example, a very positive response from both a leading religious figure (the imam) and health centre personnel, all of whom became influential opinion leaders. The Indian study reports that local providers became strong advocates of the study and its benefits for women.

Engaging both female and male community members

By far the most important stage is educating and informing community women and men of the study, what it entails and how it may benefit them. Given the unequal gender relations that prevail in all three settings, special efforts were made to involve men, convince them in the community and in the home of the rationale and need for the study, and enlist their support. In particular, efforts were made to convince men not to dissuade or forbid selected women from their families from participating in the studies, and to apprise them of the benefits of the study. In order to convey symbolically the community ownership of the study and its products, one study (India) was initiated with much fanfare at a public function involving the entire study community.

Allaying women's fears

Building and maintaining rapport with the community, particularly with women, is a continuous and multifaceted activity, and not simply a means of gaining entry into study sites. All three studies took pains to ensure that women perceived that they had a meaningful stake in activities. Objectives and research tools were explained in language women understood, with respect for cultural norms. Any study of gynaecological morbidity, reproductive tract infections and sexually transmitted infections raises anxiety in a number of ways and women must have an opportunity to allay any doubts. Common fears include who gets selected, and why have women been selected who are perceived to have engaged in premarital or extramarital relations? What might a pelvic examination reveal, and how appropriate is it for women to expose themselves to one? How confidential will the information provided remain, and similarly, the results of the clinical and laboratory tests? What is the purpose of drawing blood and how will it affect women's well-being? Also discussed with women were issues of informed consent, confidentiality and privacy. Bang and Bang report that the degree of confidentiality maintained in the India study became apparent when clinical evidence that certain adolescent females were sexually experienced was not – contrary to the fears of adolescents – disclosed to parents or other community members.

Contact with women took several forms. In the Egypt study, principal investigators and the field team spent long periods of time in the selected villages, became personally acquainted with women and their families, and were perceived as 'being a constant presence in the villages'.

Maintaining gender sensitivity

Throughout the course of the study, researchers strived to make procedures and interactions woman-centred. The field team acted as an intermediary between women and both the medical establishment in their settings and the study's clinical activities. In the Egypt study, efforts were made to improve the quality of interaction between women and health centre physicians, by sensitizing them to women's fears and concerns, and training them to ensure privacy and preserve women's dignity while conducting examinations, and by making facilities less threatening in terms of hygiene, equipment and so on. Women were clearly impressed by these changes. Field teams in Egypt spent a considerable time dispelling fears of pelvic examination, and escorted women to and from the clinic where the medical examination was conducted. In cases where women were required to seek follow-up at referral facilities, the research team routinely offered to attend the medical examination with women and act as their advocates. And finally, the use of female investigators and survey questions that use locally used terminology and are framed in culturally acceptable ways cannot be sufficiently stressed.

Minimizing inconvenience to women

Each study reports efforts designed to reduce inconvenience to women as much as possible. In the Ugandan study, self-administered vaginal swabs and field workers skilled in drawing blood enabled investigation to be conducted within women's homes. In the India and Egypt studies, investigators took pains to make appointments at convenient times for women to attend clinics, spend sufficient time in each consultation and be culturally sensitive. In the Egypt study, field teams were sensitive to and avoided certain times and days that were inconvenient to women (for example, 'cooking' day or while baking). Each study conveyed, moreover, that participation was entirely voluntary – in Egypt, many women who initially refused sought out the field staff over the course of the project and agreed to be interviewed and examined.

Dispelling rumours

Notwithstanding these efforts, some suspicion does persist, and rumours can arise. It is the continuous presence of field teams and the underlying rapport built with the community that can dispel these rumours. In the Indian study, for example, rumours abounded concerning the conduct of the pelvic examination. These were addressed through women's group meetings, one-on-one consultations with social workers, village volunteers and satisfied clients, and invitations to unconvinced women to visit clinics and attend a pelvic examination or observe surgery. In the Rakai project, rumours spread regarding the use of blood that was collected in the course of study; opening study laboratories to the community to demonstrate why blood is taken and what is done with it allayed this rumour. In Egypt, similarly, a range of rumours spread – that blood samples were to be sold and that the research team was intent on family planning and sterilization. Field teams immediately addressed these concerns in public and in one-on-one sessions.

Two of the three case studies report the importance of modest and culturally appropriate gifts as tokens of appreciation to study participants. These gifts – whether in cash or kind – are reportedly useful in motivating communities to participate in research and reassuring communities of their important role in the study. In Rakai, 'incentives' were provided to individual participant women (a bar of soap) and to communities (assistance in building a dispensary or school). In Egypt, women themselves were involved in the process of deciding on an appropriate token of appreciation: the gift comprised laundry soap powder, bars of soap and biscuits for children. While each study provided extensive treatment, this can hardly be considered an incentive, but rather an ethical obligation, as is discussed later.

Building and maintaining rapport with the community cannot be accomplished without extensive training of the entire research team. Each study focused considerable attention on the training of field teams. The Egypt study, for example, trained its field team in fieldwork techniques and reproductive health issues, as well as to act as intermediaries between the research team, medical and health professionals, and the community. Field workers were also charged with the responsibility of delivering prescribed medication and supporting women during treatment at home or in hospital. Much attention was paid to training field staff to be responsive to community needs.

Providing services

The provision of medical treatment as a part of any study of women's reproductive health problems should be considered mandatory in resource-poor settings where few women have access to quality gynaecological care. For many women, this may represent the only opportunity to address their reproductive health problems. Indeed, arranging required care may be a prerequisite for enlisting women's cooperation and participation in studies of this nature, as well as an ethical imperative. It is unlikely that many women would willingly disclose sensitive problems or agree to submit to what constitutes an invasive and embarrassing examination if effective treatment is not provided (Koenig et al., 1998).

All three case studies did indeed provide medical care to women diagnosed with an illness. For example, in Rakai, two prongs of services were provided: to women and men diagnosed or reporting a STI symptom, and general primary health care to study women and their children who experienced other health problems. Moreover, in case of an emergency or epidemic, the project became involved in services and care. In India, treatment also took several pathways. Treatment was provided to women diagnosed to have a gynaecological problem; at the same time, general services were provided for women, children and other family members. Each woman from whom blood was drawn was provided a bottle of tonic (partly to allay fears of consequent weakness and partly to address high rates of anaemia prevailing in the area). At the conclusion of the study, and in response to study findings, a number of additional interventions were undertaken: providing reproductive health education, training traditional birth attendants in reproductive tract infection diagnosis, safe delivery and referral, and training nurses in comprehensive reproductive health care; expanding services to address infertility, abortion and men's reproductive health problems; and finally, establishing a comprehensive reproductive health referral clinic.

In Egypt too, activities focused on providing timely and appropriate treatment to women diagnosed to have a gynaecological problem. Timely feedback of laboratory results and provision of required medication was a mainstay of the study. Treatment was provided to all women. Women who needed more specialized attention were referred to larger facilities; not only were all their expenses borne by the study – including surgery in a few cases – but the research team accompanied women to referral facilities and acted as intermediaries between the woman, her family and the provider. Where treatment of any kind was provided, women were monitored for compliance, and followed up during the process of recuperation from more serious treatments. Where STIs were detected, treatment was also provided for the husband.

Conclusion

These studies offer a remarkably similar set of experiences and lessons for involving communities as active participants in studies of reproductive tract and gynaecological morbidity. First, each study has stressed that building rapport takes time, and requires multi-pronged efforts and a deep understanding of the cultural context in which the study is placed. Second, each study reports the need for a wide range of actors – government officials, health service providers, key community leaders, men and other influential family members, and most of all women themselves as active participants in the research process. Finally, studies report the development of close relationships between the research team and participating women – as the Egypt study reports, field workers were perceived as family members and shared many confidences beyond gynaecological problems.

Despite the similarities in community involvement activities and the central role this played in all three studies, sociocultural factors inhibiting women in certain settings from participating in such studies of gynaecological morbidity can exert considerable influence on the participation of women in all phases of study. In the Uganda study, the use of self-administered vaginal swabs in the home setting eliminated the need for pelvic examinations or clinic visits, and resulted in a participation rate of 96 per cent. In the Egypt study, where restrictions on women's autonomy are considerable, compliance reached an impressive 91 per cent. The Indian setting was by far the most conservative and most restrictive of women, and in this setting, 59 per cent of women agreed to undergo all phases of study. Efforts, therefore, need to be made to explore creative and feasible alternatives to break through or adapt cultural barriers that can prove insurmountable, and jeopardize both women's participation in such studies and deny them the opportunity for treatment of symptoms and diseases that may otherwise be overlooked, as well as the broader generalizability of research findings.

REFERENCES

Bang RA, Bang AT, Baitule M et al. (1989) High prevalence of gynaecological diseases in rural Indian women. *Lancet*, **1**(8629): 85–88.

Koenig M, Jejeebhoy S, Singh S et al. (1998) Investigating women's gynaecological morbidity in India: not just another KAP survey. *Reproductive health matters*, **6**(11): 84–97.

Wawer MJ, Sewankambo NK, Serwadda D et al. (1999) Control of sexually transmitted diseases for AIDS prevention in Uganda: a randomised community trial. *Lancet*, **353**(9152): 525–535.

Younis N, Khattab H, Zurayk H et al. (1993) A community study of gynaecological and related morbidities in rural Egypt. *Studies in family planning*, **24**(3): 175–186.

Egypt: the Giza reproductive morbidity study

Hind Khattab

Delta Consultants Ltd, Cairo, Egypt

The objectives of the Giza reproductive morbidity study were multidimensional: to assess levels of reproductive morbidity in the study community; to test the extent to which an interview questionnaire can provide information on reproductive morbidity; and to delineate the layers of determinants of actual and perceived morbidity. The study, conducted in 1989–91, had a complex data collection strategy, which included an interview questionnaire of several components to be administered over two visits to a household, a clinical examination at the community health centre and laboratory testing at the local health centre (more specialized tests being performed at a laboratory in Cairo).

A review of previous studies involving medical examinations revealed that one of the main obstacles to obtaining credible research results was a low participation rate. Thus, defining the methodology, selecting an appropriate research team and building rapport with the community were central in overcoming the problem of a low participation rate for medical examinations in a resource-poor rural community (Bone, 1981; Fathalla et al., 1981; Wasserheit et al., 1989). The Giza study has recorded an impressive participation rate (91 and 100 per cent in the two villages studied), despite the relatively large size of the study sample and the complicated data collection process required; equally impressive rates were observed in follow-up studies in Egypt, Jordan and Lebanon based on virtually identical methodology. The high participation rates achieved in these studies provides a strong rationale for documenting the methodology used by the Giza study to build community rapport.

The objective of this case study thus is to draw lessons from the conduct of the Giza study for maximizing participation and building rapport between the study team and the community, particularly women. Maximizing community participation and building rapport requires multi-pronged action, from careful selection of study sites and research teams, to support to women to overcome fear and inhibition to participate in the study. These are outlined below.

Selection of study sites

Because of the different kinds of data to be collected in the study, the following criteria were critical in selecting the community site: logistical support, as well as the availability of clinic facilities, relatively easy physical access to the community, and an estimation of the size of the problem in terms of the expected level of prevalence of reproductive morbidity. Two adjacent villages were selected that satisfied these criteria and were fairly representative of rural communities in Giza Governorate. These villages were situated on the west bank of the Mariuttia canal in Imbaba district, 14 km from Cairo. Village A had an estimated population of 4500 and village B 12000. Both villages had Ministry of Health clinics with female physicians in charge. The proximity of the villages to Cairo simplified the logistics of daily commuting of the research team and minimized the transport time of laboratory specimens to the Cairo laboratories.

A profile of the study villages suggests a poorly educated population with a generally low income. As many as 78 per cent of females over the age of 6 years (and somewhat fewer men) had never been enrolled in school. Agriculture was the main occupation, employing some 56 per cent of husbands. Other occupations included manufacturing, transport, commerce and services, with a quarter of the sample husbands categorized as skilled labourers, 10 per cent unskilled and 8 per cent professionals. The socio-economic status of women in the sample was correspondingly low, contributing to women becoming accustomed to bearing discomfort and even pain without complaining or seeking medical help. Perceived gender roles, as well as lack of power and awareness, compounded the problem.

The research team

It was clear that the research team would need to be interdisciplinary. A medical expert, specifically one or more gynaecologists, was needed to determine the morbidities prevalent in the sample and to guide the team on signs and symptoms so that they could investigate women's experiences and perceptions of morbidities. The study also required a clinical pathologist to support and confirm, through laboratory examination, the gynaecologist's diagnosis of reproductive tract infections such as bacterial vaginosis, trichomonal vaginitis, candidiasis, gonorrhoea, chlamydia and nonspecific mucopurulent cervicitis. It was the job of the anthropologist to determine the best way to approach the women on such intimate and sensitive subjects as gynaecological symptoms, and to choose the most appropriate language to formulate the questions. A bio-statistician was needed to work in close cooperation with these specialists, and to lead the team in developing a conceptual framework, sample design and study instruments, as well as to take responsibility for analysing and presenting the data. In addition, an experienced field team was required to administer the interview questionnaire and accompany women to the medical examination. Finally, although not included in the Giza study research team, the Giza study experience suggests, in retrospect, the need for the inclusion in the research team of a psychiatrist or psychologist in future projects of this kind, given the importance of psychological aspects of disease.

As important as the composition of the research team was the nature of their interaction with one another. An exchange of expertise was needed so that a common understanding of the conceptual framework could be developed. Mutual respect and tolerance of each other's disciplines were crucial to develop a genuinely interdisciplinary team with a common goal. A readiness by each specialist to learn from the others was indispensable. The social scientists needed to learn from the medical professionals about gynaecological symptoms and diseases. The medical professionals likewise needed to learn from the social scientists the terminology used by women to express symptoms, their perceptions regarding the aetiology of these symptoms, and the sociocultural context in which they experienced morbidity conditions. The bio-statistician and the anthropologist would need to work closely to integrate quantitative and qualitative data. In short, what was required was an appreciation and respect for the interdisciplinary approach of the study, and the need for adaptability.

Finally, the field staff needed to have an in-depth knowledge of the nature of the data to be gathered and the sociocultural context in which the study was being conducted. Field staff were a vital link with the community; it was important that they acquired an in-depth knowledge of the community's cultural values, traditions, beliefs and practices in order to relate to the community in a meaningful way. Being culturally sensitive, they could interact positively with the study sample, allay their fears about participation and generally encourage their active participation in the study.

Designing the questionnaire

The second strategy that contributed to achieving high participation rates was the administration of questionnaires that were culturally sensitive and acceptable to study participants. Extensive time and effort were invested in designing the questionnaire. It was important that questions were framed using women's own terminology when referring to various conditions, that they were acceptable in terms of the cultural norms of the community and that they flowed easily (Khattab et al., 1997). Designing the questionnaire was a time-consuming exercise, lasting over a year. The research team adopted a number of methods to ascertain terminology and perceptions. In general, home visits and informal discussions with family members provided valuable information on individual perceptions, as did consultations with knowledgeable people in the village, including older women and men. Four additional activities supplemented these insights. First, an exploratory study was organized in a family planning clinic in Cairo to investigate the prevalence of gynaecological morbidity and women's perceptions of these conditions. Second, a medical workshop was conducted to clarify the medical concepts and symptomatology of reproductive morbidity. Third, a focus group session was organized in a non-study village in Giza to learn the terminology used by women and to gain an insight into the cultural norms and attitudes surrounding these conditions. Finally, pilot tests were conducted for each component of the questionnaire, followed by tests of the entire questionnaire after it was finalized.

Community-based action

The third strategy was to design and initiate community-based action. The team realized the importance of a climate of rapport and mutual trust within the study community, and the need for women to believe that they had 'a meaningful stake in what was going on' (Raeburn, 1992). Building rapport with the community involved a variety of activities:

- Field workers were key. It was important that they interacted with study participants as one woman to another, showing them that they cared about the women's well-being, treating them with respect and taking their opinions seriously. They also had to act as intermediaries between women and community medical professionals, who were often perceived as distant and patronizing (Khattab, 1992). Being sensitive to social norms and community concerns, and familiar with obstetric and gynaecological conditions, field workers were able to present medical and interview tools of research in culturally appropriate ways.

- Improving the interface between women in the community and physicians in health centres also enhanced rapport between women and the research team. For one, health centre physicians were sensitized to women's fears and concerns, and made aware of women's reluctance to undergo pelvic examinations. During special training, physicians were alerted to these problems and encouraged to improve the quality of care provided, particularly in terms of caring interaction during consultation, and ensuring privacy during examination. In addition, field team members talked to the women and reassured them about the examination procedures. At the same time, attention was paid to the physical upgrading of the health centres in terms of equipment and instruments, hygiene, cleanliness and sanitation. This served to reassure women of the quality of services that would be provided.

- A fundamental premise underlying this study was that the women were active participants in the project, not to be manipulated for research purposes, and that 'it is important that the community or population gain not only from the results of the research, but from the process itself' (Harris, 1992). To meet this objective, the research team arranged to provide treatment for all diagnosed morbidities among participating women and to refer cases that needed specialized medical investigations to the collaborating university hospital. The speed with which this was achieved in the early phase of the research served to reassure the participating women and encourage other women to participate in the study. It also helped the participating women realize that many of the symptoms they experienced could be alleviated with treatment, often quickly and at little expense.

Preparing the field team

A principal task was to have a well-prepared field team that would enter the study community, apply disciplined, appropriate and efficient procedures and tools with compassion and sensitivity, and avoid at all costs antagonizing any of the sample women. The field team had to be familiarized with the techniques of community participation since they were responsible for gaining the trust of the village community, interviewing over 500 women in the study sample, inviting each to accompany them to a medical examination, and following up on all phases of required treatment. They were also expected to smooth over problem areas, notably when dealing with apprehensive women, reluctant families or hostile husbands. Field workers would have daily and intimate contact with the two villages for a period of over a year. They were the visible face of the study project and the link between the research team, medical and health professionals, and the village community.

Six field workers, one field supervisor and one field manager, all young women, formed the field team. Each had a degree in social science and had worked in community research and development. None of them had been previously involved with the medical aspects of women's reproductive health. Training included familiarization with the objectives of the study and the details of the study instrument to be administered, as well as the medical aspects of women's reproductive health, including a review of symptoms, pelvic examination, laboratory test procedures and common treatments. Training was provided over a period of several days by the two obstetrician-gynaecologists on the research team. These specialists shared a belief (not commonly found in the medical profession) that non-medically trained persons would be able to understand and assimilate the facts of medicine and medical practice sufficiently to successfully complete the assigned research task, which included asking about medical symptoms, delivering prescribed medication to women, and supporting them during treatment at home or in hospital.

The field team was also trained by the anthropologist on the research team in communicating with the community, the women and their families. Participatory training in observation, participant observation and intensive interviews were held for almost four weeks. It was necessary to hold repeated sessions to ensure that field workers could communicate effectively with the community, particularly with the women and their families. This ability to communicate effectively proved to be important in ensuring women's full participation in the study, and enabling women to overcome the culture of silence regarding gynaecological morbidities and articulate their discomfort or suffering (Dixon-Mueller and Wasserheit, 1991). Hence, training familiarized field workers with asking sensitive questions concerning intimate details of marriage, reproductive life and health, and asking probing questions to overcome women's reluctance to acknowledge their own health needs. Even so, training stressed that it was more important to establish healthy and respectful communication with women than to emphasize participation.

In short, training of the field team cannot be over-emphasized. Training must encompass a host of features, such as:

• Study objectives.
• Details of study instruments and their administration.
• Familiarization of the medical aspects of research.
• Communicating effectively, particularly on sensitive and personal topics.
• Application of qualitative methods, such as participant observation and in-depth interviews, preferably through participatory training.

Entry into the community

Initial entry into the community required the consideration of four factors: obtaining the cooperation and participation of the physicians and staff at the two village health centres; getting official permission to implement the study and for physicians to participate; gaining the confidence and support of formal and informal village leaders; and familiarizing the village women with the field team.

Gaining community support was essential. If, for example, the participating women felt that any of the community leaders was antagonistic to the aims of the study, they would be reluctant to take part. Thus good relations between all the members of the research team and important members of the community (local doctors and village leaders) were considered vital for a successful outcome. Similarly, the men of the community, as well as the participating women, needed to be well-informed about the study, its objectives and the potential health benefits to women by participating; it was important that men would not object to the women being questioned about their gynaecological health. Having the support of the entire community also served to minimize the impact of negative rumours about the objectives of the study, which occasionally surfaced.

Cooperation of village clinic staff

The research team decided at the start that the medical examination component of the study would be undertaken at existing village health centres by the female physicians who had been in charge of the clinics for many years. Both health centres provided primary health care, and the general physician dealt with gynaecological complaints; both had basic laboratory facilities. The research team perused the facilities available and, as a first step, held informal discussions with physicians and staff of each health centre to introduce the study, its objectives, design, multidisciplinary nature, and potential health benefits. These informal visits to the two health centres, and the interest of the two physicians, served to assure the team of the appropriateness of these clinics as partners in the research study. In the course of these informal visits, the research team was also able to observe clinic facilities, check equipment and supplies, and assess the extent to which facilities would need to be upgraded.

From the study perspective, conducting the medical examination at existing facilities and through the staff of these facilities did indeed enhance community cooperation. The general physicians at both centres – both female – were well known to the village women and their familiarity made the gynaecological component of the medical examination less threatening. At the same time, participation in the study provided physicians with not only an opportunity to upgrade their skills through training and supervision, but also financial compensation within the limits imposed by government regulations. Clinic facilities also benefited from renovations to the physical infrastructure, and new equipment and instruments for the gynaecological examination.

Official permits

After these visits, the research team felt ready to take the second step to entering the community by seeking official permission and approval for the participation of the centre physicians. Obtaining a permit in Egypt is not an easy task, and it was clear that the project would have to rely on the networking skills of team members who were well known in official circles and who had some experience in dealing with the bureaucracy on other projects.

The long process of obtaining permission started in June 1989 and took five months. It is not necessary to describe all the steps involved but it is important to suggest that this period of time need not be wasted. During this time, the research and field teams began to establish rapport with village leaders and members of the community, including the men whose support is crucial to ensuring the participation of wives and daughters.

Village leaders

The experience of the Giza study highlights the importance of identifying and developing rapport with key formal and informal leaders. In the villages under study, formal leaders included members of the village council, the *omda* or village headman, and the imam or religious leader of the mosque. These leaders were visited individually, and when introducing the study, emphasis was placed on its contribution to improving women's awareness of health problems not only in the community but in Egypt as a whole, and possibly in other countries of the region. It was explained, however, that the primary responsibility was towards the village women themselves, for whom a free medical examination would be provided and free treatment offered.

Lower-level health centre personnel, both medical and paramedical, were also important local leaders. Of particular importance was the health centre registrar who was familiar with many of the women as a result of his clinic duties and because of his central role in the immunization campaigns. Also important was the *tamargiah* or female custodian at the centre, who was the confidante of most village women when they visited the health centre, discussing their problems and providing a sympathetic ear. Custodians are often sought for medical advice because of their empathy and accessibility.

Reactions of village leaders were not always positive, and scepticism was sometimes encountered. For example, the imam of one of the mosques argued that a far greater priority for the health of village residents was faulty water and sewage systems and poor living conditions, and that research findings remained unutilized, or 'thrown into drawers'. In discussions, however, he recognized the need to focus on women's health in the process of procreation, and the importance of supporting the study, reiterating that 'Islam not only elevates the status of women in the community but encourages and commends women's role as health care providers for their families' (Khattab et al., 1994: 12).

Getting to know the women

Getting to know the women in the study sample and earning their confidence was one of the field team's earliest and most pressing concerns. The first opportunity presented itself in the task of mapping the villages to select the household samples. In the course of the mapping exercise, which was conducted by the field team in co-ordination with the health centre registrar, each member of the team was personally introduced by the registrar to men and women living in the village. Such an introduction clearly lent legitimacy to the presence of team members. In the course of mapping, team members held informal discussions with women, inquiring about their health and general well-being in a friendly, non-aggressive manner, and establishing cordial community relations. This strategy may have slowed down the mapping exercise but proved extremely useful in gaining acceptance within the community.

The pre-test of the study instruments and field activities presented a second opportunity for the field team to acquaint themselves with the women. This involved interviewing selected women on the gynaecological component of the questionnaires and accompanying them to the health clinic for a medical examination and laboratory tests. During the two-week pre-test period, six women were interviewed and escorted to the health centre for a medical examination. Within three weeks, the women were presented with the results of the laboratory tests and the medical examination, and given the prescribed medication. The speed and promptness of the exercise helped to convince the villagers that the study group was serious about helping the women.

The opportunity provided during this period to learn more about the women themselves, to ask them about their reactions to the study and their response to the invitation to undertake a medical examination, proved invaluable in refining the field plan. For example, it was learned that 'Thursday is cooking day because butchers slaughter on that day . . . and women will not be free to talk'. Moreover, 'Women are usually free after 11 in the morning, because children are at school, men are at work and housework is almost done. Work activities in the fields or in peddling are also less intensive'. The team also found out that women could talk while washing, but never when baking for fear of the evil eye. These details illustrate the importance of getting to know community norms and customs for effective results.

Listening to women enabled refinement in study procedures and reaped rich rewards in terms of participation. For example, a number of comments suggested factors underlying women's reluctance to undertake a medical examination. Health professionals were perceived as insensitive. Remarks such as 'I am afraid . . . because the physician inserts a cold, hard metal object into a woman which hurts a lot', 'I feel embarrassed and very uncomfortable lying down with my legs up during the examination', and 'The last time I had a gynaecological examination, I bled and my belly hurt for a few days', were common. On probing, it became evident that some of the women's fear and discomfort was the result of previous personal experience with the health services, both public and private, although a few were based on stories related by relatives, neighbours or friends.

The pre-test also provided an opportunity for the community to assess the sincerity and commitment of the study team. Rapport built with pre-test participants was important in encouraging other women to participate in the next phase. One satisfied woman told her daughter, who was reluctant to participate, 'Look what they have done for me . . . They bought me medication from the pharmacy, which cost a lot of money. You have no excuse not to go, I'll stay with your children, I'll carry out your daily chores, just go and think about your own health'.

Such a positive attitude however, was not always observed. The team needed, therefore, to allay women's fears and concerns about pain and discomfort during examination. For example, physicians were made aware of women's fears and discomfort, and requested to be gentler during the physical examination and to give women enough time to feel relaxed and safe; another innovation was to allow a social researcher to attend the various medical investigations with women, if they so chose. Since visiting the doctor accompanied by a relative or a friend is a common practice in this culture, the suggestion was taken up by most of the women.

Women were consulted on various aspects of the study, including appropriate ways in which the study team could show appreciation to the women who chose to participate in the pre-test and in the study. A consensus was reached that the best way would be to give a small gift of two boxes of laundry soap powder, two bars of scented soap and two packets of biscuits for the children. This gift was deemed appropriate by all, since soap promoted hygiene and sanitation, and biscuits had nutritional value. At the same time, the action reinforced women's recognition of the participatory nature of the project.

In summary, gaining access into a community is a time-consuming exercise that needs to be carefully planned. The study team needs to be familiar with the layout of the study site, the characteristics of the population, the socio-economic structure, and public utilities and services, as well as the perceptions of the community with regard to women's reproductive health. The support of local leaders and educated community members is essential in securing community acceptance. At the same time, it is important that men are apprised of the study objectives and procedures, and their support is sought in convincing women to participate in the study. Equally important is the support of service providers. Ultimately however, it is women themselves with whom rapport needs to be generated, and the Giza study experience succeeded in doing so not only by listening to women but by actively involving them in, and eliciting their views on crucial aspects of the study.

Data collection phase

It is in the actual collection of data that the calibre and training of the field team plays a crucial role. Aggressive or abrupt interviewers are unlikely to be accepted by the community. Important characteristics during interviews are tact, skill and sensitivity, and a skilled interviewer can contribute to a high participation rate.

The Giza study experience suggests that the interview process requires more than a single visit. During the first visit to women in the study sample, the field worker would explain each stage of the study and seek her agreement to participate. If the woman refused, the field worker would not insist but would tell the woman that the team would be working in the village for several months, and that the same interviewer would re-visit the woman in case she had changed her mind. Over time, women exchanged experiences and the refusal rate dropped. Many women who had initially refused to take part accepted when they were approached again, or specifically sought out the interviewer when she was visiting their street. Even women who were not part of the sample visited the health centre requesting a medical examination (unfortunately, these women could not be included in the study, but were referred to available services). Once a woman agreed to join the study, two components of the survey questionnaire were administered to her, covering the socio-economic characteristics of the family and obstetric morbidity during the last pregnancy (if the last pregnancy fell in the past two years). It goes without saying that the interview would be conducted at a time that was convenient for women, even if that involved a second visit.

The field worker also made an appointment with the woman to fill in the component on gynaecological symptoms, which had to be on a day when the woman could accompany the field worker to the health unit for a gynaecological examination. Such an arrangement was necessary because the gynaecological morbidity component collected information on women's reports of current symptoms, which were to be compared with the gynaecological examination and had to take place on the same day (Zurayk et al., 1993). Every effort was made to choose a time convenient to the woman rather than the interviewer.

The third component involved an interview on gynaecological morbidity, followed by a medical examination at the health unit that included a general and a gynaecological component and the collection of specimens for laboratory tests (blood, urine, Pap smear and swab) (Younis, Khalil and Zurayk, 1994). This phase of the study required a second visit at a predetermined time. Every effort was made to reduce inconvenience or fear among women. Where necessary, transport was provided. The woman was always accompanied to and from the health centre by the field worker; the field worker played an important supportive role. At the health centre, efforts were made to reduce waiting time, and the woman received a small gift at the conclusion of the visit.

This component of the study required considerable planning on the part of the field team. Workers were expected to accompany a designated number of women to the health centre at specified times during each of an allotted three days per week. This required considerable co-ordination: the field worker had to arrange to administer the interview to the woman and take her to the health centre and back, repeating the process over and over again until the day's quota was completed. Often the field worker would arrive at a woman's house at the appointed time to find the woman otherwise engaged and unable to accompany her. Reconciling the woman's convenience with the smooth running of procedures at the health unit was sometimes a difficult balancing act. Occasionally the field worker would visit a woman three or four times before she was free to go for the medical investigation. Most of the younger women required permission from their mothers-in-law. On several occasions, the mother-in-law refused permission: 'She cannot go because she is cleaning the house', or 'She will be free in two hours, after she finishes washing and the laundry'. In one instance, a potential participant who had fixed a date for the medical examination apologized saying, 'I cannot go just yet, my mother-in-law died a few days ago, how can I think of myself when her blood is still hot?' In such cases, the field worker would have to be flexible enough to fix another appointment, adjust the day's schedule, and try to replace the cancelled appointment so that the physician's schedule would not be disrupted.

Finally, it was important that the interview process was conducted in a respectful manner, after fully apprising the woman of its content and purpose. It was important that women be informed of the various aspects of the research, informed consent obtained, and the decision respected of those who refuse to participate. Interviews needed to discuss issues on equal terms with women, on a 'woman-to-woman' basis rather than as an outsider with a patronizing attitude. And finally, it was important that survey research be supplemented by further in-depth qualitative research on the social and cultural context in which ill health occurs.

Rapport between field workers and sample women

The relationship between the field worker and women participants did not end when all the required data had been collected. Rather, field workers maintained close contact with these women whenever they were in the vicinity of their homes. This neighbourly attitude also served to maintain rapport with the community, and contributed to high participation rates. For example, on one occasion, on hearing of the death of the brother of a potential respondent, field workers visited the woman to offer their condolences. A few days later, when the field worker met the woman in the street she was asked, 'When are you coming to take me to the health centre? You know, I told my husband the other day that I cannot refuse to go with you when you cared enough to sympathize with me in my grief'.

Familiarity with the range of life-cycle events (deaths, marriages and births), economic conditions, social and family structures and cultural norms related to reproductive health enabled workers to better understand women's refusal to participate, and allay fears and misgivings about participation. In the beginning, for example, it was difficult to persuade older women or women married to older men to participate in the project. One woman said, 'I am old, such medical problems are for the sexually active, not for me'. According to another woman, 'How can I go to the health centre for gynaecological investigation when everybody knows that my husband is incapacitated. This will suggest behaviour that is incriminating. Why should I go for a gynaecological examination now? It was important that field workers were skilled in addressing perceptions of the link between symptoms and sexual activity.

Addressing rumours

The Giza study experience highlights the importance of vigilance in countering rumours that may have threatened community support and jeopardized participation. Several rumours threatened the smooth implementation of the study, for example, that there was an unidentified epidemic in the village, that the field team was taking blood samples to sell abroad, that the team was promoting family planning 'like the rest of those who come here', that they were a group of medical students using the villagers for medical training, or that the team intended to operate on women and sterilize them. The field team needed to be alert to these rumours and skilled in refuting them; this required time, effort and tact. Faced with rumours, several strategies were required:

- One response was to repeat the announcement that participants were free to refuse to give a blood sample if they wished, and given this option, the large majority of women still consented to have their blood tested.
- The strategy of including infertile as well as menopausal women in the sample helped convince women that the team was not engaged in measures to control the number of pregnancies or children families intended to have.
- The fact that the health centre physicians would themselves examine the participating women refuted rumours that villagers were being used to train students.
- The researchers requested that the Ministry of Health postpone other research or health-related projects in the area, to control for unforeseen factors that might jeopardize the study. Officials were extremely cooperative in this respect and no permits for training or research were granted during the entire course of the study period.
- The cooperation of the paramedics (nurses, laboratory technicians) working at the health centres, who were also part of the field team, provided the field workers with a great deal of support in the initial period, not only by lending legitimacy to their presence but also by refuting rumours about the project.

Treatment and referral

The study was committed to providing treatment and referral for women found to have a gynaecological disorder, and field workers were responsible for delivering medication prescribed by the physician and organizing hospital referrals and follow-up during recuperation for the few cases where this was recommended. Treatment and referral were ethical prerequisites of such a study, and were important in demonstrating the action-oriented nature of the study, and at the same time contributed to encouraging participation.

Treatment and referral were conducted as follows. Findings of medical and laboratory examinations were presented to the medical field supervisor of the research team, who would diagnose the case and prescribe medication. Field workers would buy the medication, provide it to women, along with instructions for use, and monitor compliance. Where STIs were diagnosed, medication was also provided to the husband (in one instance, upon follow-up the respondent declared that she had not dared give her husband his medicine but had taken it all herself). If further medical investigation was advised, women were referred to the collaborating university hospital, and the field worker was actively involved not only in setting up the appointment, but also in convincing and reassuring women and families about the importance of undergoing the tests or treatment (see Khattab, 1992, for details).

Conclusion and recommendations

In our discussion of the field procedures followed in the Giza morbidity study and the composition and approach of the research team, we have highlighted those aspects that contributed most to encouraging community participation, even for the medical examination and laboratory tests. As the approach has been successfully replicated in a number of studies in other countries of the region (Sudan, Jordan, Lebanon and Syria), it could be said to provide a model for achieving high participation in community-based research into gynaecological morbidity in the area. With appropriate modifications to accommodate cultural differences, this model may well be replicated in other areas of the world where gynaecological morbidity among underprivileged rural women warrants investigation.

High participation was achieved through a number of measures. Above all, the action-oriented approach of the research procedure, which offered women immediate solutions to their reproductive health problems, was not only an ethical prerequisite, but also resulted in maximizing participation. Offering treatment, whether through medication or consultations with medical professionals as an integral part of the study, enabled women to consider themselves to be valued partners rather than mere providers of data. Second, the interdisciplinary research team, working in concert using a holistic and culturally-sensitive approach, facilitated quick solutions to problems and assured women's confidence in the process; the close links established between field workers and the community provided further impetus for participation. Third, to elicit the support of a wide range of community members was essential – local leaders and professionals, informal leaders, the participating women and their menfolk, as well as the health service providers. Fourth, in preparing research instruments, care must be taken to ensure the flow of questions, the use of appropriate terminology and the framing of sensitive questions in culturally acceptable ways.

Even so, it is inevitable that some women will refuse to participate. Family pressures, fear of stigma, fear of having a medical examination, previous bad experiences or rumours can inhibit participation even among women who recognize the need. However, such measures as reinforcing the fact that participation is optional, and prompt allaying of rumours can indeed keep refusal rates at a minimum, and the experience of the Giza study observed that many women who had refused to participate later sought out the study team requesting participation.

REFERENCES

Bone MR (1981) Family formation and maternal health. In: Omran AR and Stanley CC, eds. *Further studies on family formation patterns and health*, pp. 271–302. Geneva, World Health Organization.

Dixon-Mueller R and Wasserheit J (1991) *The culture of silence: reproductive tract infections among women in the third world.* New York, International Women's Health Coalition.

Fathalla M, Hammam HM, El-Sherbini AF et al. (1981) Family formation and maternal health, Egypt. In: Omran AR and Standley CC, eds. *Further studies on family formation patterns and health*, pp. 282–287. Geneva, World Health Organization.

Harris E (1992) Accessing community development research methodologies. *Canadian journal of public health*, **83**(Suppl. 1): 862–866.

Khattab H (1992) *The silent endurance: social conditions of women's reproductive health in rural Egypt.* Amman, UNICEF and Cairo, The Population Council.

Khattab H, Zurayk H, Kamal OI et al. (1997) *An interview-questionnaire on reproductive morbidity: the experience of the Giza morbidity study.* Policy Series in Reproductive Health, No. 4. Cairo, The Population Council, Regional Office for West Africa and North Africa.

Khattab H, Zurayk H, Younis N et al. (1994) *Field methodology for entry into the community.* The Policy Series in Reproductive Health, No. 3. Cairo, The Population Council, Regional Office for West Asia and North Africa.

Raeburn J (1992) Health promotion research with heart: keeping a people perspective. *Canadian journal of public health*, **83** (Suppl. 1): 820–824.

Wasserheit J, Harris JR, Chakraborty J et al. (1989) Reproductive tract infections in a family planning population in rural Bangladesh. *Studies in family planning*, **20**(2): 69–80.

Younis N, Khalil K, Zurayk H (1994) *Learning about the gynaecological health of women.* The Policy Series in Reproductive Health, No. 2. Cairo, The Population Council. Regional Office for West Africa and North Africa.

Zurayk H, Khattab H, Younis N et al. (1993) Concepts and measures of reproductive morbidity. *Health transition review*, **3**(1): 17–40.

India: the Gadchiroli study of gynaecological diseases

Rani Bang and Abhay Bang

SEARCH, Maharashtra, India

The Gadchiroli study of gynaecological diseases was a population-based cross-sectional study of gynaecological and sexual diseases among rural women in two Indian villages (Bang et al., 1989). A high prevalence (92 per cent) of gynaecological/sexual diseases was found, with many women suffering from multiple conditions. Only a small minority (8 per cent) of the women had previously undergone a gynaecological examination. The study was conducted many years ago in 1986–87, and because it was the first study of its kind, we did not have the benefit of prior experience when designing and implementing the study. In this section, we shall discuss our experiences in the Gadchiroli study in relation to maximizing participation, and then reflect upon how it could have been done differently given what we have learned in the subsequent years (see, for example, Bang, Bang and SEARCH Team, 1989a,b).

Background

Gadchiroli is the least developed district in Maharashtra state, India, located at its eastern-most corner. It is situated about 1000 km from the state capital, Mumbai, and is 200 km from the nearest city, Nagpur. Seventy per cent of land in the district is under forest cover, inhabited by the Gond tribe. However, 60 per cent of the population is non-tribal Hindu, living in the unforested western part of the district in rural farming communities. Only 5 per cent of the population lives in towns. This study was conducted among the rural Hindu population. Agriculture, mostly paddy cultivation, is the main occupation. Irrigation is minimal and hence most farmers are able to grow only one crop in the year. There is no industry in the district. According to government estimates, 80 per cent of the population in Gadchiroli district lives below the poverty line. There is no railway in the district, and until 1986, transport and communication were poorly developed. Few villages had electricity or telephones.

Female literacy in the district was very low, at 22 per cent. Household chores, child rearing, farming or collecting firewood from the forest kept women busy from 5 in the morning to 10 at night. Practically every woman did moderately hard physical labour but received inadequate nourishment – mostly rice, a small amount of pulses and vegetables and very little fat. Not surprisingly, most women were underweight, and 82 per cent were found to be anaemic.

Health services in the district were poorly developed. Women resorted most frequently to home remedies and traditional healers, using either herbal medicines or witchcraft to treat their health problems. Traditional birth attendants (TBAs), as well as unqualified practitioners of modern medicine, were commonly used. There were three voluntary health organizations in the district. The government health care system consisted of one small hospital for the entire district located in Gadchiroli town, one primary health centre for each 30 000 population run by male doctors, and one auxiliary nurse-midwife (female paramedic worker) for every 3000 rural residents. Gynaecologists and female doctors were available only at the district hospital in Gadchiroli town. Moreover, at the time of this study, the government health care system was primarily preoccupied with the family planning programme. The official figures indicated that 56 per cent of couples in the district were protected by contraception, mostly tubectomy, vasectomy or intrauterine devices. This programme had been aggressively promoted without being accompanied by appropriate health care, and the figures of contraceptive prevalence were often inflated. The birth rate in the rural Hindu population in 1987 was 35 per 1000. Nearly 95 per cent of all deliveries occurred at home, and were attended by TBAs.

Gender discrimination, neglect of the girl child, early marriages, early and frequent pregnancies, taboos about menstruation and white discharge, and premarital and extramarital sex were common. As in most Hindu communities, each village was populated by many castes. Most numerous were the middle castes (Kunbee, Teli, Marar, Dheewar) and the lower castes (Mahar). About 10–15 per cent of the population in the Hindu villages were of tribal origin (Gond).

Maximizing participation

Maximizing participation in studies of gynaecological morbidity is important for three reasons: (a) to get unbiased information not distorted by selective participation, especially of symptomatic women; (b) to enhance the community's response to the subsequent intervention; (c) to ensure the quality of participation, especially in the interview method of data collection, so that the collected data truly reflect the beliefs and practices of women.

The Gadchiroli study of gynaecological diseases was a prevalence study of women from two Hindu villages, Wasa and Amirza, in which the prevalence was estimated by a cross-sectional survey of women. In spite of our efforts to get maximum participation, about 60 per cent of eligible women from these two villages participated in the study. Since many of the subsequent studies in India experienced serious difficulties in obtaining even this level of participation, let us reflect on what we did that might have helped to enhance participation.

Selecting the community

Selecting the right community was the most important decision. We considered various villages in Gadchiroli block, contacted community leaders, had initial dialogues with them and narrowed our choice to four villages. Of these, Wasa and Amirza were finally selected because:

- They were about 18–20 km from Gadchiroli town; hence, they were relatively unexposed and unspoilt, and yet were approachable by road.
- The population size was manageable (1500 and 2500 in Wasa and Amirza respectively, with approximately one-third being eligible women), and matched our requirement of the sample size. We had assumed a participation rate of 50 per cent.
- These two villages had a community character. In spite of factions and conflicts, the entire village would become a unified community on issues of common interest. For example, in an earlier general election, the entire village of Amirza boycotted the election because of the government's failure to build a road to the village. Such examples of village unity gave us confidence that if convinced to participate, these villages would respond magnificently as a community.
- Wasa and Amirza had village leaders who were educated, enlightened, cooperative and respected in their villages.
- We had developed good personal rapport with village leaders.
- Village leaders were enthused by the idea of the study of gynaecological problems of women.
- Wasa had a mission hospital with excellent facilities and infrastructure but poorly used, and Amirza had a primary health centre located in the village. Both provided facilities for the study.
- Village leaders were willing to take responsibility for providing the buildings to organize the study camp, and mobilizing women to participate in the study, starting with their own families.

Community involvement

A series of consultative meetings were held in each village with village elders, men, youth, women's groups (mahila mandals) and health care providers. The idea of the study, particularly how it could help them with diagnosis and treatment of diseases, and the potential to help others (research information may help in convincing the government to launch gynaecological care for all women in the district) was explained. It was made very clear that this was not a usual treatment camp, and hence not just women with symptoms but every woman in the village must participate in

the study. We explained why it was important that asymptomatic women participate, and that our condition to hold the study in their villages was the full participation of all women.

After a period of 15 days, the communities reached a collective decision to hold
such a study in the villages, accepting our conditions for participation, including
pelvic examination and blood tests. A feeling of pride developed among village
leaders: it was a privilege and honour that their villages had been selected for such
an important study. They would stand to gain the gratitude of their community
and recognition by the media, and would be considered special.

In each village, the study was inaugurated with a fanfare at a public function
attended by high-level dignitaries visiting the villages, and a community feast was
organized. This kind of social involvement was important to dispel the sense of
shame and secretiveness associated with the subject of gynaecological health.

This informal contract with the community was fundamental to the success of
the project. The study was perceived as a 'give-and-take' relationship. The communities received the benefit of participating in a study perceived to be important, and
village women were provided with gynaecological examination and treatment. In
return, the communities were expected to ensure participation and basic infrastructure facilities for the study. In order to engage the community in such negotiation, the researcher requires a position of strength. We were established in
Gadchiroli district as the source of referral care. Hence the villagers considered it a
privilege that the research team would visit their villages, examine their women,
and treat them if necessary. It was important that they perceived some benefit from
the proposed study, and a stake in participating in it. No community would permit
outside researchers to conduct pelvic examinations on women, or learn the secrets
of their private lives, unless there was some advantage perceived.

Involvement of men

The involvement of men was crucial in this setting, as they act as gatekeepers to
village women. Men in Wasa and Amirza were helpful in various ways. Because of
their higher levels of education and exposure to the modern world, they were more
receptive to appreciating the significance of the study than women were. They
assisted in organizing local hospitality and mobilization. Indeed, volunteers who
enrolled all eligible women and persuaded them to attend the study on a particular day were all young men. These volunteers were motivated and interested in participating in a project they perceived to be useful to the women in their
communities. Within the family, it was often men who were instrumental in motivating their women to participate in the study. They conveyed an interest in the
health of their women, and their own health as well. They recognized that reproductive health was a mutual concern, and hence wanted to be involved in the study.

Communication strategy

Effective communication between the researchers and community members was key to promoting participation. Community members tended not to express their real concerns at formal and public meetings. Hence, in order to assess these concerns, it was important to develop word-of-mouth, intra-community communication. For example, the study experienced an initial enthusiastic participation of women, followed by diminishing attendance. Evidently, rumours and negative reactions had begun to be spread, such as 'She [the physician] puts her entire arm inside' or 'She puts large rubber bags on her hands' and 'They ask vulgar questions'. These perceptions were rapidly spread through the communities, and women were afraid of participating in the study. In order to counter such rumours, an effective communication strategy was launched. This included dispelling rumours at various forums, such as meetings of women's clubs or groups (mahila mandals), group meetings in different wards of the villages, individual visits to reluctant women by trained social workers from the local NGO (SEARCH) and individual visits by village volunteers to explain the importance of the study to reluctant families. In group meetings, satisfied participants would share their experiences and discuss the benefits of participation. Reluctant or sceptical women were invited to visit the clinic settings, observe the conduct of examinations, and reassure themselves that 'the whole arm' was not inserted. In addition, bottles of tonic were distributed to participants who feared the loss of blood drawn for laboratory tests.

Suiting women's convenience

Every effort was made not to inconvenience women. The project could conduct interviews and tests on roughly 15–20 women daily. Using this criterion, volunteers made appointments with about 20 women, requiring women to reorganize their schedules as little as possible. Moreover, women were able to select convenient times when they would not be menstruating, and could make advance preparations prior to the appointment. It is important that the researcher consider the woman's needs and convenience if expecting her full participation in the study. Nearly a century ago, Sir Patrick Manson-Bahr advised his student Ronald Ross: 'If you want to study mosquitoes, my son, you must learn to think like a mosquito'.

Confidentiality and non-judgemental attitudes

Complete confidentiality and a non-judgemental attitude are essential ingredients for enhancing community involvement and women's participation. In this study, several adolescent females were observed to have a torn hymen or a patulous vagina, and were advised on risky sexual behaviour. The fact that researchers were able to assess loss of virginity and sexual activity through the examination raised fears among adolescent females and a reluctance to participate. The study team responded by assuring young females complete confidentiality, and demonstrated their sincerity by maintaining the confidentiality of the adolescents already participating.

Health functionaries

Recognizing that health functionaries are important opinion leaders, discussions were also held with doctors, nurses and TBAs in villages surrounding Wasa and Amirza to enlist their aid in encouraging women to participate in the study.

Sex of research team members

Women in the study villages clearly preferred a female interviewer and female doctor to conduct gynaecological examinations, and this was an obvious requirement for the study.

Health care

It is imperative that research of this nature be accompanied by treatment – not only for the gynaecological diseases detected in the study, but also for other illnesses that might be discussed in the course of the study – for children and other family members as well. Women appreciated treatment provided for their family members.

Feedback to the community

As the study proceeded, the village communities were apprised of the findings of the study – the magnitude and types of problems encountered and the treatments provided. Obviously, individual identities were never disclosed. This feedback helped to foster the perception that the study was producing positive results.

The research team

A multidisciplinary research team is important in such a study. For example, the team in the Gadchiroli study comprised a female gynaecologist, a male physician, a pathologist, a laboratory technician, two female social workers, a female nurse, a compounder and a local TBA. Village volunteers and leaders assisted this core study team.

Refusal to participate

Despite the measures discussed in the foregoing, almost 40 per cent of the sample women refused to participate in the study (see Bang, Bang and SEARCH Team, 1989b for a discussion of factors underlying women's reluctance to participate). To

Table 7.1. Characteristics of study participants and non-participants in Gadchiroli district

Indicator	% Participants ($n=650$)	%Non-participants[a] ($n=105$)
Mean age (years)	32.1	34.2
Gravidity	4.0	3.8
Gynaecological symptoms experienced:		
Vaginal discharge	13.5	8.3
Scanty periods	12.6	16.4
Irregular periods	6.9	14.9
Profuse periods	4.9	4.5
Dysmenorrhoea	15.1	13.4
Percentage experiencing obstetric morbidity	37.6	51.1
Percentage currently practising contraception (ever-married women only)	18.2	11.4

Note: [a]A random sample of 25% of all non-participants.

assess the extent to which non-participation biased final results, 25 per cent of women who refused were randomly selected and visited at home by social workers from the study team. Data were obtained on their sociodemographic characteristics, obstetric and contraceptive histories, gynaecological symptoms experienced and reasons for non-participation. Results suggested that these women were not significantly different from women who did participate (see Table 7.1).

The most frequently reported reasons for non-participation were lack of free time to participate in the study (which required nearly half a day away from work), reluctance to undergo a pelvic examination due to the sense of shame associated with the procedure, the fear of revealing their private lives, the fear of undergoing a pelvic examination and the fear of blood withdrawal. Some women were afraid that the doctor might 'introduce a family planning device without my knowledge'. Asymptomatic women were reluctant to undergo pelvic examination, and elderly women considered themselves too old to have such problems. It is important that these fears and misperceptions are fully addressed in subsequent studies in order to maximize participation. To compensate women for their loss of time, the study team did consider providing incentives, but this was eventually vetoed on ethical grounds.

Follow-up to the study

Findings of the study were conveyed to the communities involved, and indeed to the 58 other villages in Gadchiroli block. A Women's Awakening and Health Jatra (carnival) was organized to travel from village to village, and was attended by a total of nearly 25 000 people. Posters, slide shows and a play on women's reproductive life were used to disseminate findings to the local population. A series of women's camps followed, and the study team was asked about the kinds of health interventions that they proposed, now that they had established the magnitude and pattern of women's problems.

SEARCH, the NGO working in the study area, was able to develop, on the basis of community dialogue, a strategy for community-based reproductive health education and care. Activities included education on women's reproductive health, training of TBAs in the diagnosis and management of reproductive tract infections, safe delivery, education and referral, and nurses at the government primary health centres were trained in reproductive health care. Referral clinics and services for antenatal care and the diagnosis and management of gynaecological problems were established, as well as abortion services to terminate unwanted pregnancies.

Lessons learned

A review of the experience of this study underscores the importance of community involvement. Two lessons in particular need to be highlighted. First is the importance of community education efforts before beginning enrolment in the study. It is crucial that the community is well informed about the topic to be researched and the health advantages that will accrue to the communities concerned. Organizing preparatory educational sessions will generate curiosity and awareness about the subject of study among potential participants, thus improving their willingness to participate. Second, it is important that community members participate in developing the research question and perceive a stake in it. More recent experiences of the authors in participatory action research, in which the subject of study was suggested by the community itself, indicate that a study that responds to a community-defined need will have greater participation and greater potential for effective interventions. After completing the Gadchiroli gynaecological morbidity study, the men of the study villages approached the researchers to conduct another study on the reproductive health problems of men, in which 233 of 234 eligible males participated (Bang et al., 1996; Bang, Bang and Phirke, 1996). The women of the district identified alcohol abuse as a priority for study, which culminated in a mass political movement in the district for alcohol control policies (Bang and Bang, 1991; Khan, 1997). Close interaction with the community in developing study priorities will enhance participation in the research as well as in subsequent intervention programmes.

REFERENCES

Bang AT, Bang RA (1991) Community participation in research and action against alcoholism. *WHO forum*, **12**: 104–109.

Bang RA, Bang AT, Baitule M et al. (1989) High prevalence of gynaecological diseases in rural Indian women. *Lancet*, 1(8629): 85–88.

Bang AT, Bang RA, Baitule M et al. (1996) Prevalence and spectrum of reproductive morbidities in males in Gadchiroli, India. (Unpublished.)

Bang AT, Bang RA and Phirke K (1996) Do rural males see reproductive health problems as a priority, and need care? (Unpublished).

Bang RA, Bang AT and SEARCH Team (1989a) Commentary on a community-based approach to reproductive health care. *International journal of gynaecology and obstetrics* (Suppl 3): 125–129.

Bang RA, Bang AT and SEARCH Team (1989b) Why women hide them: rural women's viewpoints on reproductive tract infections. *Manushi*, **69**: 27–30.

Khan A (1997) SEARCH and the Anti-Liquor Campaign in Gadchiroli district In: *Shaping policy: do NGOs matter? Lessons from India*. PRIA, New Delhi.

Uganda: the Rakai project

David Serwadda[1] and Maria Wawer[2]

[1] Institute of Public Health, Kampala, Uganda; [2] Columbia University, New York, USA

One of the most challenging aspects of a research study is how to maximize participation, particularly in a population-based longitudinal study. Maximizing study participation is important because it enables one to attain the desired sample size, maximizes the reliability of the findings of studies, reduces biases (for example, selection bias between participants and non-participants) and improves on the validity (internal and external) of the study.

Uganda has been fortunate to have at least two population-based longitudinal studies that have been ongoing for over 10 years. The Rakai project and Medical Research Council, UK programme on AIDS in Rakai and Masaka districts, respectively, have conducted a number of population-based studies on HIV and sexually transmitted infections (STIs) (Nunn et al., 1997; Wawer et al., 1991). Most recently, the Rakai project has concluded a four-year population-based, community randomized trial to assess the effect of mass treatment of STIs on HIV transmission (Wawer et al., 1999).

The Rakai project was able to evaluate STIs and genital tract infections in depth among both women and men. A wealth of experience has been gained in implementing this study that will be of particular interest to gynaecologists and other researchers. This section is based on our experience in carrying out the Rakai project. However, the issues discussed here will be relevant to any population-based study design in developing countries.

Sociopolitical context of HIV intervention programmes in Rakai district

The first documented cases of AIDS in Uganda were reported in October 1985 from Rakai district (Serwadda et al., 1985). Since then the HIV epidemic has spread to all parts of Uganda. Currently, it is estimated that 1.5 million people out of 20 million are infected, and the average seroprevalence rate is about 10 per cent. Results from population-based studies indicate that HIV is currently the leading cause of death among adults aged 15–49 years (Sewankambo et al., 1994) and adult mortality attributable to HIV infection is as high as 50 per cent in Uganda (Mulder et al., 1994).

In 1986, President Museveni came to power, and with the new leadership the Ugandan government openly admitted that AIDS had become a major health problem. President Museveni's continued participation in delivering HIV-related health messages at every public health rally highlighted the importance of urgent action to prevent HIV transmission. It also created a positive environment to conduct intervention research programmes among the populations.

President Museveni's government has actively encouraged women's participation in local and national government. The Constitution provides affirmative action by reserving a number of seats in Parliament for women. All local councils must have a woman representative. This has assured strong women's advocacy on a number of issues that particularly affect women. In addition, these women are key entry points into the communities they represent, especially on issues that affect women.

The HIV epidemic has had a particularly devastating effect among women in Rakai district. The high HIV infection rate among girls compared to boys (Berkley et al., 1990), the excessive infant mortality rate among HIV-positive mothers (Sewankambo et al., 1994) and the reduced fertility rate among HIV-positive women (Gray et al., 1998) have increased public awareness of the risks women face in acquiring HIV.

The HIV epidemic in Rakai district is of long standing, and is perceived by the general population as a serious public health problem. As a consequence of this, together with a committed political leadership towards HIV prevention activities, the population is willing to participate in research programmes.

The Rakai study on sexually transmitted infections and HIV

The objective of the Rakai study was to evaluate whether mass treatment of STIs can reduce HIV transmission (Wawer et al., 1998). All consenting adults aged 15–59 years from 56 communities were enrolled in the study. The study populations were randomized into the intervention arm (mass treatment for STIs) and the control arm (treatment for worms and vitamin supplementation). Each arm had five study clusters, comprising four to seven contiguous communities. A total of 22 013 individuals were enrolled over five study rounds conducted at 10-month intervals, of which 11 315 (51 per cent) were women of reproductive age 15–49 years. Biological sample collection (blood, urine, self-collected vaginal swabs and genital ulcer swabs) and interviews were conducted in respondents' homes during survey visits. Pregnant women were identified through interviews and urine pregnancy tests for human chorionic gonadotropin (hCG), enrolled in a maternal–infant supplementary study (MISS) and followed until delivery. The MISS study evaluated the impact of STI treatment on the pregnancy and health of the mother and baby. Women and infants were visited after delivery for further sample collection and examinations in their home. Additional follow-up of infants was conducted on subsequent study rounds.

Points of entry into communities

Once a representative sample of the population has been drawn, the challenge is to enrol the study participants. The first step is to gain access to the study communities at various entry levels, and this involves several levels of approval that are important for participation at the household level.

Central level

How you enter into a community to carry out research is critical to the success of enrolling and maintaining a cohort in the case of a longitudinal study. In order to do this successfully, it is useful to start with relevant departments or individuals in the Ministry of Health. This serves three purposes: to explain what you intend to do and why you are doing it; to explain the implications of the study for the study population and the country as a whole; and to solicit help from the Ministry of Health officials. It is useful to involve the Ministry of Health in mobilizing the target population to increase awareness of the study. This motivates participants to enrol as it reassures respondents that the government approves of the study.

District level

Many developing countries are decentralizing health services to the district level. This means that districts are increasingly determining their health needs and priorities. Investigators should, therefore, impress upon district health officials the importance of the study in their area. The involvement of district health officials in mobilizing the population is key to success. Their participation creates a strong positive attitude towards the study among local leaders below them, for example, village leaders. The District Member of Parliament (MP), if present, should be given the opportunity to talk and explain the study to the community. MPs are also important advocates in Parliament, and with Ministry of Health officials and NGOs in facilitating the acquisition of resources for the study areas that help to complement research work (e.g. building health clinics).

Village level

Having obtained official endorsement at the higher levels, village leaders will be willing to cooperate with the investigators. Village leaders and their village committees play an important role in informing the study population of the aim of the study and what the investigators expect from them. They can help the investigators

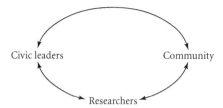

Figure 7.1   Partnership in mobilization of communities to improve participation in research.

identify other key local leaders or special target groups in the study population (e.g. commercial sex workers, long distance truck drivers).

Mobilization

Mobilization of the target population involves dynamic interaction between the researchers, the community and civic leaders (see Figure 7.1) and is a key activity in maximizing participation. It involves educating the general public and the target population about the aims of the study and how it will be conducted, and can be achieved by organizing public rallies in the study villages. Village leaders, as mentioned earlier, play a crucial role in helping the investigators encourage people to attend the rallies. Mobilization for other purposes (e.g. immunization) provides an opportunity to talk to community members, and an opportunity for district leaders to discuss the study. Other strategies include writing individual letters to each participant. This was not a useful approach in Rakai because of low literacy levels, especially among rural women. However, for those who can read, pamphlets with a description and questions and answers about the study as well as other related issues are helpful.

Mobilization in targeted populations requires discussion of the following issues that often cause anxiety among community members.

Sampling

It is worth spending time explaining the concepts of sampling and eligibility, as many respondents do not easily appreciate why some people are enrolled and others are not. This can cause confusion and suspicion.

Informed consent

This is a concept that is not easily understood in rural cultures and can cause problems if it is not carefully explained. In rural Uganda, consent is a two-stage process. First, the household head is asked to allow the study workers to visit the home, and then eligible members of the household are asked to consent to study enrolment.

Many household heads still prefer to give permission to have their wives and older children enrol, even when the children are old enough to sign a consent form on their own. Study participants are apprehensive about signing any document because they feel they may be signing away more than they are being told. It is, therefore, useful to indicate that signing a consent form does not deprive a participant of the right to withdraw from the study at any time without loss of access to medical care. Informed consent statements written by Institutional Review Boards (IRBs) often contain complex information, so it is crucial that field personnel are trained to explain issues in a locally intelligible manner and to devote time for questions, discussion and explanation. To ensure full understanding by the respondent, the process of informed consent should not be rushed.

Blood

If the study involves obtaining blood samples from respondents, then they have to be informed about what you plan to do with the blood specimens. This point cannot be overemphasized, as venepuncture is often the most important barrier to enrolment and the reason for loss of follow-up in longitudinal studies. Providing tours of the study laboratories for village leaders to demonstrate how blood and other specimens (such as urine or vaginal swabs) are processed helps to educate the population on why blood is drawn and what the investigators intend to do with it. Common concerns that too much blood is being taken, that donors will fall ill or that investigators will sell the blood need to be addressed.

Conduct of interviews

Respondents need to be reassured that interviews will be conducted in private and all the information collected will be kept confidential. Female respondents prefer to be interviewed by female interviewers as they tend to be apprehensive discussing sensitive information (such as STI symptoms and sexual behaviour) with males. All field workers must be trained in communication skills so that they can interact well with the community.

Collection of biological samples

Methods for the collection of biological samples must be simple, minimally invasive and culturally acceptable to the study population. Many women do not like to be subjected to gynaecological examination in order that biological samples can be collected. Facilities for proper examination are often lacking in developing countries, and in population-based studies, samples have to be collected in participants' homes. The advent of new technologies to preserve cells and identify microorganisms (e.g. using DNA and RNA amplification) has provided the opportunity to conduct studies of infection prevalence and incidence among non-clinic-based populations without the need for extensive gynaecological examination. It is possible to evaluate the extent of exposure to a variety of aetiological agents and intermediate outcomes of interventions using biomarkers. This makes the collection of biological samples a feasible component of population-based research in the future.

Innovative methods of sample collection may be needed to collect gynaecological specimens. In the Rakai study, women were taught for the first time how to obtain a self-collected high vaginal swab in their home. Of the 7110 women who enrolled in the study at 30 months, 95 per cent were able and willing to provide a vaginal swab.

The number and type of specimens collected from each individual can initially be a problem. If the investigators enter a community for the first time, it is advisable to start by collecting a minimal number of specimens, as many specimens may discourage enrolment. However, after working in the community for some years, the research group gains the confidence of the residents and it becomes possible to collect an extensive array of biological samples. In the Rakai study, after six years in the study community it was possible to collect blood (and in some cases saliva, for those who could not give blood for HIV testing), urine, vaginal swabs and genital ulcer swabs. During the MISS study, out of 3560 mothers, 74 per cent provided their placentas for histopathology, 94 per cent agreed to provide infant ocular swabs for gonorrhoea detection and 93 per cent agreed to provide infant blood samples.

The volume and amount of each specimen can be an important issue. Blood is not only the least acceptable specimen to collect, but the volume collected can influence enrolment and compliance with follow-up in a study. This is partly because it involves a venepuncture, which causes discomfort. Many respondents feel that the provision of blood samples depletes their nutritional reserves and leads to anaemia, so they may not permit more than a maximum of 10 ml (often explained to participants as 2 teaspoons of blood) to be drawn. In the Rakai study, compliance with blood sampling was about 90 per cent of all enrolled respondents, compared to 95 per cent for urine or vaginal swabs. The provision of repeat blood samples was approximately 85 per cent whereas compliance with repeat urine and vaginal samples was around 95 per cent. For non-invasive procedures like urine collection, it was possible to collect as much volume as needed. Women were able to provide up to four self-collected vaginal swabs on a single home visit, which allowed for diagnosis of multiple conditions, such as trichomoniasis, gonorrhoea, bacterial vaginosis, candidiasis, human papilloma virus and HIV viral shedding.

The setting in which samples are collected should be simple, yet provide privacy.

Blood collection needs the least privacy, and it is an advantage for others to see that one can have a blood sample taken with no dramatic side-effects. The collection of samples like urine and vaginal swabs needs privacy in the home. Some specimens cannot easily be collected in homes. In such cases, a predetermined site within easy walking distance can be found, and often a house within the community may serve as a temporary health unit.

Providing survey and serological results

Providing important individual test results to the study participants is a strong motivating factor for enrolment and consent. To participants, it is seen as proof that the biological samples were actually used for the purposes intended. The method chosen for the provision of individual results is also important. If a study is carried out as a household survey and investigators are able to reach each household in the village, the participants expect delivery of test results in their homes. On the other hand, if the study is based in a health clinic, then the participants are willing to collect their results from the clinic. With sensitive test results such as HIV, it is critical to provide counselling and support services. Moreover, with results for treatable infections such as syphilis, it is necessary to provide access to treatment either in the home or in a convenient clinic setting. Many participants will refuse follow-up visits until results are provided to them.

There are important ethical and legal considerations when providing HIV test results. In Uganda for example, results and counselling are provided on request, whereas in other countries, such as the US, provision of results is mandatory. In a setting where the receipt of results is voluntary, not everyone will be ready to receive their test results or they may not be at home when the counsellor visits with the results. Arrangements must be made for repeat home visits to absentees. It is possible to place results at the nearest health centre for collection, but care must be taken to ensure that confidentiality is maintained and counselling is available.

In addition to providing results from individual biological samples, the community and civic leaders expect investigators to disseminate the research findings within the community before they are published. Findings should first be discussed with the district health officers and reviewed by them. The investigators would then need to have meetings with local village leaders and their village committees to explain the research findings before community meetings can be held. Simple easy-to-read pamphlets can be distributed to households to inform the community about the research findings. This feedback to the community is greatly appreciated, and helps to convince those who earlier refused to enrol to participate in future follow-up visits.

Provision of health services

First and foremost, researchers need to provide health services in response to results from the biological samples or information gathered from study subjects. Secondly, the study participants (or their dependents, especially children in the case of women) may have health problems that are not directly related to the scientific inquiry but need to be addressed by the researchers. For example, in many developing countries malaria is a common problem that cannot be ignored. Third, the investigators may need to involve themselves in broader district-related health activities, such as assisting with the investigation of epidemics or providing health information to the Ministry of Health. All these factors act to reinforce each other and indicate to the study subjects that the investigators are interested in their health and that of the community as a whole. The provision of services helps to foster mutual trust and, as a result, the population responds by participating in the research programme. For example, over the last five years the Rakai project team has assisted the district health programme by providing personnel for the national polio immunization day and investigating a nyong-nyong epidemic in the area (Rwaguma et al., 1997).

Incentives

Providing incentives can be useful when motivating communities to participate in research. An incentive is provided to a study participant to compensate for time spent with the research team, because it is assumed that this time would otherwise have been spent on income-generating activities. Incentives can be in the form of money, services or simple gifts. The incentive should be modest, culturally acceptable and perceived to be of value. The issue of providing incentives in developing countries is complex. In economically poor settings, providing an incentive may constitute an undue inducement and may compromise voluntary participation in research. It may be difficult to find an incentive that cannot be construed as coercion. Once an incentive is provided by one group of researchers, it becomes difficult for other groups to carry out research without providing similar incentives. Furthermore, communities often demand more incentives over time. District health officers often do not like researchers to provide incentives as this compromises voluntary participation in community activities in other health-related programmes. For these reasons, some local regions or countries discourage the use of incentives.

One way of avoiding such problems is to provide incentives aimed at the household or the whole community, irrespective of individual participation in research.

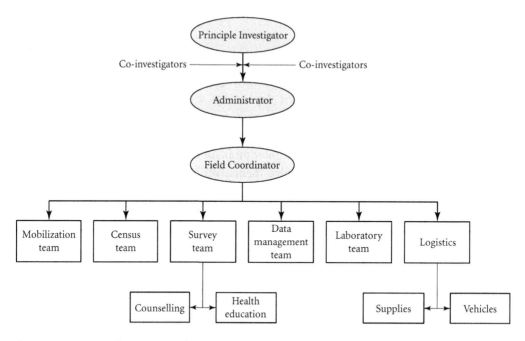

Figure 7.2   Proposed structure and composition of the research team.

For example, at the household level, if two out of three eligible participants choose to be enrolled, the entire household should benefit from an incentive. In the Rakai project, a bar of soap is given to every household member regardless of whether or not they participate. Further, all members of the household are provided treatment irrespective of whether or not they are enrolled in the study. At the community level, incentives may constitute helping the community complete a small dispensary or a school block. Depending on the particular area under study, community incentives may be more appropriate than individual incentives or vice versa.

Composition of research teams

Figure 7.2 illustrates the composition and organizational structure of a medium-to-large population-based longitudinal study team. As is often the case, such studies involve a number of collaborating institutions. Team spirit is absolutely essential among the researchers to achieve the research objectives. Co-investigators may be needed to help the principal investigator to implement the study. Often they have a specific responsibility or activity to oversee. They are usually senior members of their respective institutions. An administrator is also needed for complex studies to manage both financial and human resources. A field co-ordinator, preferably with a medical background, oversees the day to day execution of field activities. A

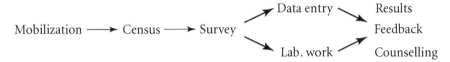

Figure 7.3   Flow of research work in the field

number of teams or departments work under the field co-ordinator, which allows for the efficient conduct of field operations. Clear delegation of responsibility and authority, and the structured flow of information is essential for the smooth running of the programmes.

Mobilization team

Figure 7.3 illustrates the sequence of activities in field operations. As mentioned earlier, the function of the mobilization team is to mobilize the study community and educate them about the aims and operation of the study. The team also provides heath education and disseminates research findings. Counsellors inform participants of the results of biological samples, particularly relating to HIV, and conduct additional counselling activities for respondents who need support. They also play a major public relations role in the community. The mobilization team is the main interface between the community and the investigation team; for example, they are involved in discussing issues of concern to the community in connection with the study. Wherever possible, information or concerns from individuals who refuse to enrol can be ascertained to help address their reservations.

Since research activities start with mobilization, it follows that the success of enrolment will depend on how well they do this job. The team should ideally be composed of a health educator and a health counsellor. The number will vary with the size of the study population and the demand for services. It is helpful to make a special effort to have females in this research team because during health education, it may be more appropriate to have special meetings to address women's concerns. It is an added advantage if some or all the team members are resident in the district or area of study. This increases acceptability of the study and improves communication with the population through the use of locally well-known and understood explanations.

Census team

The census team is principally involved in generating maps of the study area (including roads, houses and geographical landmarks) and enumerating household members. It is from this list that people eligible for enrolment can be determined. The team moves into a study area after the mobilization team has carried out its sensitization of the population. The census team should include an individual with at least a high school education, and should be headed by a graduate, preferably with an epidemiology or statistics background.

Survey team

The survey team moves into a study area after the census team has finished enumeration. Their activities include identifying and interviewing eligible individuals who have consented to be enrolled in the study, obtaining biological specimens, educating the participants about the study, answering questions that respondents may have and providing appropriate medication.

The composition of a survey team may vary depending on the particular study. It usually includes a supervisor, interviewers, biological sample collectors and field data editors. In the field, local village leaders join the team to help them locate respondents' homes. It is often useful to have interviewers who are trained to obtain biological samples like blood, as it eliminates the need to have a special phlebotomist on the team. Interviewers can come from different backgrounds but because interviews are carried out in the local language, it is a prerequisite to be able to read and speak the local language fluently. In addition, interviewers must have good communication skills. The field team is managed by a team leader. The number of interviewers and field editors depends on the sample size and the time frame. The survey team often contains more women than men because of the higher number of female respondents. Field editors play a critical role in data management. They ensure that all the questionnaires are correctly filled and that errors are rectified in the field. This is an important early step in quality control and data management.

There are several reasons for cross-training field workers so that census team members can carry out interviews and vice versa. For one, the team leader can shift workers depending on the workload, or substitute workers who leave or fall sick. Since activities are chronologically related, field workers should be able to identify inconsistencies or errors of the previous team and take appropriate action. For example, interviewers should be able to identify errors on the census list since they have also been trained in census work.

Data management team

The data management team is responsible for data entry, cleaning and analysis. The team consists of a statistician, a programmer and data entry clerks, and the number depends on the size of the research programme. The quality of the data largely depends on the effort the research team invests in data management. Field editors make sure questionnaires are properly completed. In the Rakai project, 10 per cent of respondents are re-interviewed to validate the information obtained. To minimize data entry errors, the study used data entry screens designed using Foxpro software. These screens facilitate data entry and incorporate range checks

and consistency checks to prevent data errors. Moreover, 10 per cent of questionnaires and all laboratory data are double entered to ensure accuracy.

It is important for the data management team and the survey team to work
together to resolve problems that may arise in the process of data entry or cleaning.
Data entry clerks sometimes get questionnaires that need to be sent back to the field
to clarify responses that are inconsistent with responses in another section of the
questionnaire. The data management team should regularly provide tabulations on
enrolment rates, refusals and the number of samples collected. This helps to indicate how well the research is meeting its targets.

Since the census, laboratory and mobilization teams generate data that need processing, it is more efficient to have a central data processing centre for all the departments. Special responsibilities can then be allocated within the data management
team. This allows for the optimum use of computers and permits the flexibility of
shifting personnel within the department depending on the workload.

Laboratory team

The laboratory team is composed of laboratory technicians. Depending on the type
of study, the team may need to be headed by a senior technologist, a microbiolo-
gist or virologist. The type and number of technicians will also depend on the type
of study. Laboratory technicians must process perishable biological specimens on
the day they are collected. Often samples from the field are received in the evening,
and in the Rakai study, laboratory workers have to stay as late as 10 p.m. to process
samples for which results are needed the next day. To distribute the workload in the
laboratory, samples from the morning collection are sent to the laboratory at
midday, and samples from the afternoon collection are sent early evening. This
reduces the time that samples need to be kept in cold boxes in the field. The laboratory is responsible for processing samples (e.g. separation of serum, conduct of
tests, storage and inventory of samples in freezers and shipping of samples if tests
outside the country are needed).

Logistics

Without logistical support, research teams cannot function properly. Logistical
support can be divided into supplies and transportation. The timely ordering and
distribution of research supplies can be so demanding that a department or individuals should be assigned to maintain inventories and promptly identify pending
shortages so that the continuity of supplies is maintained. Due to shipping delays,
it is critical to place advance orders for supplies that have to be imported into the
country. Clearing goods at the port of entry and maintaining refrigeration are
problems that should not be underestimated. Ideally, a logistics officer in charge of
supplies should also have some experience with store keeping in order to keep track

of stock in store. If the research project is not very large (less than 200 participants), an administrator may be able to carry out these tasks.

Transportation must be organized for the various research teams and vehicles must be maintained and serviced. Having dedicated and competent drivers will reduce the cost of maintenance and ensure longevity of the vehicles. The transport team consists of drivers and vehicle mechanics. In-house servicing and minor repairs of vehicles will reduce transportation costs compared to established repair and servicing centres.

Summary

The Rakai project has been able to achieve a high level of study participation because it was able to establish strong and mutually trusting relationships with the community and obtain samples that were minimally invasive so that sample collection and interviews could be conducted in respondents' homes. The composition and organization of the study teams depends on the size and nature of the investigation. However, the allocation of responsibilities and authority to functional units within the team provides the optimal organizational principle.

REFERENCES

Berkely SF, Naamara W, Okware S et al. (1990) AIDS and HIV infection in Uganda – are more women infected than men? *AIDS*, **4**(12): 1237–1242.

Gray R, Wawer M, Serwadda D et al. (1998) Population-based study of fertility in women with HIV-1 infection in Uganda. *Lancet*, **351**(9096): 98–103.

Mulder DW, Nunn AJ, Kamali A et al. (1994) Two-year HIV-1-associated mortality in a Ugandan rural population. *Lancet*, **343**(8904): 1021–1023.

Nunn AJ, Mulder DW, Kamali A et al. (1997) Mortality associated with HIV-1 infection over five years in a rural Ugandan population: cohort study. *British medical journal*, **315**(7111): 767–771.

Rwaguma EB, Lutwama JJ, Sempala SD et al. (1997) Emergence of epidemic of O'nyong-nyong fever in south-central Uganda after an absence of 35 years. *Emerging infectious diseases*, **3**(1): 77– 82.

Serwadda D, Mugerwa RD, Sewankambo NK et al. (1985) Slim disease: a new disease in Uganda and its association with HTLV III infection. *Lancet*, **2**(8460): 849–852.

Sewankambo N, Li C, Wabwire-Mangen F et al. (1994). Demographic impact of HIV infection in rural Rakai, Uganda: results of a population-based cohort study. *AIDS*, **8**(12): 1707–1713.

Wawer MJ, Serwadda D, Musgrave SD et al. (1991) Dynamics of spread of HIV-I infection in a rural district of Uganda. *British medical journal*, **303**(6813): 1303–1306.

Wawer MJ, Gray RH, Sewankambo NK et al. (1998) A randomized, community trial of intensive sexually transmitted disease control for AIDS prevention, Rakai, Uganda. *AIDS*, **12**(10): 1211–1225.

Wawer MJ, Sewankambo NK, Serwadda D et al. (1999) Control of sexually transmitted diseases for AIDS prevention in Uganda: a randomised community trial. Rakai Project Study Group. *Lancet*, **353**(9152): 525–535.

Definitions of clinically diagnosed gynaecological morbidity resulting from reproductive tract infection

Christopher Elias[1], Nicola Low[2] and Sarah Hawkes[3]

[1] PATH, Seattle, USA; [2] University of Bristol, Bristol, UK; [3] London School of Hygiene and Tropical Medicine, London, UK.

The importance of gynaecological morbidity resulting from reproductive tract infections among diverse populations of women in developing countries is well documented (Cates, Farley and Rowe, 1985; Koenig et al., 1998; Schulz, Cates and O'Mara, 1987; Wasserheit, 1989). Less well researched, but of growing concern, is the problem of infection-related reproductive tract morbidity among men, which is discussed in Chapter 4. Despite a growing consensus that reproductive tract infections are an important health issue, a perplexing array of problems faces those who seek to describe the extent of these conditions. The literature reveals tremendous variability in the reported prevalence of specific infections, some of which undoubtedly arises from real differences in the underlying epidemiology. Of equal importance, however, may be differences in the clinical definitions used to classify and describe various types of gynaecological morbidity, the training of the health care providers who elicit symptoms and record clinical observations, and the thoroughness with which a practitioner examines any client.

This chapter discusses the limitations of defining and observing reproductive tract morbidity in community-based research, and makes recommendations for future practice. We begin by discussing definitions of 'normality' and 'abnormality' as they apply to gynaecological morbidity, using cervical ectopy as an example. We then illustrate the problems of differences in diagnostic criteria between studies and inter-observer variation. Investigators are urged to use standardized definitions of clinically diagnosed morbidity that are both well-supported by evidence from the literature and easily applied in clinical practice. We suggest some practical definitions, but stress that these should be validated against laboratory tests, and that their reliability should be evaluated in prospective population-based studies.

Why collect clinical data on gynaecological morbidity?

Self-reported morbidity data have long been collected to determine the health care needs of populations. The methodological problems associated with such surveys are well recognized (Ross and Vaughan, 1986). Campbell and Graham (1990) have reviewed the particular problems associated with asking women about their reproductive health status, which include recall bias and lack of sensitivity and specificity of reported symptoms for predicting biomedically recognized disease states, such as reproductive tract infections. Interpreting self-reported reproductive tract symptoms is complicated by men and women's poor understanding of normal anatomy and physiology, including the cyclical and lifecourse changes associated with menstruation and hormonal fluctuations. Further confusion arises from wide variations in health care seeking behaviour and self-treatment with antibiotics, topical agents and other remedies that may alter clinical symptoms and delay encounters with the health care system. As a consequence of these factors, perceptions and self-reports by women and men of reproductive tract morbidity rarely coincide with categories of disease as defined by the biomedical community.

Clinical examination has been suggested as a more 'objective' method of describing and measuring gynaecological morbidity resulting from reproductive tract infections. The potential benefits of data from clinical observations in population-based surveys are clear. In an ideal situation, information on the presence or absence of observable clinical signs can be systematically recorded by trained health care providers using structured data collection forms. Moreover, reported symptoms and recorded signs can be compared to 'gold standard' laboratory tests and participants can receive immediate treatment for some diagnosed conditions. As discussed in Chapter 5, the availability of timely and appropriate treatment is often an essential component of population-based research efforts that seek to ensure a more representative study sample through high participation rates. In order to define clinical abnormalities of the reproductive tract, however, it is important to be clear about what constitutes normality.

What is 'normal'?

Definitions of clinical morbidity ultimately depend on our understanding of what is normal and what is abnormal. Labelling a condition as 'abnormal' has profound implications for its management and for the people thus labelled. Normality can be defined in several different and commonly used ways (Table 8.1).

Each of the definitions in Table 8.1 can be applied to reproductive tract infections. We illustrate this by using well-known examples. First, the situational

Table 8.1. Definitions of 'normality'

Term used	Properties of 'normality'	Consequences of its clinical application
Culturally acceptable	Socially and culturally appropriate	Confusion over the role of medicine in society
Risk factor	Carries no additional risk of morbidity or mortality	Assumes that altering a risk factor alters risk
Diagnostic	Range of test results beyond which a specific disease is, with known probability, present or absent	Need to know predictive values that apply in local clinical practice
Therapeutic	Range of test results beyond which therapy does more good than harm	Need to keep up with new knowledge about therapeutic interventions
Gaussian	The distribution of diagnostic test results has a certain shape	Assumes that all abnormalities have the same frequency, that is, beyond two standard deviations of the mean
Percentile	Lies within a preset percentile of previous diagnostic test results	As above. Patients are normal until tests are performed

Source: Adapted from Sackett et al. (1991): 59.

or 'cultural' acceptability of a symptom, such as vaginal discharge, influences whether it is perceived as 'normal' or 'abnormal' both by the women who experience it and the health workers who observe it. The 'culture of silence' that often surrounds women's experience of reproductive tract infections (Dixon-Mueller and Wasserheit, 1991) results in limited awareness of reproductive physiology, shame associated with genital illness, social and other barriers to accessing health care, and a reluctance to undergo a gynaecological examination. Social neglect of symptoms that cause considerable personal discomfort, but for which no care is available, is often mistakenly interpreted to be a sign of cultural acceptance or 'normality'. Given the many factors that influence individual and community perceptions of illness, local definitions of normality vary considerably between societies.

Different cultures of biomedical health practitioners also exhibit wide variation in what is accepted as 'normal'. This is perhaps most evident with regard to opinions on medical and surgical therapeutic practices, which vary across specialities and countries, and change over time as scientific knowledge accumulates. Consider, for example, the wide variation in rates of Caesarean section applied in different medical cultures for the 'normal' process of childbirth (Poma, 1999; Wilkinson et al., 1998).

Using the 'risk factor' definition of normality, a condition that is asymptomatic may be considered 'abnormal' if it increases the risk of experiencing another morbid state. For example, bacterial vaginosis, which results from a disturbance of the normal vaginal ecology, may often cause few or no symptoms. However, given recent studies suggesting that bacterial vaginosis may increase the risk of HIV transmission (Sewankambo et al., 1997), one could define bacterial vaginosis as an 'abnormal' condition simply because it increases the risk of acquiring another, very serious, morbidity.

'Diagnostic' definitions of normality are used most commonly when there is a gradient between 'normal' and 'abnormal'. Consider the 'diagnostic' definition of bacterial vaginosis. Using standardized criteria (Nugent et al., 1991) based on morphological patterns of vaginal flora, a laboratory technician can describe the gradation from normal bacterial flora characterized by a predominance of lactobacilli toward abnormality as these flora are replaced by other bacterial morphotypes. 'Abnormality' is defined if the score is above a specified cut-off point. In 'therapeutic' terms, abnormality is defined in terms of whether therapeutic intervention will do more good than harm. In the case of bacterial vaginosis, one might decide not to expend the effort of identifying and treating asymptomatic bacterial vaginosis if empirical evidence demonstrates that such treatment fails to actually reduce the risk of HIV transmission when introduced as part of a health intervention programme (Wawer et al., 1999).

Finally, quantifiable definitions of normality are most often used for laboratory tests and reflect different assumptions about the characteristics of the distribution of their normality in relation to important 'diagnostic' or 'therapeutic' criteria. For example, diagnostic test results, such as the optical density of enzyme-linked immunoassays for *Chlamydia trachomatis,* are often used to define the presence or absence of infection, although altering the cut-off point will then alter the definition of normality. The challenges of standardizing definitions of laboratory findings are addressed in greater detail in Chapters 9 and 10.

Appreciating the different ways normality is defined helps explain the confusion that often surrounds discussions of gynaecological morbidity. There are particular difficulties for clinical definitions of morbidity associated with reproductive tract infections because of conflicting ideas about the cultural, risk factor, diagnostic and therapeutic definitions of normality as they pertain to the reproductive tract. Investigators often use different terms to describe the various morbid conditions they seek to understand and, even when using the same terms, define the criteria for observing any given 'abnormality' in highly variable and imprecise ways. We will use the condition of cervical ectopy to illustrate these dilemmas.

Cervical ectopy and 'normality'

Cervical ectopy refers to the presence of columnar epithelium, present in the endocervical canal, on the visible surface of the cervix. Columnar epithelium appears red because only one layer of cells overlies the blood vessels, in comparison to the surrounding squamous epithelium. Blaustein's *Pathology of the female genital tract* definitively states that 'cervical ectopy is a normal physiologic finding and should not be construed as a pathological abnormality', and 'most women during the reproductive period' will have some cervical ectopy present (Kurman, 1994:193–95). Cervical ectopy, also referred to as cervical erosion or cervical ectropion, is, however, still listed as a cause of gynaecological morbidity in the International Classification of Diseases (World Health Organisation, 1992a).

The history of 'ubiquitous cervical erosion' (Singer and Jordan, 1976) shows how ideas on the existence, aetiology, terminology and significance of cervical ectopy developed. Initially, the term 'erosion' expressed the belief that there was actual denudation of the squamous epithelium, which persisted in the presence of infection. Subsequently, when the 'erosion' was shown to actually be columnar epithelium, squamous metaplasia of the transformation zone (the border area where the columnar epithelium is replaced by squamous epithelium) was widely thought to be a precursor to cancer (Singer, 1975). The latter concept seems to have gained importance as surgical methods to ablate the cervix by cautery and laser therapy became more widely available. In other words, the classification of an observable variation in the clinical appearance of the cervix became increasingly recognized as 'abnormal' as more options for therapeutic intervention became available.

Consequently, the 'normality' of cervical ectopy has been changing within the 'culture' of biomedicine as scientific knowledge accumulates and the incentives to provide treatment evolve. Moreover, in different medical communities the understanding of this condition and its optimal management proceeds at different paces, resulting in a large degree of variation in definition and, consequently, reported rates of gynaecological morbidity.

The 'risk' definition of abnormality introduces yet another wrinkle into our understanding of cervical ectopy, as cervical ectopy may be an independent risk factor for the acquisition of cervical infection with some pathogens, such as chlamydia, even if it is not pathological per se (Critchlow et al., 1995; Harrison et al., 1985; Johnson et al., 1990). It is biologically plausible that cervical ectopy makes it easier for cervical pathogens to be transmitted because the columnar epithelium may be more vulnerable to infection than squamous epithelium. Alternatively, any apparent association could be due to confounding by unmeasured or imprecisely measured factors. For example, unprotected sexual intercourse and, consequently, exposure to sexually transmitted pathogens are more common in the young, as is the occurrence of cervical ectopy, which is most common in women under 20 years and declines with age (Kurman, 1994). The occurrence of ectopy is also influenced by exposure to hormones in oral contraceptive pills. Studies showing an association between cervical ectopy and infection may not have controlled adequately for these factors.

It is, therefore, not surprising that the 'normality' of cervical ectopy is often in question in studies of gynaecological morbidity and, in many medical cultures, there is a tendency to treat ectopy whenever observed. However, it must be reconsidered whether the aggressive treatment of a histological condition that, at most, may be a risk factor for acquiring some cervical infections, may do more harm than good in both personal and financial terms. We concur with other authors (Goldacre et al., 1978; Hull, 1978) who recommend that cervical ectopy should not be considered a morbidity in itself, even though it should be carefully documented in studies of gynaecological morbidity. In this way, we will be able to learn more in a standardized fashion about its potential correlation with other clinical and laboratory findings and sociodemographic variables. It may also be useful in explaining some aspects of providers' presumptive diagnoses and decision-making.

Limitations of clinical diagnosis in assessing the prevalence of reproductive tract infections

Known problems with clinical diagnosis fall into the following categories: limitations in data collection; problems with the validity of clinical signs for predicting the presence of infection; and problems with the subjectivity of diagnosis leading to inter-observer variation and observer expectation.

Limitations resulting from the clinical data collection process

In order to understand problems associated with the collection and reporting of clinical data, a systematic review of published and unpublished community-based studies of gynaecological morbidity associated with reproductive tract infections was conducted by co-author Nicola Low. This review allowed us to explore the range of clinical conditions sought and the criteria used to diagnose them. It also gave us an opportunity to compare the prevalence of clinically diagnosed conditions with laboratory evidence of infection within these studies.

Inclusion criteria

We included studies (search conducted by Low, but discussed and interpreted by all) published in English and French that reported on cross-sectional studies in low- and middle-income countries, in which the study population was sampled from the general population rather than a health care setting. Studies that reported on any reproductive tract infection were eligible for inclusion if the methods section described a genital examination and specimens for laboratory testing were taken. Studies exclusively recruiting sex workers, surveys reporting only serological results and studies involving the collection of urine or genital specimens without a full genital examination were excluded.

Methods

We searched Medline (1966–99) for the medical subject headings 'sexually transmitted diseases' and 'genital diseases', combined with 'rural population', 'rural health', 'urban population' and 'urban health'. We also used EMBASE (1980–99) for the search terms 'venereal disease' and 'gynaecologic disease', in combination with 'rural population', 'rural area', 'urban population' and 'urban area'. In addition, we used references cited in the bibliographies of both included and excluded studies and data from unpublished reports, where available. For each study, information was abstracted on to a standardized spreadsheet to record geographical location, sampling strategy, and age and sex distribution of the study population. We recorded verbatim definitions given by the authors for the following clinical signs and syndromes: cervicitis (including endocervicitis and mucopurulent cervicitis), cervical ectopy or erosion, pelvic inflammatory disease, vaginal discharge, urethral discharge, epididymo-orchitis and genital ulcer disease. We also recorded the prevalence of each condition and the following laboratory diagnosed infections, where reported: bacterial vaginosis, vaginal candidiasis, trichomoniasis, gonorrhoea, genital chlamydia and syphilis. Where textbooks were cited as the source of definitions, these were also recorded (Table 8.2). No statistical pooling of the prevalence of clinical or laboratory diagnoses was attempted because of the differences between studies according to the location of study, study population and diagnostic criteria applied.

Results

A total of 45 publications reporting on 30 population-based studies of reproductive tract infections and gynaecological morbidity were identified. The electronic literature search yielded 37 publications from 21 studies (Arya , Nsanzumuhire and Taber, 1973; Arya, Taber and Nsanze, 1980; Bang et al., 1989; Belec et al., 1988; Bhatia et al., 1997; Bhatia and Cleland, 1995, 1996; Brabin et al., 1995; Bulut et al., 1997; Colvin et al., 1998; Cronje et al., 1994; Das et al., 1994; Gomo et al., 1997; Grosskurth et al., 1995, 1996; Herrero et al., 1997; Kamali et al., 1999; Killewo et al., 1994; Klouman et al., 1997; Mayaud et al., 1997; Mosha et al., 1993; Newell et al., 1993; Obasi et al., 1999; Pal et al., 1994; Pandit et al., 1995; Passey et al., 1998; Paxton et al., 1998a,b; Tiwara et al., 1996; Wagner et al., 1994; Wasserheit, 1989; Wasserheit et al., 1989; Wawer et al., 1995, 1998, 1999; Younis et al., 1993; Zurayk et al., 1995). Two studies were identified from the reference lists of these publications (Bali and Bhujwala, 1969; Ismail et al., 1990), and one paper reporting on four studies (Latha et al., 1997) and one Ph.D. thesis (Oomman, 1996) were identified from a review (Koenig et al., 1998) that also included data from two of the published studies (Bang et al., 1989; Bhatia et al., 1997). A paper presented at a conference by co-author Sarah Hawkes, was included (Hawkes et al., 1997).

Of these 30 studies, six were serological surveys in which no genital examination was carried out or reported (Belec et al., 1988; Killewo et al., 1994; Mosha et al., 1993; Obasi et al., 1999; Pandit et al., 1995; Wagner et al., 1994), five studies collected serum samples and urine (Colvin et al., 1998; Wawer et al., 1998) or genital specimens (Cronje et al., 1994; Herrero et al., 1997; Ismail et al., 1990) but did not include genital examinations, and one community-based study included only commercial sex workers (Das et al., 1994; Pal et al., 1994). Information from the remaining 18 studies is reviewed here.

Eighteen community-based studies from 10 countries were conducted between 1969 and 1996. These studies report on the prevalence of clinical signs and laboratory diagnosed infections in samples drawn from the general population (Table 8.3). Three studies included both men and women, one included only men and 14 reported results only from women.

Differences in definitions of clinically diagnosed morbidity
Taken together, the studies show that both the definitions of clinically diagnosed morbidity and the reported prevalence of infection vary widely. Whilst some of the differences in reported prevalence may, indeed, be due to geographical and

Table 8.2. Definitions and prevalence of morbidity in community-based studies

Country, setting and year of publication	Subjects	Definitions		Prevalence	
		Signs	Syndromes	Signs or syndromes[a]	Laboratory diagnoses[a]
Africa					
Teso district, Uganda, rural (Arya et al., 1973). Three parishes randomly sampled from one district. Participation rate 90%.	343 women, 15–60 years. 273 men, 15–60 years.	*Cervicitis:* No diagnostic criteria. *Epididymal thickening:* Nodular thickening of lower pole of epididymis.	*Urethral discharge:* No diagnostic criteria.	*Urethral discharge:* 32/269 (11.9%) *Epididymal thickening:* 74/269 (27.5%)	*GC, women:* 54/295 (18.3%) *GC, men:* 24/269 (8.9%)
Giza, Egypt, rural (Younis et al., 1993). One woman per household in a random sample of streets and housing blocks. Participation rate 91%.	509 women, 14–60 years.	*Abnormal vaginal or cervical discharge:* No diagnostic criteria. *Clinical cervicitis:* Mucopurulent discharge in cervix. *Cervical ectopy:* Surface layer of cervix replaced by an abnormal layer that looks red.	*Definite PID:* Uterine tenderness alone or with adnexal tenderness, together with clinical cervicitis. *Possible PID:* Uterine tenderness alone or with adnexal tenderness.	*Vaginitis (moderate discharge+):* 187/508 (36.8%) *Clinical cervicitis:* 47/485 (9.7%) *Cervical ectopy:* 108/501 (21.6%) *Definite PID:* 10/500 (2.0%) *Possible PID:* 87/500 (17.4%)	*BV:* 111/508 (21.9%) *Candida:* 56/507 (11.0%) *TV:* 93/509 (18.3%) *CT:* 43/501 (8.6%) *GC:* 0/502 (0.0%) *Syphilis:* 4/496 (0.8%)

K'Dere, Nigeria, rural (Brabin et al., 1995). All non-pregnant women. Participation rate 90%.	868 women, 10–49 years.	*Abnormal cervix:* Oedematous, friable, or mucopurulent endocervical discharge. *PID:* Lower abdominal pain and/or tenderness of fornices with adnexal tenderness.	*Mucopurulent endocervical discharge:* 45/684 (6.6%) sexually active PID: 53/684 (7.7%) sexually active	*Candida:* 269/684 (39.3%) *TV:* 56/684 (8.2%) *CT:* 40/684 (5.8%) *GC:* 11/684 (1.6%) *Syphilis:* 25/684 (3.7%)
Mwanza, Tanzania, urban and rural and roadside (Grosskurth et al., 1996). Stratified random sample. Participation rate 80%.	5876 men, 15–54 years. 1664 men with symptoms or positive urine test examined.	None reported.	*Urethral discharge:* Presence of discharge after 'milking' the urethra.	[b]*Urethral discharge:* 207/1451 (14.2%)	[b]*CT:* 39/1451 (2.7%) [b]*GC:* 128/1451 (8.8%)
Hippo Valley Estate, Zimbabwe, rural (Gomo et al., 1997). Convenience sampling of a sugar plantation. Participation rate not reported.	404 women, 15–60 years. 601 men, 15–60 years.	None reported.	*Genital ulcer disease:* No diagnostic criteria. *Inguinal lymphadenopathy:* No diagnostic criteria. *Urethral discharge:* No diagnostic criteria.	'*Signs of STIs,' women:* 153/404 (37.9%) '*Signs of STIs,' men:* 123/601 (20.5%)	*GC:* 185/1005 (18.4%), women and men combined

Table 8.2 (*cont.*)

Country, setting and year of publication	Subjects	Definitions		Prevalence	
		Signs	Syndromes	Signs or syndromes[a]	Laboratory diagnoses
Kilimanjaro, Tanzania, rural (Klouman et al., 1997). One village, whole population. Participation rate 76%.	635 women, 15–44 years. 517 men, 15–44 years.	None reported.	*PID:* Tenderness on pelvic examination with or without adnexal mass. *Genital ulcer disease:* No diagnostic criteria. *Urethral discharge:* No diagnostic criteria.	*Pelvic inflammatory disease:* 42/395 (10.6%) *Genital ulcer disease, women:* 1/398 (0.3%) *Genital ulcer disease, men:* 6/453 (1.3%) *Urethral discharge:* 4/453 (0.9%)	*Women* BV: 13/379 (3.4%) TV: 94/380 (24.7%) CT: 27/393 (6.9%) GC: 3/394 (0.8%) Syphilis: 16/628 (2.6%) *Men* CT: 43/447 (9.6%) GC: 2/457 (0.4%) Syphilis: 6/512 (1.2%)
Asia and Pacific Matlab, Bangladesh, rural (Wasserheit et al., 1989). Married women, clients of community health workers. Participation rate 95%.	2929 non-pregnant women of reproductive age included in a survey; 486 symptomatic women examined.	*Mucopurulent cervicitis:* 30 or more neutrophils per high power microscope field.	*Pelvic infection:* Uterine and/or bilateral adnexal tenderness.	*Pelvic infection:* 24/486 (4.9%) *Mucopurulent cervicitis:* 85/486 (17.5%)	*Vaginal infection (BV, candida, TV, others):* 267/486 (54.9%) NG or CT 8/472 (1.7%)

Maharashtra, India, rural (Bang et al., 1989; Koenig et al., 1998). All women, 13 years or older in two villages. Participation rate 59%.	654 women	*Vaginitis:* Vaginal wall visibly inflamed and 5+ neutrophils per high power microscope field. *Cervicitis:* Stated to be from Jeffcoate (1982) (see Table 8.3). *Cervical erosion:* Stated to be from Jeffcoate (1982) (see Table 8.3).	*PID:* Adnexae palpable and tender, with or without restricted mobility of uterus.	*Vaginitis:* Not reported. *Cervicitis:* 272/650 (48.7%) *Endocervicitis:* 67/650 (12.0%) *Cervical erosion:* 255/650 (45.7%) *PID:* 157/650 (24.2%)	*BV:* 347/558 (62.2%) *Candida:* 190/558 (34.1%) *TV:* 78/558 (14.0%) *GC:* 2/650 (0.3%) *Syphilis:* 68/650 (10.5%)
Gujarat, India, rural (Koenig et al., 1998; Latha et al., 1997). All women in 10 villages. Participation rate 49% for survey, 29% for examination.	1103 women under 35 years, ever married with a child under 6 months. 324 women examined.	*Vaginitis:* Inflammation of vaginal wall with abnormal discharge. *Cervicitis:* All diagnoses of acute and chronic cervicitis, or endocervicitis. *Cervical erosion:* No diagnostic criteria.	*PID:* Tender, palpable or thickened fornices.	*Vaginitis:* 30/293 (10.2%) *Cervicitis:* 23/293 (7.8%) *Cervical erosion:* 58/293 (19.8%) *PID:* 24/293 (8.2%)	Not reported.

Table 8.2 (*cont.*)

Country, setting and year of publication	Subjects	Definitions		Prevalence	
		Signs	Syndromes	Signs or syndromes[a]	Laboratory diagnoses
West Bengal, India, rural (Koenig et al., 1998; Latha et al., 1997). Quota sample in 8 villages. Participation rate 44%.	1130 women and unmarried girls, 13–45 years. 500 women examined.	*Vaginitis:* Inflammation of the vaginal wall with or without discharge and laboratory evidence. *Cervicitis:* All diagnoses of acute and chronic cervicitis or endocervicitis. *Cervical erosion:* No diagnostic criteria.	*PID:* Tender or palpable or thickened fornices.	*Vaginitis:* 15/395 (3.8%) *Cervicitis:* 57/395 (14.4%) *Cervical erosion:* 9/395 (2.4%) *PID:* 4/395 (1.0%)	Not reported.
Mumbai, India, urban (Koenig et al., 1998; Latha et al., 1997). 10% random sample of urban slum households in one area. Participation rate 72%.	1054 women, ever married, 15 years or older. 756 women examined.	*Vaginitis:* Inflammation of vaginal wall with discharge and itching or pain. *Cervicitis:* All diagnoses of acute and chronic cervicitis, or endocervicitis. *Cervical erosion:* No diagnostic criteria.	*PID:* Tender or palpable or thickened fornices.	*Vaginitis:* 110/715 (15.4%) *Cervicitis:* 283 (39.6%) *Cervical erosion:* 154/715 (21.5%) *PID:* 119/715 (16.5%)	Not reported.

Study	Sample	Definitions	PID definition	Clinical findings	Laboratory findings
Vadodara, India, rural (Koenig et al., 1998; Latha et al., 1997). 50% random sample from two urban slum areas. Participation rate 65%.	840 women, ever married, 18–45 years. 548 women examined.	*Vaginitis*: Inflammation of vaginal wall. *Cervicitis*: All diagnoses of acute and chronic cervicitis, or endocervicitis. *Cervical erosion*: No diagnostic criteria.	*PID*: Tender or palpable or thickened fornices.	*Vaginitis*: 62/548 (11.2%) *Cervicitis*: 74/548 (13.5%) *Cervical erosion*: 30/548 (5.5%) *PID*: 46/548 (8.4%)	Not reported
Karnataka, India, rural and urban (Bhatia et al., 1997; Koenig et al., 1998). Sample of rural and urban women. Participation rate 86%.	3600 women in original study. 440 married women under 35 years with a child under 1 year eligible for examination.	*Vaginitis*: Redness of vaginal canal, with or without discharge. *Cervicitis*: Mucopurulent discharge in cervix. *Mucopurulent cervicitis*: Numerous polymorphs with a background of fibrous material. *Cervical ectopy*: Redness of cervix. Definitions stated to be from Howkins and Bourne (1971) and Jeffcoate (1982) (see Table 8.3).	*PID*: Uterine or adnexal tenderness with clinical cervicitis and fever or history of fever.	*Vaginitis*: 52/385 (13.4%) *Cervicitis*: 92/385 (23.9%) *Mucopurulent cervicitis*: 141/385 (36.6%) *Cervical ectopy*: 39/385 (10.0%) *PID*: 41/385 (10.7%)	*BV*: 70/385 (18.2%) *Candida*: 20/385 (5.2%) *TV*: 29/385 (7.5%) *GC*: 3/385 (0.8%) *CT*: 2/385 (0.5%) *Syphilis*: 6/385 (1.5%)

Table 8.2 (*cont.*)

Country, setting and year of publication	Subjects	Definitions		Prevalence	
		Signs	Syndromes	Signs or syndromes[a]	Laboratory diagnoses
Rajasthan, India, rural (Oomman, 1996). All women volunteering participation in 40 villages. Participation rate 19% (based on 2 villages).	250 women, 15 years or older, ever married.	*Vaginitis*: Inflammation of vaginal area plus abnormal discharge. *Cervicitis*: Inflammation of cervix plus mucopurulent discharge. *Cervical ectopy*: Bright red clearly defined area on ectocervix where squamous epithelium is replaced by columnar epithelium.	*Definite PID*: Abdominal and uterine tenderness with or without adnexal tenderness, plus cervicitis. *Possible PID*: Uterine tenderness with or without adnexal tenderness.	*Vaginitis*: 74/246 (30.1%) *Cervicitis*: 48/246 (19.5%) *Cervical ectopy*: 75/246 (30.5%) *Definite PID*: 21/246 (8.5%) *Possible PID*: 67/246 (27.2%)	*BV*: 33/244 (13.5%) *Candida*: 6/244 (2.4%) *TV*: 2/244 (0.8%)
Papua New Guinea, highlands (Passey et al., 1998). Randomly selected men and women from 16 villages. Participation rate 75%.	270 women, 15 years or older.	*Vaginitis*: Vaginal erythema with or without discharge. *Visible cervicitis*: Erythema or oedema of zone of ectopy.	*PID*: Three of the following: lower abdominal tenderness, adnexal tenderness, uterine tenderness, cervical motion tenderness.	*PID*: 24/171 (14.0%) *Swab test*: 8/11 (72.7%) of CT positive and 6/11 (54.6%) of TV positive	*BV*: 18/197 (9.1%) *TV*: 92/198 (46.5%) *CT*: 53/201 (26.4%) *GC*: 3/201 (1.5%) *Syphilis*: 8/201 (4.0%)

Location (study)	Sample	Definitions	PID	Prevalence
Matlab, Bangladesh, rural (Hawkes et al., 1996). Randomly selected married women of reproductive age, from a demographic survey population. Participation rate 99%.	804 women	No clinical definitions used. All clinical signs described. *PID*: Lower abdominal pain *plus* signs of lower genital tract infection *plus* cervical/adnexal motion tenderness, *with or without* temp >38°C, palpable mass.	PID: 0/804 (0%)	BV: 28/478 (5.9%) Candida: 58/460 (12.6%) TV: 5/661 (0.8%) CT: 4/753 (0.5%) GC: 4/804 (0.5%) Active syphilis: 6/804 (0.7%) HIV: 0/458 (0%)
Europe Istanbul, Turkey, urban (Bulut et al., 1997). Women selected 'systematically' from household register. Participation rate 80%.	696 women, 15–44 years, ever users of contraception	*Vaginitis*: No definition. *Cervicitis*: Positive C. trachomatis antibodies. *Cervical erosion*: No definition. *PID*: Bilateral lower abdominal pain and supra-pubic tenderness plus cervical or adnexal tenderness.	PID: 26/696 (3.7%)	BV: 33/696 (4.8%) Candida: 36/696 (5.2%) TV: 20/696 (2.9%) CT: 34/696 (4.9%)

Notes:

Abbreviations: BV, bacterial vaginosis; CT, genital chlamydia; GC, gonorrhoea; HIV, human immunodeficiency virus; PID, pelvic inflammatory disease; TV, trichomoniasis

[a] Denominators represent number of women examined, or number for whom results are available

[b] Denominator is number of men examined

population variations, Table 8.2 highlights the lack of agreed standard terms to define clinical conditions. Some definitions of gynaecological morbidity used by these studies are based on clinical appearance alone, some require the results of laboratory tests in addition to clinically diagnosed abnormalities, whilst others are based on the presence of either clinical or laboratory findings. Clinical definitions of one or more conditions were not reported in 10 of the 18 studies. Clinical definitions that were explicitly stated to have been taken from textbooks (Howkins and Bourne, 1971; Jeffcoate, 1982) are listed in Table 8.3. For comparison, we have included a classification system from the International Classification of Diseases, 10th Revision (World Health Organization, 1992a), definitions from World Health Organization guidelines on syndromic management of sexually transmitted infections (STIs) (WHO Study Group on Management of Sexually Transmitted Diseases Patients, 1991) and a recent textbook on sexually transmitted diseases (Holmes et al., 1999).

- *Cervicitis:* A definition of cervicitis was reported in 12 of the 17 studies that included women. Terminology differed between studies, with a distinction being made between conditions referred to as cervicitis and endocervicitis in one study (Bang et al., 1989), and between clinical cervicitis and microscopically diagnosed mucopurulent cervicitis in two studies (Younis et al., 1993; Bhatia et al., 1997). The term cervicitis was used to refer to an appearance of inflammation on clinical inspection (Passey et al., 1998), cervical inflammation plus purulent discharge (Koenig et al., 1998), the presence of mucopurulent endocervical discharge alone (Younis et al., 1993) and a laboratory diagnosis of chlamydial infection (Bhatia et al., 1997; Bulut et al., 1995). Mucopurulent cervicitis was used to refer to a microscopic diagnosis in three studies, although the criteria differed in each (Bhatia et al., 1997; Wasserheit et al., 1989; Younis et al., 1993).

    Two studies in India reported a high prevalence of clinically diagnosed cervicitis – Bang et al. (1989) (48.7 per cent) and Bhatia et al. (1997) (23.9 per cent). In contrast, the prevalence of laboratory diagnosed cervical infection was below 1 per cent in both these studies. Studies conducted in African countries showed more consistent results, with clinical cervicitis diagnosed in 9.7 per cent (Younis et al., 1993) and 6.6 per cent (Brabin et al., 1995), and laboratory cervical infections diagnosed in 8.6 per cent and 7.4 per cent, respectively.

- *Cervical ectopy* or *cervical erosion:* Cervical ectopy was reported in eight studies, but was explicitly defined in only three studies as redness of the cervix (Bhatia et al., 1997), an abnormal red layer replacing the surface layer of the cervix (Younis et al., 1993) and a bright red clearly defined area on the vaginal aspect of the cervix where squamous epithelium is replaced by columnar epithelium (Oomman, 1996). The prevalence of clinically diagnosed cervical ectopy ranged from 5 per cent (Koenig et al., 1998) to 45.7 per cent (Bang et al., 1989).

- *Pelvic inflammatory disease:* A definition of pelvic inflammatory disease was given in 12 of 17 relevant studies. Signs of pelvic inflammatory disease were elicited in 0.9 per cent (Wasserheit et al., 1989) to 24.4 per cent of women (Bang et al., 1989).
- *Urethral discharge in men:* Urethral discharge was reported in three studies in Africa, of which only one provided a definition (Grosskurth et al., 1996). The prevalence of laboratory diagnosed causes of urethritis was similar to that of clinically apparent urethral discharge in two studies (Arya, Nsanzumuhire and Taber, 1973; Grosskurth et al., 1996) but the other identified the presence of gonorrhoea or chlamydia in nearly 10 per cent of men, of whom fewer than one per cent had a clinical discharge.

Differences in the prevalence of observed signs and laboratory confirmed infections
Due in part to the lack of standardization in defining clinical signs, the studies summarized in Table 8.2 provide less than complete information regarding the correlation between clinically diagnosed gynaecological morbidity and the presence of reproductive tract infection. Several studies did not fully report the results of either the clinical examination or laboratory data (Klouman et al., 1997). Others that reported the prevalence of clinically diagnosed morbidity did not specifically analyse the association between these findings with the laboratory tests performed among the same women (Gomo et al., 1997; Bang et al., 1989; Arya et al., 1973; Bhatia et al., 1997). Gomo et al. (1997) only mention that 37.9 per cent of females had 'signs of sexually transmitted infections' and, whereas Bang et al. (1989) assess the predictive value of self-reported morbidity against the aggregate presence of any gynaecological disease, they do not report the association between specific clinical signs and infections. Likewise, in the analysis conducted by Bhatia et al. (1997), both clinically diagnosed and laboratory diagnosed morbidity were classified as outcomes in the bivariate analysis and compared with sociodemographic background and self-reported morbidity variables.

Participation bias introduced through the use of clinical examinations
The results of our systematic review have highlighted additional difficulties in conducting community-based surveys that include a clinical examination. A large number of surveys identified by the literature search (12 of the 31) collected samples of blood, urine, or both, but did not examine the participants, perhaps for fear of lowering participation rates. There is a well-founded belief that many women may decline to take part in surveys that involve a full gynaecological examination. In the studies in the systematic review, participation rates ranged from 19 to 99 per cent. High refusal rates result in diminished power to detect associations and, more importantly, introduce selection bias. Women who consent to take part may be those who either have symptoms that they wish to be

Table 8.3. Definitions of clinical morbidity in the international classification of diseases, WHO technical report and selected textbooks

Textbook authors	Vaginitis or vaginal discharge	Cervicitis	Cervical ectopy	Pelvic inflammatory disease	Urethritis	Epididymitis
World Health Organization (1992a). ICD–10 International Classification of Diseases and Health Related Problems.	A54.0: Gonococcal vulvo-vaginitis NOS; A56.0: Chlamydial vulvo-vaginitis; N76: Other inflammation of vagina and vulva; N76.0: Acute vaginitis; N76.1: Subacute and chronic vaginitis; N77.1[a]: Vaginitis, vulvitis and vulvo-vaginitis in candidiasis, herpes simplex, pinworm infection.	A54.0: Gonococcal cervicitis NOS; A56.0: Chlamydial cervicitis; N72: Inflammatory disease of cervix uteri: Cervicitis, Endocervicitis Exocervicitis (excludes erosion and ectropion without cervicitis).	N86: Erosion and ectropion of cervix uteri: Decubitus ulcer and eversion (excludes erosion and ectropion with cervicitis).	A54.2[b]: Gonococcal female pelvic inflammatory disease; A56.1[b]: Chlamydial female pelvic inflammatory disease; N70: Salpingitis and oophoritis; N70.0: Acute; N70.1: Chronic; N70.9: Unspecified.	A54.0: Gonococcal urethritis NOS; A56.0: Chlamydial urethritis; N34.1: Nonspecific urethritis.	A54.2[b]: Gonococcal epididymitis and orchitis; A56.1[b]: Chlamydial epididymitis and orchitis; N45: Orchitis and epididymitis.
World Health Organization (1992b). The Management of Sexually Transmitted Diseases.	*Vaginal discharge:* STD-related discharges are abnormal in colour, odour and/or amount. The discharge may be accompanied by pruritus, genital swelling, dysuria or lower abdominal pain.	Mucopurulent discharge exuding from the endocervix.	Not described.	Lower abdominal tenderness and/or vaginal discharge and/or fever and/or risk factors for PID.	*Urethral discharge:* Exudate present in the anterior urethra. It may be necessary to 'milk' the urethra in order to see the discharge or re-examine after the patient has held urine for at least 3 hours.	*Scrotal swelling:* Inflammation of the epididymis is usually accompanied by pain, oedema and erythema ...Evidence of urethral discharge should be sought.

Reference					
Jeffcoate (1982). Principles of Gynaecology.[a]	No generic definition. Clinical features of infantile, senile, trichomonal, candidal and non-specific vaginitis described. *Leucorrhoea:* An excessive amount of the normal discharge, consists mainly of the cervical component.	*Acute cervicitis:* Cervix congested and enlarged with swollen mucous membrane pouting at the external os. Tender when touched or moved. Profuse purulent discharge exudes from the cervical canal. *Chronic cervicitis:* The end result of injury and inflammation usually a histopathologic diagnosis without clinical significance.	*Erosion:* The squamous covering of the vaginal aspect of the cervix is replaced by columnar epithelium. An erosion was formerly thought to predispose to cancer of the cervix but this view is no longer acceptable. Once regarded as indicative of chronic cervicitis. This is pure theory and out of keeping with the known natural life history of erosion.	*Acute salpingo-oophoritis:* Toxic; generalized tenderness on bimanual examination; pain on rocking the cervix from side to side; brisk polymorphonuclear leucocytosis. *Chronic salpingo-oophoritis:* Generalized tenderness and fixation of the pelvic organs on bimanual palpation.	Not applicable.	Not applicable.
Howkins and Bourne (1971). Shaw's Textbook of Gynaecology.[a]	No generic definition. *Leucorrhoea:* Normal vaginal secretion increased in amount. Non-pathogenic leucorrhoea can be classified as cervical or vaginal.	*Acute cervicitis:* Cervix reddened, swollen with oedema and mucopus discharged through the cervical canal. *Chronic cervicitis:* A discharge of mucus and pus must be present.	Reddened area slightly raised above the level of the squamous epithelium of the vaginal portion of the cervix. May be congenital, associated with chronic cervicitis or due to hyperplasia of mucous membrane.	*Salpingo-oophoritis:* Severe bilateral lower abdominal pain, fever, leucocytosis, vaginal discharge.	Not applicable.	Not applicable.

Table 8.3 (cont.)

Textbook authors	Vaginitis or vaginal discharge	Cervicitis	Cervical ectopy	Pelvic inflammatory disease	Urethritis	Epididymitis
Holmes et al. (1999). Sexually Transmitted Diseases.	No generic definition.	*Mucopurulent endocervical discharge.* Yellow endocervical exudate or increased numbers of neutrophils in endocervical mucus. *Mucopurulent endocervicitis:* Inflamed endocervical appearance with yellow discharge, oedema, erythema of zone of ectopy and easily induced bleeding. *Endocervicitis:* Histopathologic features of endocervical inflammation.	Endocervical columnar epithelium extending out beyond the external os. Squamocolumnar junction visible on vaginal surface of cervix.	Low abdominal pain plus signs of lower genital tract infection on wet-mount examination of vaginal fluid plus one or more of ESR (erythrocyte sedimentation rate) greater than or equal to 15 mm/hr, temperature >38°C, palpable adnexal mass.	Presence of urethral discharge and Gram stained slide of discharge with >4 polymorphonuclear lymphocytes in five randomly selected high power microscope fields.	Severe scrotal pain, redness and oedema of scrotum, with or without swelling and tenderness of spermatic cord.

Notes:

[a] References cited as source of clinical definitions by Bhatia et al. (1997).

[b] References cited as source of clinical definitions by Bang et al. (1989).

treated or may be less subjected to social and cultural pressures that exclude, for example, younger unmarried women and adolescents. The studies in Bangladesh were specifically precluded from interviewing unmarried women (Hawkes et al., 1997; Wasserheit et al., 1989), who may be at highest risk of morbidity.

Overcoming such participation bias has been made easier in recent years with the development of a greater understanding of ways of working with communities to build rapport and trust, as well as the emergence of new laboratory techniques that may preclude the need for genital examination. For example, it is now possible to screen urine samples for some pathogens with high sensitivity and specificity (Crotchfelt et al., 1997; Davies, Low and Ison, 1998; Schachter, 1998). Specimens retrieved from self-administered vaginal or vulval swabs (Stary et al., 1997) or tampons (Tabrizi et al., 1998) can also be used to diagnose both vaginal and cervical infections. These developments are reviewed more fully in Chapters 9 and 10.

Limitations resulting from the validity of self-reported symptoms and clinical signs for predicting reproductive tract infection

Few community-based studies included in our systematic review calculated the sensitivity and specificity of observed clinical signs in predicting the presence or absence of laboratory confirmed infection. In a survey carried out in rural Bangladesh by Hawkes (1997), the presence of cervical mucopus or friability had a sensitivity of 12.5 per cent, specificity of 98.7 per cent and a positive predictive value of 9.1 per cent for predicting cervical infection (gonorrhoea or chlamydia). This is because of the low prevalence of laboratory-diagnosed infections despite high levels of reported symptoms. Over 37 per cent reported an abnormal vaginal discharge on the day of the interview and trained primary health care workers reported cervical mucopus or cervical friability in 6.5 per cent of the sample; however, only one woman with a cervical infection was correctly identified and treated. Endogenous infections were more likely to be correctly identified, helped by using pH paper and potassium hydroxide staining (sensitivity 82.1 per cent and specificity 97.8 per cent for bacterial vaginosis, and sensitivity 15.1 per cent and specificity 94.5 per cent for candidiasis).

Studies that examined associations between clinically diagnosed morbidity and the presence of reproductive tract infection showed weak and inconsistent findings. In the Turkish study, the only clinical sign strongly associated with genital chlamydial infection in univariate analysis was cervical ectopy (odds ratio 3.24, 95 per cent, confidence intervals 1.45 to 7.25) (Ronsmans et al., 1996). Multivariable analyses controlling for age and contraceptive method were not reported. Passey et al. (1998) examined the association between a variety of clinical signs and reproductive tract infections among a rural population in Papua New Guinea. Only the 'swab test', positive if a white cotton tipped swab of endocervical secretions appeared 'yellow' in colour (Brunham et al., 1984), was predictive of the presence of cervical chlamydia infection in a multivariable analysis (odds ratio 4.73, 95 per cent confidence intervals 1.32 to 16.88). In Giza, Egypt, Zurayk et al. (1995) found that despite substantial agreement between women's reports of discharge and the physician's observations, neither were good predictors of reproductive tract infection.

Given the recent interest in developing syndromic management flowcharts and the greater ease of conducting studies in health care settings, more information about the associations between symptoms, signs and laboratory tests for reproductive tract infections among both symptomatic and asymptomatic women is available. Comprehensive reviews of these studies have recently been published (Dallabetta et al., 1998; Haberland et al., 1999). Data from clinic-based studies corroborate the findings from community-based studies, showing a lack of consistent correlation between observable clinical signs and the presence of specific reproductive tract infections. Caution in using such signs in presumptive diagnosis and syndromic treatment has, therefore, been advised. Furthermore, the predictive value of an observed clinical sign decreases with the prevalence of infection. Consequently, in community-based samples where prevalence rates are generally lower than in clinic-based studies of symptomatic individuals, the poor predictive value of clinical signs is unacceptably low.

Limitations resulting from differences in observers' assessment of clinical morbidity
Inter-observer variation in the performance of clinical examinations

We have already seen how the lack of a global standard for defining clinical conditions results in wide variations in recorded prevalence between studies, over and above expected variations from different settings and study populations. Part of the variation is a result of the use of different diagnostic criteria between studies. An equally important source of variation, however, arises when diagnoses are based on the clinical impression of the person conducting the examination. Two investigators applying the same diagnostic criteria to an examination of the same person will often differ, particularly if the criteria are largely subjective. Such 'inter-observer variation' can be measured by comparing the observed level of agreement between observers with the level that would be expected by chance (Altman, 1991). We are not aware of any published studies of inter-observer variation in the diagnosis of gynaecological morbidity associated with reproductive tract infections. A recent study of two cities in the Philippines, where the clinical examination of sex workers was carried out by different groups of health care workers, stressed the need for training to standardize the recognition of mucopurulent cervicitis (Wi et al., 1998). The study found that the sensitivity of a clinical algorithm for the diagnosis of cervical infection was 42 per cent when applied by doctors in Manila with specialist training in gynaecology, but only 12 per cent when used by non-specialist clinicians in Cebu. Other physical differences in the setting in which the examination was conducted, or differences in the use of antibiotics prior to examination, could also have contributed to the observed discrepancy. We examined inter-observer variation in diagnosis using data from a study carried out in the Matlab area of rural Bangladesh in 1995 and 1996.

Methods

The study was conducted by Sarah Hawkes to evaluate the training needs of primary health care workers in using the recommended syndromic management guidelines to treat women with symptoms suggestive of a reproductive tract or STI. As part of the study, over 90 women complaining of abnormal vaginal discharge were seen by both a physician and a primary health care worker. The same physician saw each woman, but a number of different primary health care workers took part in the survey. Each woman underwent a speculum examination and full laboratory testing.

All levels of health care workers in Matlab had participated in a training programme for syndromic management early in 1995. Their diagnoses were based upon the recommended syndromic management guidelines summarized in Table 8.3 (WHO Study Group on Management of Sexually Transmitted Diseases Patients, 1991). The doctor and primary health care worker recorded their diagnoses independently of each another. At the end of the study, the diagnoses recorded by the physician and the primary health care worker were compared both with each other and with the laboratory findings.

Results

Of the 94 women seen, laboratory results indicated that 22 per cent had bacterial vaginosis, 15 per cent had candida and none had evidence of a STI (*Trichomonas vaginalis, Neissera gonorrhoeae* or *C. trachomatis*). Over-diagnosis was common among all health care workers, especially for STIs. The main difference between the physician and primary health care worker was that the specificity of the physician's diagnosis of endogenous infection, bacterial vaginosis and candidiasis was better. The sensitivity of clinical diagnosis by both groups was low, resulting in under-treatment of women with laboratory diagnosed infections.

This small study shows that agreement for clinical diagnoses between different levels of health care workers was only fair. If comparisons are to be made between studies conducted in different settings, then the amount of variation in the reported prevalence of conditions associated with reproductive tract infections between studies that is likely to be due to inter-observer variation needs to be known. For diagnoses based on clinical examinations, the level of training that each observer has received and the duration of clinical experience will have an important impact on the findings (Holmes and Stamm, 1999). This is not to suggest that only highly trained personnel should undertake clinical surveys. It may be important, however, to consider which practitioner carried out the clinical examinations when analysing survey results, and to try, wherever possible, to limit the number of clinical staff carrying out examinations. Larger studies designed to validate standardized clinical definitions should include a prospective evaluation of inter-observer variation.

Observer expectation and its influence on clinical diagnosis of reproductive tract infection

In resource poor settings, women are most often treated on the basis of history and clinical signs without access to laboratory test results. Observer expectations, based on information elicited from the clinical and sexual history and on observed clinical findings, strongly influence treatment norms and, consequently, patterns of antibiotic use and misuse. Unfortunately, as we have shown, these signs often correlate poorly with the actual presence of reproductive tract infection. In the absence of definitive aetiologic diagnoses, clinicians' presumptive treatment will always be a balance between under- and over-treatment of specific reproductive tract infections.

Recently, co-author Chris Elias participated in a study of reproductive tract infection prevalence in Hue, Vietnam, where the investigators sought to understand the criteria clinicians use to arrive at presumptive diagnoses of vaginal discharge syndromes in the absence of advanced laboratory tests or standardized case management guidelines (Lien et al., 1998).

Methods

Speculum examinations for 600 women attending a maternal and child health/family planning centre were carried out where the clinician recorded the presence or absence of the following clinical signs: vaginal discharge; redness of the cervix (and the percentage of the area of the cervix affected); mucopus in the cervical canal; and cervical contact bleeding. The clinician was also asked to make a note of whether or not she believed that there was a reproductive tract infection present before the results of any laboratory tests (other than the potassium hydroxide 'whiff test' and vaginal pH) were available. If a reproductive tract infection was presumed to be present, the clinician also recorded her impression of whether it was vaginal, cervical and/or pelvic in nature. Specimens for laboratory diagnosis of bacterial vaginosis, *Candida albicans, T. vaginalis, N. gonorrhoeae* and *Chlamydia trachomatis* were taken.

Results

The prevalence of any reproductive tract infection was 21.2 per cent, of which only 28 cases (4.7 per cent) were due to a STI. The prevalence of cervical infection was very low. Five cases of chlamydia (0.8 per cent) and one case of gonorrhoea (0.2 per cent) were diagnosed.

Presumptive diagnosis of infections
Clinicians commonly made a presumptive diagnosis of vaginal infection (42.8 per cent) and cervical infection (43.5 per cent), but pelvic infection was considered rare (2.3 per cent). A significant proportion of all women (24.3 per cent) were considered by the clinician to have both cervical and vaginal infection. These figures were considerably higher than the prevalence of laboratory confirmed infection. This was particularly true of cervical infections, for which a presumptive diagnosis was made in 43.5 per cent of women whereas the combined prevalence of gonorrhoea and chlamydia was only 1 per cent. Therefore, over-diagnosis and presumptive treatment of cervical infection was more than 40-fold.

Criteria used by clinicians for presumptive diagnosis
Three symptoms were found to be significantly associated with the positive diagnosis of 'any reproductive tract infection' or 'cervical infection' by clinicians in this study. The presence of an observed vaginal discharge was most strongly associated with a positive presumptive diagnosis of 'any reproductive tract infection', while cervical 'redness' and contact bleeding influenced the clinicians' presumptive diagnosis of cervical infection. Significantly, the identification of cervical 'redness' was based on minimal clinical signs. When asked to estimate what percentage of the cervix displayed 'redness' among women exhibiting this sign, the modal figure given was only 5 per cent. The presence of cervical mucopus was found to be unrelated to either the presence of infection or clinicians' presumptive diagnoses in this study.

Thus, the indicative signs used by the clinicians did not correlate well with the actual presence of an infection. Although the vast majority of actual reproductive tract infection cases were accompanied by observed vaginal discharge (96.9 per cent), only 29.9 per cent (123/595) of all women observed to have a discharge actually had a reproductive tract infection. For example, despite the fact that in 100 per cent of the cases where a reproductive tract infection was correctly identified by the clinician a vaginal discharge was observed, such discharge was also observed in 249 (95.8 per cent) of the 260 women for whom infection was erroneously diagnosed when compared to laboratory testing. These data suggest that clinicians strongly believe that some observable clinical signs reliably predict the presence of treatable causes of gynaecological morbidity despite the fact that their expectations are not supported by epidemiological data. This has significant implications for clinical practice, especially with regard to antibiotic usage and over-usage.

Non-infectious gynaecological morbidity

So far, this chapter has focused exclusively on definitions of clinically diagnosed gynaecological morbidity related to reproductive tract infection. This is because there are even less data (and less standardized recording of data) for non-infectious gynaecological morbidities, such as genital prolapse. Almost all the studies listed in Table 8.2, for example, provide no information on the definition or prevalence of non-infectious conditions. In the Giza study by Younis et al. (1993), genital prolapse was defined as 'anterior vaginal wall', 'posterior vaginal wall' and/or 'uterine' prolapse when these structures 'descended below their normal position'. Genital prolapse was found to be a common cause of gynaecological morbidity (56.4 per cent) in this study. Related anthropological research revealed that prolapse also often had wide-ranging personal and social consequences for the women (Khattab, 1992). Unfortunately, most studies focus only on infectious and/or potentially transmissible conditions and, consequently, there is a need to clearly define and better document clinical findings potentially related to non-infectious gynaecological morbidities in future population-based studies.

Recommendations

We have seen in this chapter that the lack of standardized definitions for clinical observations can lead to wide variations in the reported prevalence of infection-related gynaecological morbidity. Even when clinical definitions are standardized, the correlation between recorded clinical signs and the laboratory-diagnosed presence of infection is often poor. Furthermore, inter-observer variation and observer expectations may have an important impact on the recorded prevalence of clinical signs and presumptive diagnosis and treatment practices. The lack of well-standardized definitions and the potential for large degrees of inter-observer variation also applies to non-infectious conditions, such as genital prolapse. This situation obviously has important and somewhat daunting implications for researchers undertaking community-based surveys of gynaecological morbidity, as well as those using such study results to plan appropriate interventions and assess service requirements.

Given the difficulties outlined in the foregoing, we suggest five guidelines for researchers considering future community-based studies of gynaecological morbidity.

The necessity of obtaining data from a population-based sample should be critically assessed. Studies conducted in health care settings may be easier to execute and provide adequate data for decision making.

As discussed in greater length in Chapter 5, carefully executed community-based surveys of gynaecological morbidity are difficult and expensive. Given the commitment of human and financial resources required to undertake a rigorous community-based study, there are significant opportunity costs involved in a decision to proceed with this type of investigation. Other methodological approaches may provide more timely and appropriate data for addressing reproductive health programme and policy needs.

Pilot studies should be undertaken before proceeding with a large-scale community-based survey of gynaecological morbidity. In particular, the sample participation rate should be greater than 75 per cent and must be sustainable beyond the pilot phase.

Given the inherent variation that exists in the measurement of gynaecological morbidity, investigators planning this type of study must take measures to reduce further threats to validity by ensuring that population-sampling procedures are representative and participation is maximized. Our figure of 75 per cent was arbitrarily chosen but, in our systematic review, participation rates were 75 per cent or below in half the included studies, introducing the possibility of significant selection bias. Careful pilot studies will help to refine budget calculations for the full-scale study, including the costs of gaining and sustaining community trust and rapport. If this recommendation were to be applied, the non-feasibility of many proposed community-based surveys of gynaecological morbidity would become apparent.

All community-based studies of gynaecological morbidity should use standardized terminology and criteria for defining clinically diagnosed morbidity.

Given the data reviewed for this chapter, we feel it is imperative that investigators use a standardized set of definitions for clinically diagnosed morbidity. Standardization will improve comparability between studies and may, ultimately, facilitate meta-analysis of data from combinable studies. Drawing from our systematic review as well as from field experience in a wide variety of cultural and geographic settings, we have proposed a simple core set of terms and definitions that can be adopted for observing and describing clinical conditions (Table 8.4). We have suggested unambiguous definitions that are easily applied in clinical practice with a minimum of training and equipment. Our proposed list does not seek to include all pathological conditions of the reproductive tract that might be of interest and, consequently, observed or recorded. The proposed definitions are guidelines for researchers and require validation in a variety of contextual settings.

Some studies may use more sophisticated equipment and procedures such as colposcopy or cervicography. It is beyond the scope of this paper to recommend standard methods for such techniques but we urge the use of internationally standardized definitions, whenever possible. For example, the World Health Organization has previously produced guidelines for recording the observations of colposcopic findings (World Health Organization, 1995).

Table 8.4. Suggested guidelines for observing and recording clinically diagnosed morbidity

Condition	Definition and rationale	Guidelines for recording observations
Vaginal discharge	*The presence of vaginal secretions that are malodorous, excessive in amount, or yellow/green in colour.* This term is preferred to vaginitis or vaginal infection since the presence of observable discharge cannot be consistently correlated with either vaginal inflammation or infection.	Record characteristics of vaginal secretions as follows: Odour: (a) Normal (b) *Malodorous* Amount: (a) Scanty (b) Normal c) *Profuse* Colour: (a) Clear (b) White (c) Bloody (d) *Yellow/Green* Abnormal vaginal discharge is present if results highlighted in *italics* are found or if there is a bloody discharge in a non-menstruating woman.
Endocervical discharge	*The presence of secretions from the endocervical canal that are yellow/green in colour or excessive in amount.* This term is preferred to cervicitis or cervical infection since the presence of observable discharge cannot be consistently correlated with either cervical inflammation or infection. Indeed, cervical infection is often not associated with *any* clinical symptoms or signs. Yellow/green cervical secretions are typically referred to as mucopus. This term may be interpreted in a variety of ways, however, hence we recommend standardizing this observation in terms of the colour of the endocervical secretions/exudate.	Record characteristics of cervical secretions as follows: Amount: (a) Absent (b) Normal (c) *Profuse* Colour: (a) Clear (b) White (c) Bloody (d) *Yellow/Green* Cervical discharge is present if results highlighted in *italics* are found or if there is a bloody discharge in a non-menstruating woman. *Important*: Endocervical secretions should be observed and, hence, the coloration of secretions should be standardized by collecting a swab specimen from the endocervix (after gently removing vaginal secretions from the surface of the cervix with a large swab, if necessary). The swab should then be held against a white background (such as a gauze) to determine if the secretions are yellow/green in colour.[a]

Cervical ectopy	*The presence of a distinct area of erythema or redness surrounding the endocervix.*	Record characteristics of cervical ectopy as follows:
	This term is preferred to cervical erosion or cervical ectropion as the erythema most often results simply from the increased vascularity of the columnar epithelium of the transformation zone and not from an 'erosive' process. The zone of cervical ectopy surrounding the endocervix may be either symmetrical or asymmetrical.	Cervical Ectopy: (a) Absent (b) Present Approximate percentage of cervix that appears 'red': (a) < 25% (b) 25–75% (c) >75% Draw a picture of the cervical appearance (optional).
	Note: The observation of cervical ectopy, while important to observe and record, does NOT necessarily indicate the presence of a gynaecological morbidity.	
Contact bleeding	*The presence of easily induced cervical bleeding (e.g. using a cotton swab lightly pressed against the cervix).*	Record characteristics of contact bleeding as follows:
	This term is preferred to cervical friability, which may be variably interpreted in different medical cultures.	Contact bleeding of cervix: (a) Present (b) Absent
Mucosal ulceration	*The presence of any lesion(s) resulting from disruption of the mucosal or epithelial lining of the genital tract.*	Record the characteristics of genital ulceration as follows:

	Ulceration can occur throughout the genital tract (from cervix to external labia). Thorough and systematic examination of the entire reproductive tract is essential for clinical observation.	Was any epithelial disruption noted on the vulva/labia?
		
		  (a) Absent (b) Present
		
		If present, quantify number of ulcerations observed:
		
		  (a) 1 (b) 2–5 (c) >5
		
		If present, estimate average size of lesion:
		
		  (a) < 5mm (b) 5–10 mm (c) >10 mm
		
		If present, describe location: _____
		
		Was any mucosal disruption noted in the vagina?
		
		  (If present, note details as above)
		
		Was any mucosal disruption noted on the cervix?
		
		  (If present, note details as above)

Table 8.4 (*cont.*)

Condition	Definition and rationale	Guidelines for recording observations
Pelvic tenderness	*The presence of pain (as evidenced by changes in facial expression or muscle tone and/or bodily motion) during pelvic examination.* To minimize variation in the occurrence of mild discomfort or pain, this definition excludes pain verbally reported by the woman being examined unless it is accompanied by an observable reaction.	Record the occurrence of pelvic tenderness as follows: Was pain experienced by the woman during bimanual examination? (a) No (b) Yes If yes, could the pain be localized? (a) No (b) Yes If yes, was the pain localized to: (a) Cervical motion tenderness (b) Uterus (c) Right adnexa (d) Left adnexa (e) Other, specify _____
Genital prolapse	*A disturbance of genital tract structure noted by the clinician during pelvic examination.*	Record the presence of genital prolapse as follows: Was prolapse of genital structures noted? (a) No (b) Yes If yes, indicate which structure(s) exhibited prolapse: (a) Vaginal (anterior) (b) Vagina (posterior) (c) Uterus Did prolapsed tissue protrude past the introitus? (a) No (b) Yes, but only with increased intra-abdominal pressure (c) Yes, at all times

Pelvic masses	*The presence of abnormal, palpable pelvic masses noted by the clinician during pelvic examination.*
	
	Palpation of normal genital structures (i.e. ovaries or pregnant uterus) should not be recorded. While describing the more subtle characteristics of any given abdominal mass will certainly inform individual client management, for population-based research emphasis is limited to occurrence, size, and involved organ.
		Record the occurrence of a pelvic mass as follows:
		
		Was a pelvic mass noted by the clinician during bimanual examination?
		
		  (a) No (b) Yes
		
		If yes, could the mass be localized?
		
		  (a) No (b) Yes
		
		If yes, was the mass localized to the:
		
		  (a) Cervix (b) Uterus (c) Right adnexa (d) Left adnexa
		  (e) Vagina (f) Vulva (g) Other, specify _____
		
		Estimate approximate size of the mass: _____ cm × _____ cm

pH	*The pH of vaginal secretions as measured by the clinician immediately following specimen collection.* A specimen of vaginal secretions should be sampled from the posterior fornix and immediately applied to a strip of pH paper.	Record the results of the vaginal pH as follows: (a) < 4.5 (b) >= 4.5 OR pH = _____

Notes:

[a](Brunham et al., 1984).

Table 8.4 attempts to standardize key findings observable on clinical examination that may be related to gynaecological morbidity. It is important to note that some observations, for example cervical ectopy, do not necessarily indicate the presence of morbidity. The guidelines for recording observations emphasize easily verifiable characteristics such as their presence, colour and size, instead of diagnostic entities such as 'mucopus' and 'cervicitis', which allow for considerable variation resulting from differences in observer judgement. A major advantage of the proposed definitions and guidelines is that they can be used to standardize training and monitoring and, consequently, be subjected to external quality control during the course of the study. We have added one simple diagnostic test (vaginal pH) to be performed by the practitioner at the time of the examination as this test may provide important additional information, and can be easily and cheaply collected in all clinic settings. Familiarity with this test may also facilitate the future introduction of rapid diagnostic tests.

The number of study personnel conducting and recording clinical examinations should be kept to a minimum, with consistency of personnel throughout the study. Clinical observers should receive training in the application of examination procedures and means of recording observations. Inter-observer variation and reliability should be formally documented.

Given the variation that often exists between clinical observers, the reliability of recorded clinical data must be seen as an important threat to the internal validity of the research enterprise. We recommend reducing the potential for inter-observer variation by minimizing the number of observers and providing rigorous training on study procedures. As inter-observer variation is a potential source of explanation for abnormal patterns of results, its occurrence should be assessed. Further operational research is needed to determine the most appropriate means of training and ensuring clinician participation to reduce inter-observer variation.

Validate the presence of clinically diagnosed gynaecological morbidity related to reproductive tract infection through the routine inclusion of adequate laboratory testing.

Given the lack of consistent correlation between clinically diagnosed morbidity and the presence of laboratory diagnosed reproductive tract infection, we recommend that laboratory testing for a core group of reproductive tract pathogens be considered an essential component of all community-based studies of gynaecological morbidity. Laboratory validation and quality control should also be included in the study design. As a minimum, we recommend 'gold standard' laboratory testing for the following pathogens: *N. gonorrhoeae, C. trachomatis, T. vaginalis, Candida spp*, bacterial vaginosis and syphilis (see Chapter 9).

Conclusions

In the immediate future, the standardization of clinical observations and their routine validation against laboratory tests for the most important reproductive tract pathogens in community-based surveys of gynaecological morbidity will fill important gaps in our knowledge about the associations between clinical and laboratory measures of morbidity. This work is needed to improve the current evidence base, which suffers from a legacy of studies with low sample participation rates that used non-standardized criteria for recording clinical findings. We should be prepared, however, for the possibility that better quality data will simply confirm the available evidence that clinically diagnosed conditions do not adequately predict infection-related gynaecological morbidity. This may be particularly true if the reason we consider these conditions 'abnormal' is because they are risk markers for associated conditions such as pelvic inflammatory disease, infertility or HIV transmission. In this situation we must, at some point, consider the ethics and acceptability of collecting clinical morbidity data using genital examinations that entail significant participant discomfort. These decisions will also be influenced by the increasing affordability and availability of new reproductive tract infection diagnostic technologies and non-invasive sample collection techniques.

Irrespective of technological advances, we feel that the use of a standardized set of clinical definitions will, with appropriate training, lead to more systematic genital examination and thorough observation by individual practitioners and, thereby, reduce inter-observer variation and improve the comparability of studies conducted among diverse populations.

REFERENCES

Altman DG (1991) *Practical statistics for medical research*. London, Chapman & Hall.

Arya OP, Nsanzumuhire H, Taber SR (1973) Clinical, cultural, and demographic aspects of gonorrhoea in a rural community in Uganda. *Bulletin of the World Health Organization*, **49**: 587–595.

Arya OP, Taber SR, Nsanze H (1980) Gonorrhoea and female infertility in rural Uganda. *American journal of obstetrics and gynecology*, **138**: 929–932.

Bali P, Bhujwala RA (1969) A pilot study of clinico-epidemiological investigations of vaginal discharges in rural women. *Indian journal of medical research*, **57**: 2289–2301.

Bang RA, Bang AT, Baitule M et al. (1989) High prevalence of gynaecological diseases in rural Indian women. *Lancet*, **1**(8629):85–87.

Belec PL, Gresenguet G, Georges-Courbot MC et al. (1988) Sero-epidemiologic study of several sexually transmitted diseases (including HIV infection) in a rural zone of the Central

African Republic (in French). *Bulletin de la Societe de Pathologie Exotique et de Ses Filiales*, **81**: 692–698.

Bhatia JC, Cleland J (1995) Self-reported symptoms of gynecological morbidity and their treatment in south India. *Studies in family planning*, **26**: 203–216.

Bhatia JC, Cleland J (1996) Obstetric morbidity in south India: results from a community survey. *Social science and medicine*, **43**: 1507–1516.

Bhatia JC, Cleland J, Bhagavan L et al. (1997) Levels and determinants of gynecological morbidity in a district of south India. *Studies in family planning*, **28**: 95–103.

Brabin L, Kemp J, Obunge OK et al. (1995) Reproductive tract infections and abortion among adolescent girls in rural Nigeria. *Lancet*, **345**: 300–304.

Brunham RC, Paavonen J, Stevens CE et al. (1984) Mucopurulent cervicitis – the ignored counterpart in women of urethritis in men. *New England journal of medicine*, **311**: 1–6.

Bulut A, Filippi V, Marshall T et al. (1997) Contraceptive choice and reproductive morbidity in Istanbul. *Studies in family planning*, **28**: 35–43.

Bulut A, Yolsal N, Filippi V et al. (1995) In search of truth: comparing alternative sources of information on reproductive tract infection. *Reproductive health matters*, **6**: 31–39.

Campbell OMR, Graham WR (1990) *Measuring maternal mortality and morbidity: levels and trends*. Maternal and Child Epidemiology Unit, Publication Number 2. London, London School of Hygiene and Tropical Medicine.

Cates W, Farley TM, Rowe PJ (1985) Worldwide patterns of infertility: is Africa different? *Lancet*, **2**(8455): 596–598.

Colvin M, Abdool KS, Connolly C et al. (1998) HIV infection and asymptomatic sexually transmitted infections in a rural South African community. *International journal of STD and AIDS*, **9**: 548–550.

Critchlow CW, Wolner-Hanssen P, Eschenbach DA et al. (1995) Determinants of cervical ectopia and of cervicitis: age, oral contraception, specific cervical infection, smoking, and douching. *American journal of obstetrics and gynecology*, **173**: 534–543.

Cronje HS, Joubert G, Muir A et al. (1994) Prevalence of vaginitis, syphilis and HIV infection in women in the Orange Free State. *South African medical journal*, **84**: 602–605.

Crotchfelt KA, Welsh LE, DeBonville D et al. (1997) Detection of Neisseria gonorrhoeae and Chlamydia trachomatis in genitourinary specimens from men and women by a coamplification PCR assay. *Journal of clinical microbiology*, **35**: 1536–1540.

Dallabetta GA, Gerbase AC, Holmes KK (1998) Problems, solutions, and challenges in syndromic management of sexually transmitted diseases. *Sexually transmitted infections*, **74**(Suppl. 1): S1–11.

Das A, Jana S, Chakraborty AK et al. (1994) Community based survey of STD/HIV infection among commercial sex-workers in Calcutta (India). Part-III: Clinical findings of sexually transmitted diseases (STDs). *Journal of communicable diseases*, **26**: 192 196.

Davies PO, Low N, Ison CA (1998) The role of effective diagnosis for the control of gonorrhoea in high prevalence populations. *International journal of STD and AIDS*, **9**: 435–443.

Dixon-Mueller R, Wasserheit JN (1991) *The culture of silence: reproductive tract infections among women in the Third World*. New York, International Women's Health Coalition.

Goldacre MJ, Loudon N, Watt B et al. (1978) Epidemiology and clinical significance of cervical erosion in women attending a family planning clinic. *British medical journal*, 1: 748–750.

Gomo E, Ndamba J, Nhandara C et al. (1997) Prevalence of gonorrhoea and knowledge of sexually transmitted infections in a farming community in Zimbabwe. *Central African journal of medicine*, **43**: 192–195.

Grosskurth H, Mayaud P, Mosha F et al. (1996) Asymptomatic gonorrhoea and chlamydial infection in rural Tanzanian men. *British medical journal*, **312**: 277–280.

Grosskurth H, Mosha F, Todd J et al. (1995) A community trial of the impact of improved sexually transmitted disease treatment on the HIV epidemic in rural Tanzania: 2. Baseline survey results. *AIDS*, **9**: 927–934.

Haberland N, Winikoff B, Sloan N et al. (1999) Case finding and case management of chlamydia and gonorrhoea infections among women: what we do and do not know. The Robert H Ebert Program on Critical Issues in Reproductive Health. New York, The Population Council.

Harrison HR, Costin M, Meder JB et al. (1985) Cervical Chlamydia trachomatis infection in university women: relationship to history, contraception, ectopy, and cervicitis. *American journal of obstetrics and gynecology*, **153**: 244–251.

Hawkes SJ, de Francisco A, Chakraborty J et al. (1997) Using the results of the Matlab RTI/STI study to develop suitable STI control programmes in Bangladesh. Oral presentation at the Sixth Annual Scientific Conference of ICDDR, Bangladesh. Dhaka, March.

Herrero R, Schiffman MH, Bratti C et al. (1997) Design and methods of a population-based natural history study of cervical neoplasia in a rural province of Costa Rica: the Guanacaste Project. *Pan American journal of public health*, 1: 362–375.

Holmes KK, Sparling PF, Mardh P-A et al., eds. (1999) *Sexually transmitted diseases*, 3rd edn. New York, McGraw-Hill, Inc.

Holmes KK, Stamm WE (1999). Lower genital tract infection syndromes in women. In: Holmes KK, Sparling PF, Mardh P-A et al., eds. *Sexually transmitted diseases*, pp. 761–781. New York, McGraw-Hill, Inc.

Howkins J, Bourne G (1971) *Shaw's textbook of gynaecology*, 9th edn. Edinburgh, Churchill Livingstone.

Hull MG (1978) Cervical 'erosion' [letter]. *British medical journal*, 1: 1143.

Ismail SO, Ahmed HJ, Jama MA et al. (1990) Syphilis, gonorrhoea and genital chlamydial infection in a Somali village. *Genitourinary medicine*, **66**: 70–75.

Jeffcoate N (1982) *Principles of gynaecology*, 4th edn. London, Butterworths.

Johnson BA, Poses RM, Fortner CA et al. (1990) Derivation and validation of a clinical diagnostic model for chlamydial cervical infection in university women. *Journal of the American Medical Association*, **264**: 3161–3165.

Kamali A, Nunn AJ, Mulder DW et al. (1999) Seroprevalence and incidence of genital ulcer infections in a rural Ugandan population. *Sexually transmitted infections*, **75**: 98–102.

Khattab H (1992) The silent endurance: social conditions of women's reproductive health in rural Egypt. Amman, UNICEF Regional Office; Cairo, The Population Council.

Killewo JZJ, Sandstrom A, Raden UB et al. (1994) Prevalence and incidence of syphilis and its association-with-HIV-1 infection in a population-based study in the Kagera region of Tanzania. *International journal of STD and AIDS*, 5: 424–431.

Klouman E, Masenga EJ, Klepp K-I et al. (1997) HIV and reproductive tract infections in a total village population in rural Kilimanjaro, Tanzania: women at increased risk. *Journal of Acquired Immune Deficiency Syndromes and human retrovirology*, 14: 163–168.

Koenig M, Jejeebhoy S, Singh S et al. (1998) Investigating gynecological morbidity in India: not just another KAP survey. *Reproductive Health Matters* 6(11): 84–97.

Kurman RJ (1994) *Blaustein's pathology of the female genital tract*, 4th edn. New York, Springer-Verlag New York Inc.

Latha K, Kanani SJ, Bhatt RV et al. (1997) Prevalence of clinically detectable gynaecological morbidity in India: results of four community-based studies. *Journal of family welfare*, 43: 8–16.

Lien PT, Elias CJ, Uhrig J et al. (1998) The prevalence of reproductive tract infections at the MCH/FP center in Hue, Vietnam: a cross-sectional descriptive study. Conference report. Hanoi, Population Council.

Mayaud P, Mosha F, Todd J et al. (1997) Improved treatment services significantly reduce the prevalence of sexually transmitted diseases in rural Tanzania: results of a randomized controlled trial. *AIDS*, 11: 1873–1880.

Mosha F, Nicoll A, Barongo L et al. (1993) A population-based study of syphilis and sexually transmitted disease syndromes in north-western Tanzania. 1. Prevalence and incidence. *Genitourinary medicine*, 69: 415–420.

Newell J, Senkoro K, Mosha F et al. (1993) A population-based study of syphilis and sexually transmitted disease syndromes in north-western Tanzania. 2. Risk factors and health seeking behaviour. *Genitourinary medicine*, 69: 421–426.

Nugent RP, Krohn MA, Hillier SL (1991) Reliability of diagnosing bacterial vaginosis is improved by a standardized method of gram stain interpretation. *Journal of clinical microbiology*, 29: 297–301.

Obasi A, Mosha F, Quigley M et al. (1999) Antibody to herpes simplex virus type 2 as a marker of sexual risk behavior in rural Tanzania. *Journal of infectious diseases*, 179: 16–24.

Oomman N (1996) *Poverty and pathology: comparing rural Rajasthani women's ethnomedical models with biomedical models of reproductive morbidity: implications for women's health in India*. Ph.D. thesis, Baltimore, Johns Hopkins School of Hygiene and Public Health.

Pal NK, Chakraborty MS, Das A et al. (1994) Community based survey of STD/HIV infection among commercial sex workers in Calcutta (India). Part-IV: sexually transmitted diseases and related risk factors. *Journal of communicable diseases*, 26: 197–202.

Pandit DD, Angadi SA, Chavan MK et al. (1995) Prevalence of VDRL sero-positivity in women in reproductive age group in an urban slum community in Bombay. *Indian journal of public health*, 39: 4–7.

Passey M, Mgone CS, Lupiwa S et al. (1998) Community based study of sexually transmitted diseases in rural women in the highlands of Papua New Guinea: prevalence and risk factors. *Sexually transmitted infections*, 74: 120–127.

Paxton LA, Kiwanuka N, Nalugoda F et al. (1998a) Community based study of treatment seeking among subjects with symptoms of sexually transmitted disease in rural Uganda. *British medical journal*, 317: 1630–1631.

Paxton LA, Sewankambo N, Gray R et al. (1998b) Asymptomatic non-ulcerative genital tract infections in a rural Ugandan population. *Sexually transmitted infections*, **74**: 421–425.

Poma PA (1999) Effects of obstetrician characteristics on cesarean delivery rates. a community hospital experience. *American journal of obstetrics and gynecology*, **180**: 1364–1372.

Ronsmans C, Bulut A, Yolsal N et al. (1996) Clinical algorithms for the screening of Chlamydia trachomatis in Turkish women. *Genitourinary medicine*, **72**: 182–186.

Ross DA, Vaughan JP (1986) Health interview surveys in developing countries: a methodological review. *Studies in family planning*, **17**: 78–94.

Sackett DL, Haynes RB, Guyatt GH et al. (1991) *Clinical epidemiology: a basic science for clinical medicine*, 2nd edn. Boston, Little, Brown and Company.

Schachter J (1998) Chlamydia trachomatis: the more you look, the more you find – how much is there? *Sexually transmitted diseases*, **25**: 229–231.

Schulz KF, Cates WJ, O'Mara PR (1987) Pregnancy loss, infant death, and suffering: legacy of syphilis and gonorrhoea in Africa. *Genitourinary medicine*, **63**: 320–325.

Sewankambo N, Gray RH, Wawer MJ et al. (1997) HIV-1 infection associated with abnormal vaginal flora morphology and bacterial vaginosis. *Lancet*, **350**: 546–550.

Singer A (1975) The uterine cervix from adolescence to the menopause. *British journal of obstetrics and gynaecology*, **82**: 81–99.

Singer A, Jordan JA (1976) The anatomy of the cervix. In: Jordan JA and Singer A, eds. *The cervix*, pp. 13–36. London, WB Saunders Company Ltd.

Stary A, Najim B, Lee HH (1997) Vulval swabs as alternative specimens for ligase chain reaction detection of genital chlamydial infection in women. *Journal of clinical microbiology*, **35**: 836–838.

Tabrizi SN, Paterson BA, Fairley CK et al. (1998) Comparison of tampon and urine as self-administered methods of specimen collection in the detection of Chlamydia trachomatis, Neisseria gonorrhoeae and Trichomonas vaginalis in women. *International journal of STD and AIDS*, **9**: 347–349.

Tiwara S, Passey M, Clegg A et al. (1996) High prevalence of trichomonal vaginitis and chlamydial cervicitis among a rural population in the highlands of Papua New Guinea. *Papua New Guinea medical journal*, **39**: 234–238.

Wagner HU, Van Dyck E, Roggen E et al. (1994) Seroprevalence and incidence of sexually transmitted diseases in a rural Ugandan population. *International journal of STD and AIDS*, **5**: 332–337.

Wasserheit JN (1989) The significance and scope of reproductive tract infections among third world women. *Supplement to International journal of gynecology and obstetrics*, **3**: 145–168.

Wasserheit JN, Harris JR, Chakraborty J et al. (1989) Reproductive tract infections in a family planning population in rural Bangladesh. *Studies in family planning*, **20**: 69–80.

Wawer MJ, McNairn D, Wabwire-Mangen F et al. (1995) Self-administered vaginal swabs for population-based assessment of Trichomonas vaginalis prevalence [letter]. *Lancet*, **345**: 131–132.

Wawer MJ, Gray RH, Sewankambo NK et al. (1998) A randomized, community trial of intensive sexually transmitted disease control for AIDS prevention, Rakai, Uganda. *AIDS*, **12**: 1211–1225.

Wawer MJ, Sewankambo NK, Serwadda D et al. (1999) Control of sexually transmitted diseases for AIDS prevention in Uganda: a randomised community trial. *Lancet*, **353**: 525–535.

WHO Study Group on Management of Sexually Transmitted Diseases in Patients (1991) *Management of patients with sexually transmitted diseases.* Geneva, World Health Organization.

Wi T, Mesola V, Manalastas R et al. (1998) Syndromic approach to detection of gonococcal and chlamydial infections among female sex workers in two Philippine cities. *Sexually transmitted infections*, **74**(Suppl. 1): S118–S122.

Wilkinson C, McIlwaine G, Boulton-Jones C et al. (1998) Is a rising caesarean section rate inevitable? *British journal of obstetrics and gynaecology*, **105**: 45–52.

World Health Organization (1992a) *ICD-10. International statistical classification of diseases and related health problems*, 10th Revision. Geneva, World Health Organization.

World Health Organization (1992b). *The management of sexually transmitted diseases.* WHO Technical Report Series 810. Geneva, World Health Organization.

World Health Organization (1995). *Manual for the standardization of colposcopy for the evaluation of vaginally administered products.* Geneva, World Health Organization.

Younis N, Khattab H, Zurayk H et al. (1993) A community study of gynecological and related morbidities in rural Egypt. *Studies in family planning*, **24**: 175–186.

Zurayk H, Khattab H, Younis N et al. (1995) Comparing women's reports with medical diagnoses of reproductive morbidity conditions in rural Egypt. *Studies in family planning*, **26**: 14–21.

9

Laboratory tests for the detection of reproductive tract infections

Jane Kuypers[1] and World Health Organization Regional Office for the Western Pacific[2]

[1] University of Washington, Seattle, USA; [2] WHO, Manilla, Philippines

Valid laboratory assays for the detection of reproductive tract infections are necessary to confirm suspected reproductive tract infections in symptomatic individuals, identify infections in asymptomatic individuals, investigate cases of resistance to usual treatment, monitor the evolution of pathogen sensitivity to antimicrobial agents and conduct research on reproductive tract infection prevalence and incidence. An optimal laboratory test for the diagnosis of infection should be simple to perform, sensitive, specific, reproducible, objective, rapid, inexpensive and should require no special equipment.

In recent years, new methods to detect reproductive tract infections have been developed using sophisticated molecular biology techniques. Molecular detection techniques do not rely on the ability to culture or directly observe intact organisms but are designed to detect specific cellular antigens or nucleic acids. Therefore, because viable and nonviable microorganisms can be detected, stringent transport requirements for clinical samples are no longer needed. The development of molecular detection assays has led to the ability to use one sample for the detection of many organisms, to test for multiple organisms in one assay and to automate assays. Due to their extreme sensitivity, newly developed nucleic acid amplification systems allow the use of samples obtained by noninvasive methods, including patient self-sampling and urine collection. In addition, certain assays are used to determine the number of nucleic acid copies in a sample. Some of these new molecular methods meet many of the criteria for optimal tests and have improved the diagnosis of reproductive tract infections. In other cases, older, conventional assays (for instance, microscopy, culture and antibody detection) remain valid and should still be used. Deciding which tests to perform depends on many factors, including the facilities and funds available for specimen collection, transport and analysis, the expertise of the laboratory personnel and the research goals.

This chapter is a summary of up-to-date, state-of-the-art laboratory methods that are useful for the detection of 11 reproductive tract infections.[1] The types of assays described fall into several categories, including detection of organisms by direct microscopy and culture, detection of metabolic products, and the detection of specific antibodies, antigens, DNA or RNA. Not all organisms can be detected using all types of assays, nor can all laboratories perform all types of assays. For each organism discussed, a table is included that describes its sensitivity and specificity, advantages and disadvantages, and the appropriate level of use of each method. The level of use has been divided into four settings, including the exam room, on-site lab, intermediate lab and referral lab, and is based on the complexity of the training and equipment required, and on the ease of performance. Each table also includes the indicative cost of reagents (at current rates in the US) for each method. The sensitivity and specificity of an assay will vary depending on the method used as the 'gold standard'. The assay sensitivity and specificity figures in this chapter are based on a range of values taken from many different sources, including all types of patient populations.

The general techniques for the molecular assays described in this chapter are included as footnotes. Detailed instructions for carrying out each test can be found in the manufacturer's manual accompanying each test kit and should be strictly adhered to. Specific kits are used as examples of particular types of assays; however, their inclusion in this chapter does not indicate an endorsement of the product.

Laboratory tests for specific diseases

Candidiasis

Candida is a commensal yeast commonly found in the normal vaginal microbial flora. While most colonized women show no symptoms of infection, in some, colonization progresses to symptomatic disease. Laboratory confirmation is often necessary to diagnose vaginal candidiasis in cases where symptoms are nonspecific. Infection is usually, but not always, associated with higher numbers of yeast organisms and the presence of the mycelial form, together with an inflammatory response. However, the relationship between the number of organisms and infection is not clear (Evans, 1990). Although the number of yeast organisms may be changed, the normal microbial flora of Gram-positive rods of lactobacillus and diptheroid species remain unchanged.

Detection by microscopy

A swab of the vaginal secretions is placed in saline and the evaluation for yeast is carried out immediately by adding a drop to a slide and mixing it with a drop of potassium hydroxide solution. The potassium hydroxide lyses the patient's cells,

---

[1] An earlier version of this summary was published by the WHO Regional Office for the Western Pacific in 1999.

making the yeast easier to see. Alternatively, the swab is rolled onto a slide, which is fixed and Gram stained. This slide does not have to be stained or evaluated immediately. Both slides are examined under a light microscope for the presence of the yeast or mycelial form of candida and for an inflammatory response. Both the wet mount and Gram stain of vaginal secretions can also be used for the detection of other organisms (see the sections on trichomoniasis and bacterial vaginosis). While microscopy is rapid and inexpensive, it is also insensitive and subjective.

Detection by culture

A swab of the vaginal secretions or an aliquot of a vaginal wash is inoculated onto agar within a few hours of collection and incubated for up to two days at 37 °C. Colonies are identified as yeast by performing a Gram stain. The quantity of yeast is determined, with more than 10^3 colony-forming units (cfu)/ml of vaginal secretions usually being associated with disease. Culture takes longer than microscopy but is more sensitive for the detection of disease.

Detection of candida antigen

A swab of vaginal secretions or a drop of vaginal wash is mixed on a slide with a commercially available solution of latex beads that are coated with an antibody to the major constituent of the candida cell wall, which is found in the vagina when candida are present (SuperDuo, Mercia Diagnostics, Guildford, England). The antigen–antibody complexes are observed as agglutination of the suspension. Although this kit is more expensive than microscopy and culture, it is rapid and simple to use and contains latex beads for the detection of *Trichomonas vaginalis* from the same sample.

Detection of candida DNA

Candida DNA is directly detected in a vaginal swab sample using a commercially available, 40-minute, automated DNA probe hybridization assay (Affirm VP3 Microbial Identification Test, Becton-Dickinson Diagnostic Systems, Sparks, MD, USA) (DeMeo et al., 1996; Table 9.1). *Trichomonas vaginalis* and *Gardnerella vaginalis* DNA can also be detected in the same sample.[2] Samples are collected with a swab, placed in the collection tube supplied in the kit, stored at 4 °C and tested within 24 hours. This method is both rapid and objective, and the automation allows easy testing of large numbers of samples for three different organisms.

---

[2] Pathogen-specific, oligonucleotide DNA probes are coupled to nylon beads, which are embedded in a dipstick to form a probe-analysis card. The sample is placed in a lysis solution and heated to release DNA into the solution. A hybridization buffer is added and the sample solution is hybridized to the probe that is attached to the beads on the card. The card is moved through wells containing a wash buffer, a second probe that is biotin-labelled and hybridizes to the target DNA captured on the beads, and reagents that react with the biotin to produce a colour change in positive samples.

Table 9.1. Characteristics of candida detection assays

	Microscopy	Culture		DNA detection
	Wet mount	>10^3 cfu/ml	Antigen detection	Affirm VP3
Sensitivity[a]	35–45%	67%	61–81%	80%
Specificity[a]	99%	66%	97%	98%
Advantages	Rapid, inexpensive	Sensitive	Rapid, also detects trichomonas	Rapid, objective, also detects trichomonas and gardnerella
Disadvantages	Subjective	Requires 24 hours	Expensive	Expensive, requires special equipment and test read immediately after completion
Level of use	Exam room, on-site lab.	On-site lab., intermediate lab.	Exam room, on-site lab.	Intermediate lab., referral lab
Training	Moderate	Moderate	Minimal	Moderate
Equipment	Light microscope	Incubator, light microscope	None	Heat block, special processor
Ease of performance	Easy	Moderate	Easy	Easy to moderate, automated
Cost	US$1.00	US$2.00	US$12.00 (includes detection of trichomonas)	US$12.00 (includes detection of trichomonas and gardnerella

Note:
[a] Sensitivity and specificity are for clinical signs and symptoms of vulvovaginal candidiasis.

Trichomoniasis

Trichomonas vaginalis is a parasitic protozoan that causes vaginal inflammation. Infection with trichomonas can range from severe vaginitis with discharge to asymptomatic carriage. Since asymptomatic carriage can account for as many as 50 per cent of cases, diagnosis cannot be made solely on the basis of clinical presentation (Petrin et al., 1998). Laboratory detection of the parasite is required to confirm diagnosis.

See Table 9.2 for a summary of characteristics of trichomonas detection assays.

Table 9.2. Characteristics of trichomonas detection assays

	Microscopy	Culture	Antigen detection		DNA detection	
			Immunoassay	Latex agglutination	Hybridization assay Affirm VP3	Polymerase chain reaction
Sensitivity[a]	38–82%	98%	86%	80–85%	88–91%	93%
Specificity[a]	100%	100%	99%	99%	100%	96%
Advantages	Rapid, inexpensive	Sensitive diagnosis in men	Rapid	Rapid	Rapid, objective, also detects gardnerella and candida	Very sensitive, allows patient self-sampling
Disadvantages	Low sensitivity, must be performed immediately, subjective	Takes 1–4 days	Expensive	Expensive	Expensive, requires special equipment and test read immediately after completion	Expensive, requires expertise
Level of use	Exam room on-site lab.	On-site lab, intermediate lab.	On-site lab.	Exam room, on-site lab.	Intermediate, referral lab.	Referral lab.
Training	Moderate	Moderate	Moderate	Minimal	Moderate	Extensive
Equipment	Light microscope	Incubator, light microscope	Light or fluorescent microscope	None	Heat block, special processor	Thermal cycler, microwell plate reader
Ease of performance	Easy	Easy	Moderate	Easy	Easy to moderate automated	Complex, automated
Cost	US$1.00	US$3.00	US$6.00	US$12.00 (includes detection of candida)	US$12.00 (includes detection of candida and gardnerella)	US$11.00

Note:

[a] Sensitivity and specificity are for detection of *Trichomonas vaginalis* by combined wet prep and culture results.

Detection by microscopy

Direct microscopic observation of characteristic motile parasites is made from a swab of vaginal secretions, which is placed in a saline solution. A drop of the solution is immediately placed on a slide with a coverslip and observed under a light microscope. As with microscopy for candidiasis, this method is rapid and inexpensive but has low sensitivity.

Detection by culture

A swab of secretions taken from the posterior vaginal fornix is used within 6 hours of sample collection to inoculate a tube of Trichosel or modified Diamond's culture medium. The culture is incubated at 35 °C for up to 4 days with daily examination by wet mount (see the section on Detection by Microscopy for Motile Trichomonads). A commercially available culture system (InPouch TV Culture System, Biomed, San Jose, CA, USA) with a self-contained, two-chambered bag permits, after inoculation with the swab, both incubation of the culture and an immediate wet mount by microscopic examination through the upper chamber of the bag (Levi et al., 1997). Although culture is both sensitive and specific, the disadvantage is that it can take up to 4 days to obtain a result.

Detection of *T. vaginalis* antigens

Trichomonas vaginalis antigens are detected using the Trichomonas Direct Enzyme Immunoassay or Direct Fluorescent Immunoassay (California Integrated Diagnostics, Bernicia, CA, USA). A swab of vaginal secretions is rolled onto a glass slide and air-dried in the examination room. In this one-hour procedure, labelled antibodies to various *T. vaginalis* antigens are added to the slide and detected using substrates that change colour or fluoresce. Slides are examined under a light microscope for the colorimetric assay and under a fluorescent microscope for the fluorescent assay.

Another method uses a swab of vaginal secretions or a drop of vaginal wash mixed on a slide with a commercially available solution of latex beads that are coated with antibodies to *T. vaginalis* antigens (SuperDuo). The antigen–antibody complexes are observed as agglutination of the suspension. The kit also contains latex beads for the detection of candida antigens in the same sample.

Detection of *T. vaginalis* DNA

Trichomonas vaginalis DNA is directly detected in a vaginal swab sample using a commercially available, 40-minute, automated DNA probe hybridization assay (Affirm VP3 Microbial Identification Test) (DeMeo et al., 1996). The assay will also detect candida and a high level of *G. vaginalis* DNA in the same sample.[3] The

---

[3] See note 12.

sample is collected with a swab and placed in the collection tube supplied by the kit, stored at 4°C and tested within 24 hours.

Amplification and detection of *T. vaginalis* DNA

A polymerase chain reaction (PCR) DNA amplification assay[4] for *T. vaginalis* has been reported (van Der Schee et al., 1999) but is not yet commercially available. Several sample collection methods have been tested including urine from men and women, a self-administered swab of the vaginal introitus, and a technique in which the patient inserts, then immediately withdraws, a tampon (commercially available). The swab and tampon samples are placed into transport media and can be tested for up to one month following collection. The *T. vaginalis* DNA fragment is labelled during amplification and detected using hybridization with a DNA probe in a semi-automated assay (Enzymun-Test DNA Detection Assay, Boehringer Mannheim, Mannheim, Germany).[5] The use of PCR amplification and detection methods, although very sensitive, requires extensive training and special equipment.

Bacterial vaginosis

Bacterial vaginosis is a condition in which the natural balance of organisms found in the vagina is changed from a predominance of lactobacillus to an overgrowth of other bacteria including *G. vaginalis*, mobiluncus and other anaerobes (Hillier, 1993).

See Table 9.3 for a summary of the characteristics of bacterial vaginosis detection assays.

Detection by microscopy and/or metabolic products

The most widely accepted method for diagnosis of bacterial vaginosis is the presence of three of the following four criteria: a homogeneous vaginal discharge; a vaginal pH of greater than 4.5; clue cells; and a fishy odour after the addition of

---

[4] A PCR mix contains salts, magnesium, *Taq* DNA polymerase, deoxynucleotide triphosphates (dNTP) and paired oligonucleotide DNA primers designed so that they hybridize to opposite strands of the target DNA, usually between 100 to 800 base-pairs apart. For some procedures, degenerate primers are used. These are mixtures of oligonucleotides the sequences of which differ from each other by one or more bases. They are used to amplify consensus regions of DNA found among related strains or variants of microorganisms. The PCR takes place in a thermal cycler that incubates the reaction mix through 30 to 40 cycles of three temperature steps of denaturation, annealing and extension. DNA is synthesized in both directions to produce a double-stranded piece that has one primer sequence on each end. One of the primers or one of the dNTPs can be labelled with a protein to facilitate later detection of the synthesized fragment (amplicon). Each time a cycle is repeated, the number of amplicon copies is doubled. In this way, one copy of a target DNA can be amplified over a million-fold. The reaction can include a second primer pair to amplify a human DNA sequence (internal control, such as β-globin) to determine if the sample has an adequate amount of DNA for analysis and if the sample contains inhibitors of PCR. Amplicons are usually detected using oligonucleotide probes that bind to sequences on the amplicon that are internal to the primers.

[5] The DNA detection assay uses digoxigenin-labelled dUTP in the reaction mixture to label the amplicons during PCR amplification. The labelled amplicons are hybridized with a target-specific biotin-labelled probe, captured in microwells coated with streptavidin, and detected with an enzyme-labelled anti-digoxigenin antibody and a colorimetric substrate to the enzyme. The absorbance values of the wells are read in a microwell plate reader. The detection can be automated using the ES 300 analyzer.

potassium hydroxide to the vaginal secretions (the amine test) (Hillier, 1993). After evaluation of discharge and pH, a swab of vaginal fluid is obtained from the posterior fornix, placed in saline and used immediately for the following two tests.

- A drop is placed on a slide and examined under a light microscope for the presence of clue cells, which are epithelial cells heavily coated with bacteria so that the peripheral borders are obscured. Samples are generally considered positive for bacterial vaginosis if clue cells comprise more than 20 per cent of all epithelial cells.
- A drop is placed on a slide with a drop of potassium hydroxide solution. The release of amines produces a fishy odour.

A simpler and more specific assay is a Gram stain of a vaginal smear. A swab of vaginal secretions is rolled onto a glass slide and air-dried. The sample is stable for days at ambient temperature. The slide is Gram stained and a standardized 0–10 point scoring method is used to evaluate the smear (Nugent, Krohn and Hillier, 1991). Points are given by estimating the number of three different bacterial morphotypes from 0 to 4+, including large Gram-negative rods, small Gram-negative/variable rods and curved Gram-negative/variable rods. The biggest disadvantage of the Gram stain technique is that interpretation of the slides is subjective and learning to read them accurately requires careful training.

The proline aminopeptidase test (Schoonmaker et al., 1991) is an indirect test for a chemical produced by the organisms associated with bacterial vaginosis. A vaginal swab from the posterior fornix is placed into normal saline and can be held at 4°C for up to 4 hours and then frozen until testing. Samples can be shipped on ice. Vaginal secretions are added to a substrate and incubated for 4 hours. A colour change denotes the test result. This assay, which is not commercially available, is less subjective than Gram stain but takes longer to obtain a result.

Detection of *G. vaginalis* DNA

High concentrations of *G. vaginalis* DNA are directly detected in a vaginal swab sample using a commercially available, 40-minute, automated DNA probe hybridization assay (Affirm VP3 Microbial Identification Test) (Briseldon and Hillier, 1994). The assay will also detect candida and *T. vaginalis* DNA in the same sample.[6] Samples are collected with a swab and placed in the collection tube supplied with the kit, stored at 4°C and tested within 24 hours.

Chlamydiosis

Chlamydia trachomatis is an important cause of urethritis and cervicitis. Laboratory detection of *C. trachomatis* is necessary because as many as 70–80 per cent of women and up to 50 per cent of men who are infected do not experience

---

[6] See note 12.

Table 9.3. Characteristics of bacterial vaginosis detection assays

	Microscopy and metabolic product detection			DNA detection
	3 of 4 criteria	Gram stain	Proline aminopeptidase	Hybridization assays Affirm VP3
Sensitivity[a]	81%	89%	93%	94%
Specificity[a]	94%	93%	93%	81%
Advantages	Rapid, inexpensive	Reproducible, standardized, inexpensive	Objective	Objective, can also detect candida and trichomonas
Disadvantages	Subjective, some criteria nonspecific	Requires expertise	Takes longer than wet mount or stain	Expensive, requires special equipment, test read immediately after completion
Level of use	Exam room, on-site lab.	On-site lab.	On-site lab., intermediate lab.	Intermediate lab., referral lab.
Training	Moderate	Moderate	Minimal	Moderate
Equipment	Light microscope	Light microscope	Centrifuge, incubator	Heat block, special processor
Ease of performance	Easy	Easy	Easy	Easy to moderate, automated
Cost	US$1.00	US$0.50	US$1.00	US$12.00 (includes detection of candida and trichomonas)

Note:

[a] Sensitivity and specificity are for the diagnosis of bacterial vaginosis by the presence of three or four criteria and/or positive Gram stain.

any symptoms. Untreated, infected individuals transmit chlamydial infections to sexual partners and are at risk for sequelae such as epididymitis in men and pelvic inflammatory disease and infertility in women (Black, 1997).

Detection by culture

The conventional method for the laboratory diagnosis of *C. trachomatis* has been inoculation of a cell culture with a genital specimen. This method is expensive, labour-intensive and time-consuming. It requires considerable expertise to perform correctly and meticulous handling of the specimen during transport to maintain viable organisms. For these reasons, culture tests are now used less frequently and antigen and nucleic acid detection techniques, which do not require viable organisms, have become common methods for the detection of *C. trachomatis* infection, allowing testing in laboratories that lack the facilities for tissue cell culture (Black, 1997).

Detection of host response

The leukocyte esterase (LE) assay is a rapid, nonspecific urine dipstick test for the presence of inflammation. The LE test can diagnose urethritis but cannot identify the specific cause of the infection. The sensitivity and specificity of LE for the detection of chlamydial and gonococcal infections vary widely from 54–97 per cent and 36–95 per cent, respectively. The LE test performs best as a screening test for chlamydial infection in asymptomatic adolescent and young men with positive tests confirmed by enzyme immunoassay for chlamydial antigen (see section on Dectection of *C. trachomatis* antigens) (Bowden, 1998).

Detection by microscopy (Table 9.4)

In the direct immunofluorescence assay (DFA), urethral or endocervical epithelial cells collected on swabs are rolled onto glass slides and stained with labelled antibodies specific for *C. trachomatis*. DFA allows for the visualization of the distinctive morphology and staining characteristics of chlamydial inclusions and elementary bodies. It also permits simultaneous assessment of the specimen adequacy. For all chlamydial detection assays, samples must contain urethral or endocervical cells and not exudate. The presence of 10 or more elementary bodies is generally accepted for the test to be positive. DFA is useful as a confirmatory test for samples found positive by antigen and nucleic acid detection assays (see sections on Detection of *C. trachomatis* antigens, and DNA and RNA) (Black, 1997).

Detection of *C. trachomatis* antigens (Table 9.4)

A common test for genital *C. trachomatis* infection is the detection of chlamydial specific antigens in cervical and urethral swab specimens using any of several

Table 9.4. Characteristics of *Chlamydia* detection assays

	Microscopy	Antigen detection		RNA detection	DNA amplification and detection	
	DFA	EIA	Rapid	PACE 2C	PCR	LCR
Sensitivity[a]	74–90%	71–87%	52–85%	75–85%	99%	90–97%
Specificity[a]	98–99%	97–99%	>95%	98–99%	99–100%	99–100%
Advantages	Rapid, easy	Can batch samples	Rapid, easy	Automated	Internal control for inhibitors; Allow noninvasive sampling from both men and women	Less affected by inhibitors
Disadvantages	Labour-intensive, subjective	Requires confirmation	Insensitive, requires confirmation	Less sensitive than PCR, requires confirmation	False positives and negatives	No test for sample inhibitors
Level of use	On-site lab., intermediate	Intermediate, referral lab.	Exam room, on-site lab.	Intermediate, referral lab.	Intermediate, referral lab.	Intermediate, referral lab.
Training	Moderate to extensive	Moderate	Minimal	Moderate	Moderate to extensive	Moderate
Equipment	Fluorescent microscope	Microwell plate reader	None	Heat block, luminometer	Thermal cycler, incubator, microwell plate reader	Thermal cycler, LCx processor
Ease of performance	Moderate	Moderate	Easy	Moderate	Moderate to difficult, automated	Moderate, automated
Cost	US$6.00	US$6.00	US$13.00–16.00	US$8.00	US$1.00 (US$14.00 for *Neisseria gonorrhoeae* detection also)	US$16.00

Note:

[a] Sensitivity and specificity are for detection of *Chlamydia trachomatis* by culture or by DNA amplification.

commercially-available enzyme immunoassay (EIA) kits (Black, 1997). Because chlamydial antibodies may cross-react with other bacteria to give false-positive results, blocking assays are needed to confirm positive EIA results and thus improve specificity.[7] Confirmation can also be done by performing a direct fluorescent antibody assay on the centrifuged specimen.

Rapid immunodot or latex agglutination assays are simple tests in which the swab sample is mixed with chlamydia antibody-coated particles on a membrane or card. The antigen–antibody complexes are observed visually as agglutination. These tests are rapid and easy to perform. However, they are subject to the same potential for false-positive results due to cross-reactivity with other bacteria, and are generally less sensitive and specific than EIA (Black, 1997).

Detection of *C. trachomatis* RNA and DNA (Table 9.4)

Chlamydia trachomatis RNA is detected by hybridization with a DNA probe (PACE 2C, GenProbe, San Diego, CA, USA).[8] A probe competition assay has been developed to confirm positive samples. The kit can be used to detect *Neisseria gonorrhoeae* RNA in the same sample. Endocervical swabs and urethral swabs can be tested. Specimen collection kits containing swabs and transport medium, which lyse the organisms and release the RNA, are provided by the manufacturer. No stringent transportation conditions are required and the samples are stable at ambient temperature for one month (Black, 1997).

Chlamydia trachomatis DNA is detected by hybridization with an RNA probe using a new nucleic acid signal amplification-based test (Hybrid Capture II, Digene Diagnostics, Gaithersburg, MD, USA) (Schachter et al., 1999). The assay simultaneously detects *N. gonorrhoeae* DNA in the same sample. Positive specimens are then retested with individual probes. This test employs a special conical shaped brush for cervical specimen collection.

Amplification and detection of *C. trachomatis* DNA and RNA (Table 9.4)

A PCR amplification assay for *C. trachomatis* DNA is commercially available (AMPLICOR, Roche Diagnostics, Branchburg, NJ, USA) (Puolakkainen et al.,

---

[7] In direct EIA, LPS (lipopolysaccharide) extracted from elementary bodies in the specimen binds to microwells. The bound antigen is detected with enzyme-labelled antibodies that recognize all species of chlamydia. In indirect EIA, a primary mouse anti-LPS antibody is used to bind the LPS extracted from the sample and then a second enzyme-labelled anti-mouse IgG antibody is added to the wells. Detection of the enzyme-labelled antibodies is performed using a substrate that changes colour and by measuring the absorbance in a spectrophotometer. To confirm a positive test, the EIA is repeated in the presence of non-labelled monoclonal antibodies to chlamydial LPS, which block LPS binding to the enzyme-labelled antibody. A reduced signal with the addition of the blocking antibody is interpreted as confirmation of the positive EIA result.

[8] Cells in the swab samples are lysed to release 16S rRNA that is hybridized to an acridine ester-labelled single-stranded DNA probe. Unhybridized probe is hydrolyzed in a hybridization protection assay. The chemiluminescence of the hybridized sample is read in a luminometer.

1998). The kit also amplifies *N. gonorrhoeae* DNA from the same sample and detects it in a separate hybridization well. To prevent false-negative results due to inhibitors of the amplification reaction in the patient samples, this kit includes an internal standard that is amplified in the same reaction tube and detected in a separate hybridization well.[9]

Another DNA amplification technique for *C. trachomatis* detection is ligase chain reaction (LCR) (Abbott Laboratories, Abbott Park, IL, USA).[10] The amplified products are detected in an automated instrument that is designed to minimize false-positive samples due to contamination from carry-over (Puolakkainen et al., 1998). The enzymes used in LCR are not as sensitive as the enzymes in PCR to inhibitors in the sample. A kit is available that also amplifies *N. gonorrhoeae* DNA from the same sample.

A third amplification assay for *C. trachomatis* uses transcription-mediated amplification (TMA) of RNA (GenProbe).[11] Amplification and product detection take place in one tube (Pasternak, Vuorinen and Miettinen, 1997). This method can also be automated and contains an internal control to test for reaction inhibitors.

PCR, LCR and TMA are excellent tests for the detection of *C. trachomatis* not only in endocervical and urethral swabs but also in urine samples from both men and women. In addition, other noninvasive specimen collection methods such as self-collected vaginal introitus swabs or tampons can be tested. Specimen collection

---

[9] The PCR mixture contains two biotinylated primer pairs, one each for amplification of *C. trachomatis* and *N. gonorrhoeae* DNA. The internal control DNA, which is a synthetic DNA fragment containing identical primer binding sequences and an internal sequence distinct from the *C. trachomatis* amplicon, is added to each reaction. The amplicons are detected in three separate microwells, each containing an immobilized oligonucleotide probe that captures a specific amplicon. The detection kits are purchased separately. The biotinylated captured amplicons are detected using enzyme-labelled avidin and a colorimetric substrate. A positive signal in the well containing the internal control DNA probe indicates that the sample does not contain inhibitors of the polymerase enzyme. To minimize carry-over contamination of the samples with previously amplified DNA, the kit also contains uracil-N-glycosylase (UNG). During amplification, uracil is incorporated into the amplicons instead of thymidine. During the first step of the amplification reaction, UNG cleaves the uracil-containing DNA so that it cannot be used as a template for DNA synthesis. If the sample is contaminated with DNA from a previous reaction, it will be destroyed and not available for amplification. Both the chlamydia and the CT/NG kits are available in a microwell format and a fully automated format that performs amplification, detection and results reporting.

[10] In the LCR test, two labelled oligonucleotide probes bind to adjacent sites on one strand of the target DNA and two other labelled probes bind to adjacent sites on the opposite strand. One probe of each pair is labelled with fluorescein and the other is labelled with biotin. The gap of one to two nucleotides between the adjacent probes is filled by DNA polymerase and the two probes are joined by ligase. The two ligated probe pairs anneal to each other and form the templates for successive reactions. The reaction is done in a thermal cycler for 30–40 cycles of denaturation, annealing and ligation to produce a logarithmic amplification of the target sequences. The products are detected in an automated instrument. Anti-fluorescein antibody-coated microparticles capture the amplicons that are labelled at one end with fluorescein. Anti-biotin antibody conjugated to an enzyme binds to the opposite, biotin-labelled end of the captured amplicons. A fluorescent substrate is added and the samples are read in the automated processor.

[11] TMA is very similar to NASBA (see note 26). The reaction contains RNA polymerase, reverse transcriptase and two primers to amplify specific sequences of RNA. After initial heating to melt the nucleic acids in the sample, the reaction is isothermal. The RNA amplicons are detected in the same tube as the amplification reaction using a hybridization protection assay in which a single-stranded chemiluminescent DNA probe is added and the RNA:DNA hybrids are protected from hydrolysis (see note 8).

kits are provided by the manufacturers. Swab and tampon samples can be kept at ambient temperature, but urine samples should be refrigerated and are stable for up to 4 days. They will remain stable for up to 60 days when frozen. Although the commercially available PCR and TMA assays have internal controls to identify negative results due to inhibitors, none of the commercial kits provide assessment of specimen adequacy (i.e. a sufficient number of cells for amplification). Nucleic acid amplification assays can usually be automated to facilitate testing large numbers of specimens. A disadvantage of these tests is the high cost for reagents and equipment, especially in low volume settings. PCR, LCR and transcription-mediated amplification (TMA) are all highly sensitive assays. Unless specimens are carefully collected in the clinic, appropriately transported and handled carefully in the laboratory, they are susceptible to contamination and may give false-positive results. For kits, the manufacturer's instructions must be carefully followed and adhered to. For example, to ensure no contamination at the laboratory level, positive-displacement pipettes or plugged pipette tips should be used. For 'in-house' assays, there should be physical separation (in separate rooms) for the various steps of PCR, such as the nucleic acid extraction process, preparation of master mixes and product detection.

Gonorrhoea

Infection of the genital tract with *N. gonorrhoeae* can cause urethritis, cervicitis, proctitis or Bartholinitis. Complications of untreated disease include epididymitis, prostatitis and infertility in men, and pelvic inflammatory disease and infertility in women. Because most cases in females are asymptomatic, detection of infection using laboratory tests is needed to prevent sequelae and transmission to sexual partners and, for pregnant women, to neonates (Gaydos and Quinn, 1999).

See Table 9.5 for a summary of the characteristics of *N. gonorrhea* detection assays.

Detection by microscopy

A smear is made immediately after collecting the specimen by rolling the swab onto a slide, which is Gram stained and viewed under an oil immersion microscope lens. The presence of Gram-negative diplococci inside polymorphonuclear leukocytes in urethral smears from symptomatic men is diagnostic for presumptive gonorrhoea. However, the Gram stain is not as useful for endocervical smears (sensitivity of 50–70 per cent) because the presence of other Gram-negative diplococci makes interpretation difficult (Davies, Low and Ison, 1998).

Detection by host response

The LE is a rapid, nonspecific urine dipstick test for the presence of inflammation. The LE test can diagnose urethritis but cannot identify the specific cause of the

Table 9.5. Characteristics of *Neisseria gonorrhoeae* detection assays

| | Microscopy | Culture | RNA detection | DNA amplification and detection | |
			PACE 2C	PCR	LCR
Sensitivity[a]	90–95%[b]	81–100%	86–100%	89–97%	95–100%
Specificity[a]	98–100%[b]	100%	99%	94–100%	98–100%
Advantages	Rapid, inexpensive	Gold standard, isolates available for further testing	Rapid, viable organisms not required	Viable organisms not required, extremely sensitive, allow non-invasive sampling, can detect *Chlamydia trachomatis* in same sample	
Disadvantages	Insensitive for females	Stringent handling, requires up to 3 days	Expensive	Expensive, requires expertise.	No test for sample inhibitors
Level of use	On-site lab.	On-site lab., intermediate lab.	Intermediate, referral lab.	Intermediate, referral lab.	Intermediate, referral lab.
Training	Moderate	Moderate	Moderate	Moderate to extensive	Moderate
Equipment	Light microscope	Incubator, light microscope	Water bath, luminometer	Microfuge, thermal cycler, incubator, microwell reader	Heat block, thermal cycler, microfuge, Imx processor
Ease of performance	Easy	Moderate	Moderate	Moderate to difficult, automated	Moderate, automated
Cost	US$0.50	US$1.00 (1 to confirm positive isolates)	US$6.00	US$11.00 (US$14.00 for *C. trachomatis* detection also)	US$14.00

Notes:
[a] Sensitivity and specificity are for the detection of *N. gonorrhoeae* in urethral and endocervical samples by culture except for microscopy.
[b] Sensitivity and specificity are for the detection of *N. gonorrhoeae* in urethral and samples by culture of symptomatic men.

infection. The sensitivity and specificity of LE as a marker for chlamydial and gono-coccal infection are 54–97 per cent and 36–95 per cent, respectively. The LE test performs best as a screening test for gonococcal infection in asymptomatic men, with positive tests confirmed by DNA detection, discussed in the section on Detection of *N. gonorrhoeae* DNA (Bowden, 1998).

Detection by culture

The endocervical or urethral swab is used immediately after collection to inoculate a plate of selective media. The agar plate is placed into a plastic, zip-lock bag with a CO_2 generating tablet, rapidly transported to the laboratory and incubated at 35°C for up to 3 days. Typical colonies are tested with a Gram stain, and oxidase and catalase or superoxal tests for presumptive identification of *N. gonorrhoeae* (Davies, Low and Ison, 1998).

To confirm a presumptive culture, the isolated organism is tested for sugar fer-mentation by growth in standard carbohydrate fermentation tubes, or by using any of several rapid, nongrowth methods for confirmation of *N. gonorrhoeae* isolates, including detection of preformed enzymes and agglutination with antibodies. The biggest advantage of performing culture is the ability to assess the antibiotic sus-ceptibility of the isolated organisms.

Detection of *N. gonorrhoeae* antigen

Gonococcal antigen is detected by an enzyme immunoassay that is similar to a Gram stain in sensitivity and specificity for presumptive diagnosis in men, but is less sensitive for endocervical swabs (Davies, Low and Ison, 1998).

Detection of *N. gonorrhoeae* RNA and DNA

Neisseria gonorrhoeae RNA is detected using a 2-hour, DNA probe hybridization assay (PACE 2C, GenProbe) (Ciemens et al., 1997).[12] A probe competition assay has been developed to confirm positive samples. The kit can be used to detect *C. tra-chomatis* RNA in the same sample. Endocervical swabs and urethral swabs can be tested. Specimen collection kits that contain swabs and transport medium, which lyse the organisms and release the RNA, are provided by the manufacturer. *Neisseria gonorrhoeae* DNA is detected by hybridization with an RNA probe using a new nucleic acid signal amplification-based test (Hybrid Capture II, Digene Diagnostics) (Schachter et al., 1999). The assay will simultaneously detect *C. tra-chomatis* DNA in the same sample. Positive specimens are then retested with indi-vidual probes. This test uses a special conical shaped brush for cervical specimen collection from nonpregnant women and swabs from pregnant women. While

[12] See note 8.

these assays are as sensitive as culture, they have the added advantages of being faster and requiring no stringent specimen transportation conditions (samples are stable at ambient temperature for one month). However, they are more expensive, require special equipment and antibiotic susceptibility testing cannot be performed on positive specimens.

Amplification and detection of *N. gonorrhoeae* DNA

A PCR amplification assay for *N. gonorrhoeae* is commercially available (AMPLI-COR, Roche Diagnostics) (Gaydos and Quinn, 1999). The kit also amplifies *C. trachomatis* DNA from the same sample and detects it in a separate hybridization well.[13] To prevent false-negative results due to inhibitors of the amplification reaction in the patient samples, the kit includes an internal standard that is amplified in the same reaction tube and detected in a separate hybridization well.

Another DNA amplification technique for *N. gonorrhoeae* detection is LCR (LCR, Abbott Laboratories).[14] The amplified products are detected in an automated instrument that is designed to minimize false-positive samples due to contamination from carry-over. The enzymes used in LCR are not as sensitive as the enzymes in PCR to inhibitors in the sample (Birkenmeyer and Armstrong, 1992). A kit is available that also amplifies *C. trachomatis* DNA from the same sample.

LCR and PCR are excellent tests for the detection of *N. gonorrhoeae* not only in endocervical and urethral specimens, but also in urine samples from both men and women. In addition, other noninvasive specimen collection methods such as self-collected vaginal introitus swabs or tampons can be tested. Specimen collection kits are provided by the manufacturers. Swab samples and tampons can be kept at ambient temperature, but urine samples should be refrigerated and are stable for up to four days. They will remain stable for up to 60 days when frozen. The same advantages and disadvantages described for the nucleic acid amplification assays used to detect *C. trachomatis* apply to the DNA amplification assays used for *N. gonorrhoeae* detection. As discussed in the section on *C. trachomatis* detection, due to the high sensitivity of DNA amplification methods, special precautions must be taken when collecting, transporting and analyzing specimens to avoid contamination that may give false-positive results.

Syphilis

Syphilis, a chronic infection with clinical manifestations occurring in distinct stages, is caused by the spirochaete *Treponema pallidum*. Since untreated infection can be important in patient outcome (e.g. pregnancy), laboratory tests are essential in the diagnosis of patients with syphilis. This bacterium cannot be cultured in

---

[13] See note 9.   [14] See note 10.

vitro or stained using standard techniques. The rabbit infectivity test is the oldest and most sensitive method to identify infection with *T. pallidum*. While it is not practical for routine laboratory use, it is the standard for measuring the sensitivity of other methods. Routine laboratory methods rely on demonstrating the presence of *T. pallidum* in a characteristic lesion or the presence of antibodies in serum. Not all methods can be used to diagnose all stages of syphilis. For example, the tests for *T. pallidum* are only relevant when lesions are present in primary and secondary syphilis, and antibodies are not present early in disease (1–4 weeks after a primary lesion has formed).

See Table 9.6 for a summary of the characteristics of syphilis detection assays.

Detection by microscopy

Treponema pallidum is detected in primary or secondary lesions by dark-field microscopy. A glass slide is touched to fluid expressed from a lesion or node aspirate, coverslipped, and examined immediately under a light microscope fitted with a dark-field condenser. *Treponema pallidum* is identified by its characteristic morphology and motility. Specimens from oral lesions are not suitable for this method because other spirochaetes normally present in these specimens cannot be distinguished from *T. pallidum* (Larsen, Steiner and Rudloph, 1995).

The direct fluorescent antibody assay detects *T. pallidum* by an antigen–antibody reaction. The organism does not have to be motile for identification. The specimen is obtained in the same way as for dark-field microscopy but the smear is air-dried and fixed. A labelled antibody to *T. pallidum* is added to the smear, which is examined for treponemes displaying typical morphology using a fluorescent microscope (Larsen, Steiner and Rudloph, 1995).

Detection of nontreponemal antibodies

Nontreponemal antibody tests, which are used to screen patients for syphilis, are based on detection of antibodies to a cardiolipid–cholesterol–lecithin antigen (reagin). Undiluted or serial twofold dilutions of patient specimen are added to the antigen on a slide or card. The reagents are then mixed and observed for flocculation. The rapid plasma reagin (RPR) test, in which the antigen is mixed with charcoal so the antigen–antibody complexes can be seen without a microscope, is the most commonly used test for antibodies in serum or plasma. The Venereal Disease Research Laboratory (VDRL) slide test, which is read microscopically, is used to detect antibodies in cerebral-spinal fluid.

For some immunoassays, the reagin is coated onto microwells to capture the antibodies in the patient serum, which are then detected using other antibodies that are labelled with an enzyme (Larsen, Steiner and Rudloph, 1995) or coated onto erythrocytes (Stone et al., 1997).

Table 9.6. Characteristics of syphilis detection assays

	Microscopy	Antibody detection				DNA amplification and detection
	Dark-field	Nontreponemal RPR	Treponemal TP-PA	Antigen detection		Multiplex PCR
Sensitivity[a]	74–86%[b]	72–100%[c, d]	69–90%[c]	81%[b]		91%[b]
Specificity[a]	97–100%[b]	93–98%	98–100%	89%[b]		99%[b]
Advantages	Positive, early, rapid, specific, inexpensive	Inexpensive, rapid, easy, antibody titer to follow treatment	Specific, confirms nontreponemal tests	Detects *Treponema pallidum* before antibodies are positive		Sensitive, specific, allows self-collected sample
Disadvantages	Insensitive, no oral sample	False positives, less sensitive for early disease	More difficult, more expensive	Time consuming, expensive		Inhibitors of PCR reaction cause false-negative results, complex, expensive
Level of use	Exam room, on-site lab.	On-site lab., intermediate lab.	Intermediate lab., referral lab.	Intermediate lab., referral lab.		Referral lab.
Training	Extensive	Minimal	Moderate	Moderate		Extensive
Equipment	Light microscope with dark-field condenser	Centrifuge, rotator	Centrifuge	Spectrophotometer		Microfuge, thermal cycler, incubator, microwell plate reader
Ease of performance	Easy	Easy	Moderate	Moderate		Complex
Cost	US$0.40	US$0.50	US$1.40	US$3.00		US$14.00 (includes detection of *Haemophilus ducreyi* and HSV)

Notes:

[a] Sensitivity and specificity are for the detection of primary syphilis.

[b] The tests for *T. pallidum* are only relevant when lesions are present in primary and secondary syphilis.

[c] The sensitivity of both nontreponemal and treponemal antibody detection increases for the detection of secondary syphilis.

[d] The sensitivity of nontreponemal antibody detection decreases for detection of latent and tertiary syphilis.

A positive nontreponemal antibody test provides a presumptive diagnosis for syphilis and must be confirmed using a specific treponemal antibody test. In addition to their use as screening tests, nontreponemal antibody tests are useful to gauge response to appropriate treatment, as specific treponemal antibody tests, once positive, usually remain so for life. The sensitivity of nontreponemal antibody detection decreases during latent and tertiary syphilis. However, treponemal antibodies are detectable during these stages of infection when lesions are not present (Larsen, Steiner and Rudloph, 1995).

Detection of treponemal antibodies

The fluorescent treponemal antibody absorption test (FTA-ABS) and the *T. pallidum* particle agglutination assay (TP-PA) detect specific antibodies to *T. pallidum*. For FTA-ABS, *T. pallidum* is fixed on a slide and patient serum is added. Labelled antibodies are added and the slide is examined for spirochaetes using a fluorescent microscope.

In TP-PA, gelatin particles are coated with *T. pallidum* antigen, mixed with patient serum or plasma and observed for agglutination.

Immunoassays have also been developed that use *T. pallidum* antigen-coated microwells to capture specific antibodies from the patient serum, which are detected with labelled antibodies (Silletti, 1995).

Detection of *T. pallidum* antigens

Treponema pallidum antigens are detected using an enzyme immunoassay (Cummings et al., 1996). Antigens are extracted within 72 hours of collection from swabs containing lesion exudate.

Amplification and detection of *T. pallidum* DNA and RNA

Treponema pallidum DNA is amplified in a PCR and the specific amplified products detected in a microwell plate hybridization assay.[15] This assay has been described as a multiplex-PCR for the simultaneous amplification of herpes simplex virus and *Haemophilus ducreyi* DNA in the same sample (Orle et al., 1996). Each specific amplified product is detected in a separate well using a different probe.

A highly sensitive reverse transcriptase-PCR assay has been described for the amplification and detection of *T. pallidum* ribosomal RNA. This technique, though not commercially available, is especially useful for the diagnosis of neurosyphilis, where very low numbers of organisms are found (Centurion-Lara et al., 1997).

---

[15] See note 4.

Genital herpes

Herpes simplex virus (HSV) is one of the major causes of genital ulcer disease. Genital herpes infection is usually caused by HSV type 2. Primary infection is followed by latency and variable periods of reactivation. Although clinical diagnosis may be accurate if based on the presence of typical vesicles, up to two-thirds of individuals acquire HSV asymptomatically. Since most infected persons shed the virus during latent, asymptomatic periods, laboratory diagnosis is necessary to detect HSV in asymptomatically infected people to prevent transmission to sexual partners and to children born to infected mothers (Woods, 1995).

See Table 9.7 for a summary of the characteristics of genital herpes detection methods.

Detection by culture

The standard method of HSV detection in symptomatic patients is to inoculate cells in tissue culture with patient specimens. To obtain a specimen, intact vesicles are broken and the lesions are rubbed at their base with a swab, or fluid is extracted from vesicles and immediately placed in transport medium. The sample can be stored at 4 °C for up to 5 days before it is used to inoculate a cell line, although ideally this should be done as soon after collection as possible. Diagnosis is made by observation of a characteristic effect on the cells after incubation for up to one week. The presence of the virus is confirmed by staining the infected cells with antibodies specific for HSV.

A rapid culture and stain method uses a genetically engineered cell-line that is inoculated with a clinical specimen, incubated for 16–24 hours and stained with a solution that causes HSV infected cells to turn blue (Turchek and Huang, 1999). Cells are visualized by light microscopy. This rapid culture method is as sensitive and specific as conventional culture. Although the rapid culture method is faster than the conventional method, it is as expensive, labour-intensive and requires considerable expertise to perform.

Detection of HSV antibodies

Serology is an effective way to diagnose asymptomatic HSV-2 infection. Newly developed enzyme immunoassays are commercially available that specifically detect the presence of HSV-2 antibodies in serum (HSV Type 2 Specific IgG ELISA, Gull Laboratories, Inc., Salt Lake City, UT, USA) (Eis-Hubinger et al., 1999). However, antibody detection is not sensitive during primary infection before the patient has seroconverted.

Detection of HSV antigen

In the DFA and the indirect immunoperoxidase assays, cells are collected from a lesion by rubbing the base well with a swab, concentrated and spotted onto a slide

Table 9.7. Characteristics of genital herpes detection methods

	Culture	Antibody detection EIA	Antigen detection EIA	DNA amplification and detection Multiplex PCR
Sensitivity[a]	Gold standard	96–98%	70–95%	More sensitive than culture
Specificity[a]	100%	96–97%	90–100%	98–100%
Advantages	Sensitive, specific	Detects asymptomatic infection	Rapid, relatively inexpensive, more sensitive than culture for detection in late-stage lesions	Very sensitive, specific, allows self-collected sample
Disadvantages	Expensive, time-consuming, requires expertise	False negative in primary infection before seroconversion	Needs blocking assay to confirm positive results	Inhibitors of PCR cause false-negative results, complex, expensive
Level of use	Referral lab.	Intermediate lab.	Intermediate lab.	Referral lab.
Training	Extensive	Moderate	Moderate	Extensive
Equipment	CO_2 incubator, microscope	Centrifuge, microwell plate reader	Incubator, microwell plate reader	Microfuge, thermal cycler, incubator, microwell plate reader
Ease of performance	Complex	Moderate	Moderate	Complex
Cost	US$40.00	US$4.00–8.00	US$4.00–8.00	US$14.00 (includes detection of *Treponema pallidum* and *Haemophilus ducreyi*)

Note:

[a] Sensitivity and specificity are for the detection of HSV by conventional cell culture.

that is incubated with labelled antibodies. In the DFA, the slide is observed under a fluorescent microscope for the presence of intracellular fluorescence. In the indirect immunoperoxidase assay, the slide is observed under a light microscope. These procedures are insensitive for the detection of HSV compared to culture (Sanders et al., 1998).

An enzyme immunoassay for the detection of HSV antigen is commercially available (HerpChek Direct Herpes Simplex Virus Antigen Test, DuPont Medical Products) (Cone et al., 1993). This assay is as sensitive as culture for HSV detection and much easier to perform. The assay has also been reported to be more sensitive than culture for detection in late-stage lesions. The specimens are collected and transported in a medium supplied by the manufacturer, and the assay can be performed in about 4 hours. Positive specimens should be confirmed using a blocking assay.

Amplification and detection of HSV DNA

HSV DNA is amplified in a PCR and the HSV specific products detected in a microwell plate hybridization assay.[16] This assay is described as a multiplex-PCR for the simultaneous amplification of *T. pallidum* and *H. ducreyi* DNA in the same sample (Orle et al., 1996). Each specific amplified product is detected in a separate well using a different probe. The sensitivity of this method allows for self-collected specimens to be accurately analyzed.

Chancroid

Chancroid is a genital ulcer disease caused by the bacterium *H. ducreyi*. As is also seen in other genital ulcer diseases, inguinal lymphadenopathy is present in about 50 per cent of cases, which sometimes progresses to an inguinal bubo. The accuracy of clinical diagnosis varies due to the atypical presentation of the ulcer.

See Table 9.8 for a summary of the characteristics of chancroid detection assays.

Detection by culture

Before obtaining material for culture, the ulcer base should be exposed and free of pus. Culture material should be obtained from the base or margins of the ulcer with a swab and immediately inoculated directly onto culture plates. *Haemophilus ducreyi* is a fastidious organism and requires special media for growth. Plates are incubated for up to 3 days at 33–35 °C in 5 per cent CO_2 atmosphere. A Gram stain is performed on suspected colonies (Ballard and Morse, 1996). Gram-negative bacilli from colonies compatible with *H. ducreyi* can be identified, based on their growth requirements, by using fluorescent antibodies (see section on Detection of

---

[16] See note 4.

Table 9.8. Characteristics of chancroid detection methods

	Culture	Antigen detection	DNA amplification and detection PCR
Sensitivity	56–90%[a]	Not determined	77–98%[b]
Specificity	100%	Not determined	98–100%
Advantages	Isolates available for further testing	Faster	Very sensitive
Disadvantages	Insensitive, proper medium difficult to obtain	Not commercially available	Inhibitors of PCR cause false-negative results, complex, expensive
Level of use	On-site lab.	Referral lab.	Referral lab.
Training	Moderate	Moderate	Extensive
Equipment	Incubator, light microscope, candle jar	Fluorescent microscope or microwell plate reader	Microfuge, thermal cycler, incubator, microwell plate reader
Ease of performance	Difficult	Moderate	Complex
Cost	US$2.00 (without confirmation)	Not available	US$14.00 (also detects *Treponema pallidum* and HSV)

Note:

[a] The sensitivity of culture varies depending on the type of medium used and can only be estimated since there is no gold standard on which to base the diagnosis of chancroid.

[b] Resolved sensitivity of PCR vs *Haemophilus ducreyi* culture.

H. ducreyi antigen) or by DNA hybridization (Totten and Stamm, 1994). Culture is an insensitive method because of the fastidious growth requirements of this bacterium. However, organisms that are successfully cultured are available for antimicrobial susceptibility testing.

Detection of *H. ducreyi* antigen

Haemophilus ducreyi can be detected in fixed smears of lesional material with an antibody specific for this organism. A second, labelled antibody is added and the slide is examined under a fluorescent microscope (Ballard and Morse, 1996). Other antibodies can detect the organism in genital lesion specimens using an enzyme immunoassay (Roggen et al., 1993). These assays are not commercially available and the sensitivity and specificity for the detection of *H. ducreyi* have not yet been determined.

Amplification and detection of *H. ducreyi* DNA

> *Haemophilus ducreyi* DNA is amplified in a PCR (Orle et al., 1996) and the specific products detected in a microwell plate hybridization assay.[17] Swab samples collected from the genital ulcer or aspirated from the bubo are placed in specimen transport medium and frozen until ready to test. The assay has been described as a multiplex-PCR for the simultaneous amplification of *T. pallidum* and HSV DNA in the same sample. Each specific amplified product is detected in a separate well using a different probe. The PCR assay, unlike culture, does not require meticulous handling of the specimens and in some settings has been shown to be more sensitive than culture.

Donovanosis

> Donovanosis, or granuloma inguinale, is one cause of genital ulcer disease. The disease is caused by *Calymmatobacterium granulomatis*, which can be seen in infected tissue as intracellular bacterial inclusions known as Donovan bodies (Joseph and Rosen, 1994) but cannot be cultured on artificial media. Donovanosis is likely to be confused with other diseases affecting the genital region, making clinical diagnosis difficult. A limited number of laboratory techniques are available to aid in the diagnosis. Some such as immunofluoresence and PCR are not commercially available but are promising methods for future development.
>
> See Table 9.9 for a summary of the characteristics of donovanosis detection assays.

Detection by microscopy

> Diagnosis of donovanosis is made by direct visualization, under a light microscope, of Donovan bodies present in stained tissue sections made from formalin-fixed biopsy specimens (VanDyck and Piot, 1992).
>
> Alternatively, a piece of clean granulation tissue is removed from the leading edge of the genital ulcer with a scalpel and crushed and spread on a slide. A smear can also be made by rolling a swab firmly over the ulcer surface. The collected material is deposited by rolling the swab across a glass slide. The slide is air-dried and stained with Wright-Giemsa stain or a rapid (one minute) staining technique called RapiDiff (Clinical Science Diagnostics Ltd., Booysens, South Africa) (O'Farrell et al., 1990). This technique, although slightly less sensitive, is much faster and easier than examining a formalin-fixed tissue section.

---

[17] See note 4.

Table 9.9. Characteristics of donovanosis detection assays

	Microscopy		Antibody detection	DNA amplification and detection
	Tissue	Swab RapiDiff		PCR
Sensitivity	70–90%	60–80%	Not yet determined	Not yet determined
Specificity	100%	100%	Not yet determined	Not yet determined
Advantages	Very specific	Very specific, rapid	Sensitive	Objective
Disadvantages	Sample collection painful, lengthy	Slightly less sensitive than tissue	Limited sensitivity for early detection	Complex procedure, time-consuming, usefulness not yet determined
Level of use	Intermediate lab., referral lab.	On-site lab., intermediate lab.	Referral lab.	Referral lab.
Training	Extensive	Moderate	Extensive	Extensive
Equipment	Microtome, light microscope	Light microscope	Microtome, fluorescent microscope	Thermal cycler, PAGE apparatus, equipment for DNA sequencing
Ease of performance	Difficult	Easy	Difficult	Complex
Cost	US$7.00–8.00	US$0.50	Not available	Not available

Detection of *C. granulomatis* antibodies

An indirect immunofluorescence technique has been developed (Freinkel et al., 1992). Serological tests are not available for routine use but, when validated, could be used as epidemiological tools.

Amplification and detection of *C. granulomatis* DNA

DNA extracted from biopsy specimens is added to PCR mixtures[18] (Bastian and Bowden, 1996). Detection of *C. granulomatis* by PCR is currently only available as a research tool. It is a complex procedure and its usefulness has not yet been determined.

Human papillomavirus

Human papillomavirus (HPV), a common infection of several genital sites, causes anogenital cancers, most frequently cervical cancer. Although over 80 distinct types of HPV have been identified, only 12–15 types are detected in the majority of genital precancerous and cancerous lesions. The detection of HPV is complicated by the fact that it cannot be identified by conventional viral detection methods such as growth in tissue cell culture or with serological assays. Cytological and histological staining methods have traditionally provided indirect evidence of HPV infection in cervical cell or tissue samples by demonstrating cellular dysplasia, the result of an HPV infection. The most accurate way to demonstrate the presence of an HPV infection is by detection of the viral DNA in the clinical sample. The detection of DNA from HPV types that cause cancer (high risk types) has been shown to be as sensitive, but not as specific, as a Papanicolaou smear for the detection of high-grade cervical dysplasia, the precursor lesion to cervical cancer (Trofatter, 1997).

See Table 9.10 for a summary of the characteristics of HPV detection assays.

Detection by cellular morphology

Epithelial cells are collected from the endocervix and ectocervix using a plastic or wooden spatula, a nylon brush or a Dacron swab. Cells are either rolled onto a glass slide, which is fixed and transported to the laboratory, or placed in a liquid cytology medium (PreservCyt, Cytyc Inc., Boston, MA, USA) and sent to the laboratory for processing into a Thin-prep slide using a special instrument (Cytyc Inc.). Cervical cell samples are stained with the Papanicolaou stain and read by a cytotechnologist and/or pathologist. Particular abnormal cellular morphology is indicative of an HPV infection. To confirm an abnormal smear, a cervical biopsy is obtained that is fixed in formalin and embedded in paraffin. Thin sections are cut, mounted on a slide, stained and examined for abnormal histological morphology.

---

[18] See note 4.

Table 9.10. Characteristics of human papillomavirus (HPV) detection assays

				High-risk HPV DNA detection	
	Cellular morphology	Hybrid capture II		In situ hibridization	PCR + SHARP
Sensitivity	62–85%[a]	64–93%[a]		60–80%[b]	75–95%[a]
Specificity[c]	33–96%	64–68%		80–90%	40–61%
Advantages	Detects HPV disease	Objective		Confirm equivocal histological evaluation	Very sensitive
Disadvantages	False-negative results, expertise required	No cellular morphology		Labour-intensive, low sensitivity	Low specificity for disease
Level of use	Intermediate lab., referral lab.	Intermediate lab., referral lab.		Referral lab.	Referral lab.
Training	Extensive	Moderate		Extensive	Extensive
Equipment	Light microscope	Water bath, shaker, luminometer		Oven, slide incubator, light microscope	Heat block, microcentrifuge, thermal cycler, microwell plate reader
Ease of performance	Difficult	Moderate		Complex	Complex
Cost	US$7.00–8.00	US$22.00		US$26.00	US$8.00

Note:

[a] Sensitivity is for detection of biopsy-confirmed high-grade dyplasia.

[b] Sensitivity is for detection of HPV in tissue confirmed by PCR amplification.

[c] Sensitivity is for detection of biopsy-confirmed high-grade dyplasia.

Both the liquid cytology medium and the formalin-fixed tissue can be used for HPV DNA detection (see following section on Detection of HPV DNA).

Detection of HPV DNA

HPV DNA present in epithelial cells can be detected using a solution hybridization assay. The kit detects DNA from 18 types of HPV using one probe mix that contains probes to five low-risk HPV (not usually found in precancerous lesions) and another probe mix that contains probes to 13 high-risk HPV (associated with precancerous and cancerous lesions) (Hybrid Capture II, Digene Diagnostics).[19] For specimen collection, cervical epithelial cells collected on a swab or conical cytology brush are placed in a tube of transport medium provided with the kit or in a liquid cytology medium (Peyton et al., 1998). Both samples are stable for days at room temperature. Detection of a high-risk HPV type is only predictive of dysplasia. The presence of cervical dysplasia must still be confirmed with histological testing (see section on Detection by cellular morphology).

HPV DNA present in formalin-fixed, paraffin-embedded tissue sections mounted on slides can be detected using an in situ hybridization assay.[20] Individual labelled, high-risk type HPV DNA probes are commercially available for in situ hybridization assays (Dako Corp., Carpinteria, CA, USA). A kit that provides two probe mixes for five high-risk HPV types and the in situ assay reagents is also available (Enzo Diagnostics, Farmington, NY, USA).

Amplification and detection of HPV DNA

For PCR amplification, DNA is extracted from the cervical cell sample and amplified using primers that will amplify most known genital HPV types. After amplification, the products are captured in microwells and identified using two mixtures of DNA probes specific for five low-risk HPV types and nine high-risk HPV types (SHARP Signal System, Digene Diagnostics) (Lorincz, 1996).[21] Because

---

[19] Hybrid Capture II uses full-length genomic HPV RNA probes to hybridize to denatured target HPV DNA sequences in solution. Two probe mixes are supplied. Probe A consists of RNA transcripts of low-risk HPV types 6, 11, 42, 43 and 44. Probe B consists of RNA transcripts of high-risk HPV types 16, 18, 31, 33, 35, 39, 45, 51, 52, 56, 58, 59 and 68. The RNA:DNA hybrids are captured by antibodies immobilized in tubes. The captured hybrids are detected using antibodies conjugated to alkaline phosphatase and the enzyme is detected using a chemiluminescent substrate. The results are read as light units in a luminometer.

[20] Formalin-fixed, paraffin-embedded tissue is dewaxed and rehydrated, then permeabilized with protease. The probe, which is labelled with biotin, is added and allowed to hybridize. The biotin is detected using avidin conjugated to horseradish peroxidase, which is detected using a colorimetric substrate. The rest of the tissue is counterstained. HPV-DNA-positive cells are visualized using a light microscope.

[21] The biotin-labelled PCR amplicons are denatured and added to a tube containing hybridization buffer and either of the two probe mixes. Probe A consists of full-length genomic HPV RNA transcripts of HPV types 6, 11, 42, 43 and 44. Probe B consists of full-length genomic HPV RNA transcripts of HPV types 16, 18, 31, 33, 35, 45, 51, 52 and 56. After hybridization, each sample is transferred to a microwell coated with streptavidin. The streptavidin captures biotin-labelled amplicons and those that are hybridized to an RNA probe are detected using an anti-RNA:DNA antibody that is conjugated to alkaline phosphatase. The enzyme is reacted with a colorimetric substrate and the absorbance values in the wells are read on the microwell plate reader.

of the high analytical sensitivity of the PCR assay, a cervical/vaginal swab or tampon obtained by the patient can be used for specimen collection, eliminating the need for a cervical swab obtained with a speculum in place (Moscicki, 1993). As described earlier, detection of DNA from a high-risk HPV type is predictive of the presence of dysplasia, which must be confirmed by obtaining a cervical biopsy.

Human immunodeficiency virus

Most individuals can be diagnosed as infected with human immunodeficiency virus (HIV) using an assay based on the detection of HIV specific antibodies. For the detection of early infection, before seroconversion occurs, or to detect HIV infection in neonates, assays that detect HIV antigen or HIV DNA or RNA are used. Quantitative HIV RNA assays, while not necessary for the diagnosis of infection, are useful for monitoring disease progression and treatment.

See Table 9.11 for a summary of the characteristics of HIV detection assays.

Detection of HIV antibodies (screening and confirmation assays)

HIV antibodies can be detected in serum samples using any of more than 100 commercially available tests from more than 40 manufacturers. The problems of the 'window phase' of early HIV infection, during which antibodies are not detectable, and the antigenic diversity of the virus strains, have resulted in continual improvements in HIV antibody detection tests since 1985, with some assays being marketed as third and fourth generation (Weber, 1998).

Screening assays for HIV antibody detection include enzyme immunoassays (EIA)[22] and a variety of rapid, simple test devices such as immunodot, line immunoassay, particle agglutination and dipstick.[23] The most sensitive HIV antibody screening tests are antigen sandwich EIA. Most detect both HIV-1 and HIV-2 antibodies in one assay using mixtures of recombinant antigens and synthetic peptides common to all HIV strains. Some EIA not only detect but also differentiate the type

---

[22] Several variations of the sandwich-type capture EIA have been developed for HIV-antibody-detection assays. Second generation assays are usually indirect assays in which the microwells are coated with anti-human IgG antibodies that capture all IgG antibodies from the sample. The HIV-specific antibodies are detected using HIV antigens that are conjugated to an enzyme. The enzyme is detected using a colorimetric substrate and the absorbance is read in a microwell plate reader. Third-generation tests are usually direct sandwich EIA in which the microwells are coated with HIV recombinant antigens and synthetic peptides from the core, env and p24 proteins. The immobilized antigens capture HIV-specific antibodies from the sample, which are then detected using enzyme-labelled antigens or anti-human IgG antibodies. In a double-antigen sandwich EIA, HIV antibodies bind to biotin-labelled and digoxygenin-labelled antigens in solution. The immunocomplexes then bind to streptavidin-coated microwells and are detected with an anti-digoxygenin antibody conjugated to an enzyme.

[23] Rapid simple dot, strip or line immunoassays use membranes, nylon strips or disks that are impregnated with HIV-1 and HIV-2 recombinant antigens and synthetic peptides. The antigens can be combined into a screening assay for the simultaneous detection of antibodies against HIV-1 and HIV-2 or coated separately onto the membrane to distinguish between the types. The HIV antibodies in the sample bind to the antigens and are detected in the same way as for a western blot using enzyme-labelled anti-human IgG.

Table 9.11. Characteristics of HIV detection assays

| | Antibody detection | | Antigen detection | DNA amplification and detection | RNA amplification and detection |
	EIA	Rapid		PCR	Quantitative
Sensitivity	100%	100%	Detect earlier than antibody tests	As sensitive as culture	Earliest detection
Specificity	95.8–100%	99–100%	100%	100%	100%
Advantages	Sensitive, inexpensive, automated	Rapid, no equipment needed	Early detection	Perinatal diagnosis, sensitive	Monitor HIV levels
Disadvantages	False-positive results, no serotyping	Expensive	Insensitive	Expensive, time-consuming	Expensive, time-consuming
Level of use	Intermediate lab.	On-site lab., intermediate lab.	Referral lab.	Intermediate lab., referral lab.	Referral lab.
Training	Moderate	Minimal	Moderate	Moderate	Extensive
Equipment	Centrifuge, microwell plate reader	Centrifuge	Centrifuge, microwell plate reader	Microfuge, thermal cycler, microwell plate reader	Depends on method[a]
Ease of performance	Moderate	Easy	Moderate	Moderate	Extensive
Cost	US$2.00–3.00	US$6.00–7.00	US$4.00–5.00	US$12.00	US$60.00

Note:

[a] For RT-PCR: microfuge, thermal cycler, incubator, microwell plate reader. For DNA: ultracentrifuge, luminometer. For NASB: microfuge, luminometer.

of HIV antibodies present. New fourth generation screening EIA, which permit the simultaneous detection of HIV antigen and antibodies, have been developed, reducing the diagnostic window for HIV infection (Weber et al., 1998).

Simple and rapid immunoassays for HIV antibody detection have been developed that require no special equipment and provide results in a very short time. The majority of these tests are not as sensitive as the best commercial EIA but provide adequate sensitivity. Although rapid, simple tests have not traditionally been used to screen clinical specimens, they can be useful for small-scale testing (Giles, Perry and Parry, 1999).

The western blot (WB) assay has been the standard method for confirmation of specimens positive by screening assays. However, carefully chosen screening assays used in pairs (either a combination of monospecific EIA or EIA plus a rapid test) have been shown to perform at least as well as a screening assay supplemented by WB (Nkengasong et al., 1998).

HIV antibody assays provide sensitivities and specificities with oral specimens comparable to those achieved with serum samples. Oral fluid is collected by dribbling or using one of several commercially available devices that use a chemically treated cotton fibre pad that is placed between the lower gum and cheek. Comparative studies have shown no significant differences in sensitivity between these two methods of oral fluid collection. A special EIA called IgG antibody capture EIA (GAC-EIA) has been developed to optimize antibody detection from oral fluid (Granade et al., 1998).

Whole blood can be collected and dried on filter paper and stored for up to 6 weeks before testing for HIV antibodies. The blood is eluted from the paper and analysed using an EIA (Pappaioanou et al., 1993).

Detection of HIV antigen

The presence of the p24 antigen of HIV-1 in serum is detected by EIA. The specificity of the assay is increased by including an antigen neutralization test to confirm all positive specimens. The p24 antigen assay becomes positive approximately 16 days after the subject becomes infectious (Weber et al., 1999).

Amplification and detection of HIV DNA

A PCR assay is used to detect HIV-1 DNA present in peripheral blood mononuclear cells, which are pelleted from whole blood that is collected in tubes containing EDTA anticoagulant.[24] This assay is as sensitive as HIV culture for diagnosing perinatal HIV infection, and much faster. The assay can be performed on as little as

---

[24] See note 4.

0.1 ml of blood and on dried blood spots. Two commercially-available HIV-1 DNA detection assays use primers and probes that target a highly conserved region of the HIV-1 genome (Fiscus, 1999).[25]

Amplification and quantification of HIV RNA

Several commercial assays are available for the quantification of HIV-1 RNA in peripheral blood. These assays are based on different techniques, including competitive reverse transcriptase-PCR, nucleic acid sequence-based amplification and branched-chain DNA assay.[26] The limit of detection of these assays is 200, 400 and 500 HIV RNA copies/ml of plasma, respectively. All the assays have similar reproducibility and equal reliability and give similar results for HIV-1 clade B subtypes. However, some do not recognize the subtype A or E viruses with equal efficiency. Plasma is a better sample to use than serum, and acid citrate dextrose and EDTA are better anticoagulants in which to collect blood than is heparin (Fiscus, 1999).

[25] One test kit uses biotinylated primers that amplify a 124 base pair region of the HIV-1 *gag* gene. Detection of amplicons is carried out in microwell plates coated with a probe that hybridizes to the HIV-1 *gag* sequences, which are detected using an enzyme-linked colorimetric absorbance assay. Another test detects PCR-amplified HIV-1 *gag* sequences using a hybridization protection assay in which a chemiluminescent acridine ester-labelled RNA probe binds to the amplicons. After hybridization, a base is added, which hydrolyzes any probe that is not hybridized to target DNA, destroying its ability to luminesce. The intensity of the chemiluminescent signal, measured in a luminometer, is proportional to the number of probe:target hybrids.

[26] The RT-PCR assay uses r*Tth* polymerase to reverse transcribe HIV RNA into cDNA and PCR-amplify a 124 base pair fragment of the HIV-1 *gag* gene in the same reaction tube. Quantification is accomplished using a competitive assay in which a known amount of an internal control RNA (IQS) is added to the sample prior to RNA extraction. The HIV-1 primers amplify a similar size fragment from the IQS cDNA but the internal sequences are different. Detection of amplicons is done in separate microwells containing probes for the HIV-1 fragment and for the IQS fragment. The absorbance values of the HIV and IQS wells for each sample are compared and the amount of HIV RNA in the sample can be calculated.

For the branched-chain DNA assay, the virions in the sample are formed into pellets by ultracentrifugation. They are then lysed and the HIV-1 RNA is captured using a probe that hybridizes to the HIV-1 *pol* gene sequences. The signal is amplified by hybridizing branched DNA-amplifier molecules to the immobilized hybrids, then hybridizing multiple enzyme-labelled probes to each branched DNA molecule. Detection is based on light emission of a chemiluminescent substrate.

The nucleic acid sequence-based amplification reaction (NASBA) is able to directly amplify specific sequences of single-stranded RNA. The NASBA reaction mixture contains T7 RNA polymerase, RNase H, reverse transcriptase, nucleoside triphosphates and two specific primers. One end of the first primer is complementary to the target sequence while the other end contains a promoter for the T7 RNA polymerase. In the reaction, the target RNA is transcribed into cDNA, from which the RNA hybrid is hydrolyzed. The cDNA is synthesized to double-stranded DNA and as many as 100 copies of RNA are transcribed from the T7 promoter. The reactions take place at one temperature and become cyclic when each new RNA molecule is available to begin the cycle again. The reaction is made quantitative by adding known amounts of internal standard RNA to the sample. Amplified RNA is detected using labelled probes in a chemiluminescent reaction. The amount of HIV-1 RNA in the sample is calculated from the ratio of the target signal to the signal of the standards.

REFERENCES

Ballard R, Morse S (1996) Chancroid. In: Morse SA, Moucland AA, Holmes KK, eds. *Atlas of STD and AIDS*, pp. 47–63. Baltimore, MD, Mosby-Holtz.

Bastian I, Bowden FJ (1996) Amplification of klebsiella-like sequences from biopsy samples from patients with donovanosis. *Clinical microbiology and infection*, 23: 1328–1330.

Birkenmeyer L, Armstrong AS (1992) Preliminary evaluation of the ligase chain reaction for specific detection of Neisseria gonorrhoeae. *Journal of clinical microbiology*, 30: 3089–3094.

Black CM (1997) Current methods of laboratory diagnosis of *Chlamydia trachomatis* infections. *Clinical microbiology reviews*, 10: 160–184.

Bowden FJ (1998) Reappraising the value of urine leukocyte esterase testing in the age of nucleic acid amplification. *Sexually transmitted diseases*, 25: 322–326.

Briseldon AM, Hillier SL (1994) Evaluation of Affirm VP microbial identification tests for *Gardnerella vaginalis* and *Trichomonas vaginalis*. *Journal of clinical microbiology*, 32: 148–152.

Centurion-Lara AC, Castro C, Shaffer JM et al. (1997) Detection of *Treponema pallidum* by a sensitive reverse transcriptase PCR. *Journal of clinical microbiology*, 35: 1348–1352.

Ciemens EL, Borenstein LA, Dyer IE (1997) Comparisons of cost and accuracy of DNA probe test and culture for the detection of *Neisseria gonorrhoeae* in patients attending public sexually transmitted disease clinics in Los Angeles County. *Sexually transmitted diseases*, 24: 422–428.

Cone RW, Swenson PD, Hobson AC et al. (1993) Herpes simplex virus detection from genital lesions: a comparative study using antigen detection (HerpChek) and culture. *Journal of clinical microbiology*, 31: 1774–1776.

Cummings MC, Lukehart SA, Marra C et al. (1996) Comparison of methods for the detection of Treponema pallidum in lesions of early syphilis. *Sexually transmitted diseases*, 23: 366–369.

Davies PO, Low N, Ison CA (1998) The role of effective diagnosis for the control of gonorrhoea in high prevalence populations. *International journal of STD and AIDS*, 9: 435–443.

DeMeo LR, Draper DL, McGregor JA et al. (1996) Evaluation of a deoxyribonucleic acid probe for the detection of *Trichomonas vaginalis* in vaginal secretions. *American journal of obstetrics and gynecology*, 174: 1339–1342.

Eis-Hubinger AM, Daumer M, Matz B et al. (1999) Evaluation of three glycoprotein G2-based enzyme immunoassays for detection of antibodies to herpes simplex virus type 2 in human sera. *Journal of clinical microbiology*, 37: 1242–1246.

Evans EGV (1990) Diagnostic laboratory techniques in vaginal candidosis. *British journal of clinical pathology*, 71(Suppl.): 70–72.

Fiscus S (1999) Molecular diagnosis of HIV-1 by PCR. In: Peeling RW, Sparling PF, eds. *Sexually transmitted diseases: Methods and protocols*, pp. 129–139. Totowa, NJ, Humana Press.

Freinkel AL, Dangor Y, Koornhof HJ et al. (1992) A serological test for granuloma inguinale. *Genitourinary medicine*, 68: 269–272.

Gaydos CA, Quinn TC (1999) *Neisseria gonorrhoeae*: detection and typing by probe hybridization, LCR and PCR. In: Peeling RW, Sparling PF, eds. *Sexually transmitted diseases: methods and protocols*, pp.15–32. Totowa, NJ, Humana Press.

Giles RE, Perry KR, Parry JV (1999) Simple/rapid test devices for anti-HIV screening: do they come up to the mark? *Journal of medical virology*, 56: 104–109.

Granade TC, Phillips SK, Parekh B et al. (1998) Detection of antibodies to human immunodeficiency virus type 1 in oral fluids: a large-scale evaluation of immunoassay performance. *Clinical and diagnostic laboratory immunology*, 5: 171–175.

Hillier SL (1993) Diagnostic microbiology of bacterial vaginosis. *American journal of obstetrics and gynecology*, **169**: 455–459.

Joseph AK, Rosen T (1994) Laboratory techniques used in the diagnosis of chancroid, granuloma inguinale and lymphogranuloma venereum. *Dermatologic clinics*, 12: 1–8.

Larsen SA, Steiner BM, Rudolph AH (1995) Laboratory diagnosis and interpretation of tests for syphilis. *Clinical microbiology reviews*, **8**: 1–21.

Levi MH, Torres J, Pina C et al. (1997) Comparison of the InPouch TV culture system and Diamond's modified medium for detection of *Trichomonas vaginalis*. *Journal of clinical microbiology*, **35**: 3308–3310.

Lorincz AT (1996) Molecular methods for the detection of human papillomavirus infection. *Obstetrics and gynecology clinics of North America*, **23**: 707–730.

Moscicki AB (1993) Comparison between methods for human papillomavirus DNA testing: a model for self-testing in young women. *International journal of infectious disease*, **167**: 723–725.

Nkengasong JN, Maurice C, Koblavi S et al. (1998) Field evaluation of a combination of monospecific enzyme-linked immunosorbent assays for type-specific diagnosis of human immunodeficiency virus type 1 (HIV-1) and HIV-2 infections in HIV-seropositive persons in Abidjan, Ivory Coast. *Journal of clinical microbiology*, **36**: 123–127.

Nugent RP, Krohn MA, Hillier SL (1991) Reliability of diagnosing bacterial vaginosis is improved by a standard method of Gram stain interpretation. *Journal of clinical microbiology*, **29**: 297–301.

O'Farrell N, Hoosen AA, Coetzee K et al. (1990) A rapid stain for the diagnosis of granuloma inguinale. *Genitourinary medicine*, **66**: 200–201.

Orle KA, Gates CA, Martin DH et al. (1996) Simultaneous PCR detection of Haemophilus ducreyi, Treponema pallidum, and herpes simplex virus types 1 and 2 from genital ulcers. *Journal of clinical microbiology*, **34**: 49–54.

Pappaioanou M, Kashamuka M, Behets F et al. (1993) Accurate detection of maternal antibodies to HIV in newborn whole blood dried on filter paper. *AIDS*, 7: 483–488.

Pasternak R, Vuorinen P, Miettinen A (1997) Evaluation of the Gen-Probe Chlamydia trachomatis transcription-mediated amplification assay with urine specimens from men. *Journal of clinical microbiology*, **35**: 676–678.

Petrin D, Delgaty K, Bhatt R et al. (1998) Clinical and microbiologic aspects of *Trichomonas vaginalis*. *Clinical microbiology reviews*, **11**: 300–317.

Peyton CL, Schiffman M, Lorincz AT et al. (1998) Comparison of PRC- and hybrid capture-based human papillomavirus detection systems using multiple cervical specimen collection strategies. *Journal of clinical microbiology*, **36**: 3248–3254.

Puolakkainen M, Hiltunen-Back E, Reunala T et al. (1998) Comparison of performances of two commercially available tests, a PCR assay and a ligase chain reaction test, in detection of urogenital *Chlamydia trachomatis* infection. *Journal of clinical microbiology*, **36**: 1489–1493.

Roggen EL, Pansaerts R, VanDyck E et al. (1993) Antigen detection and immunological typing of *Haemophilus ducreyi* with a specific rabbit polyclonal serum. *Journal of clinical microbiology*, 31: 1820–1825.

Sanders C, Nelson C, Hove M et al. (1998) Cytospin-enhanced direct immunofluorescence assay versus cell culture for detection of herpes simplex virus in clinical specimens. *Diagnosis of microbial infectious diseases*, 32: 111–113.

Schachter J, Hook EW 3rd, McCormack WM (1999) Ability of the Digene hybrid capture II test to identify *Chlamydia trachomatis* and *Neisseria gonorrhoeae* in cervical specimens. *Journal of clinical microbiology*, 37: 3668–3671.

Schoonmaker JN, Lunt BD, Lawellin DW et al. (1991) A new proline aminopeptidase assay for diagnosis of bacterial vaginosis. *American journal of obstetrics and gynecology*, 165: 737–742.

Silletti RP (1995) Comparison of CAPTIA Syphilis G enzyme immunoassay with rapid plasma reagin test for detection of syphilis. *Journal of clinical microbiology*, 33: 1829–1831.

Stone DL, Moheng MC, Rolich S (1997) Capture-S, a non-treponemal solid phase erythrocyte adherence assay for serological detection of syphilis. *Journal of clinical microbiology*, 35: 217–222.

Totten PA, Stamm WE (1994) Clear broth and plate media for culture of *Haemophilus ducreyi*. *Journal of clinical microbiology*, 32: 2019–2023.

Trofatter KF (1997) Diagnosis of human papillomavirus genital tract infection. *American journal of medicine*, 102: 21–27.

Turchek BM, Huang YT (1999) Evaluation of ELVIS HSV ID/Typing System for the detection and typing of herpes simplex virus from clinical specimens. *Journal of clinical virology*, 12: 65–69.

van Der Schee C, van Belkum A, Zwijgers L et al. (1999) Improved diagnosis of *Trichomonas vaginalis* infection by PCR using vaginal swabs and urine specimens compared to diagnosis by wet mount microscopy, culture, and fluorescent staining. *Journal of clinical microbiology*, 37: 4127–4130.

VanDyck E, Piot P (1992) Laboratory techniques in the investigation of chancroid, lymphogranuloma venereum and donovanosis. *Genitourinary medicine*, 68: 130–133.

Weber B (1998) Multicenter evaluation of the new automated Enzymun-Test Anti-HIV 1 + 2 + Subtyp O. *Journal of clinical microbiology*, 36: 580–584.

Weber B, Fall EHM, Berger A et al. (1998) Reduction of diagnostic window by new fourth-generation human immunodeficiency virus screening assays. *Journal of clinical microbiology*, 36: 2235–2239.

Weber B, Muhlbacher A, Michl U et al. (1999) Multicenter evaluation of a new rapid automated human immunodeficiency virus antigen detection assay. *Journal of virological methods*, 78: 61–70.

Woods GL (1995) Update on laboratory diagnosis of sexually transmitted diseases. *International journal of gynecological pathology*, 15: 665–684.

10

Laboratory methods for the diagnosis of reproductive tract infections and selected conditions in population-based studies

Mary Meehan,[1] Maria Wawer,[1] David Serwadda,[2] Ronald Gray[3] and Thomas Quinn[3]

[1] Columbia University, New York, USA; [2] Institute of Public Health, Kampala, Uganda; [3] Johns Hopkins University, Baltimore, USA

This chapter focuses on advances in reproductive health research that permit sample and data collection within population-based studies in a wide range of non-clinical settings, including the home. Areas of interest are assessment of classical sexually transmitted infections (STIs) and other reproductive tract infections, including oncogenic human papillomavirus (HPV), the principal causal agent of cervical cancer. Assessment of pregnancy loss is also addressed. The importance of linking behavioural data with biological sampling, in order to provide interpretable information for the development and evaluation of disease prevention and control programmes, is discussed. Finally, a number of strategies are proposed for the incorporation of biological sampling into survey research.

The study of reproductive morbidity in population-based studies was hindered for many years by the difficulty of diagnosis and the selectivity of the populations studied. Biological samples to assess many reproductive tract infections and STIs could only be obtained through genital and/or pelvic examination. In addition, available tests for many conditions required specialized handling of samples (in the case of gonorrhoea culture, for example) or immediate testing (such as wet mounts for trichomonas). Thus, studies were largely restricted to selected clinic-based populations, including users of antenatal or STD (sexually transmitted diseases) clinics, and results could not be generalized to the population as a whole. These limitations were particularly acute in rural settings with poor access to clinical services and laboratories, to say nothing of basics such as water and electricity.

In view of these limitations, symptoms, as reported by study participants, have been used in the evaluation of STIs in population-based studies. Using pre-established algorithms, the symptoms are then used to establish probable diagnoses for survey or treatment purposes, with a prescribed sequence of treatment if the first intervention does not prove to be successful. Symptom reporting may be supplemented by simple physical examination conducted by health or survey personnel. Limitations of the symptom-based approach include the high frequency of asymptomatic or unrecognized infections (Dallabetta, Gerbase and Holmes, 1998; Grosskurth et al., 1996; Kapiga et al., 1998; Paxton et al., 1998), differing perceptions of normality in various cultural settings (particularly common with respect to genital discharge in women) and the frequency of polymicrobial infections which may lead to complex symptom manifestations. Symptom-based algorithms also lack specificity, since conditions such as vaginal discharge can be the result of several different cervicovaginal pathogens. Thus, interview-based studies are likely to miss and/or misdiagnose many reproductive tract infections and STIs.

New diagnostic technologies that have been recently developed have greatly improved our ability to conduct field studies of STIs, reproductive tract infections and other selected reproductive conditions. Many of these methods rely on noninvasive specimen collection (urine, self-administered vaginal swabs) permitting sampling in diverse settings, including the home. Although some of the available tests are still fairly costly research tools, costs are likely to decline over time, as will the complexity of some assay techniques.

It should be noted that this chapter cannot present a summary of every potential test that may be included in population-based studies. Technological progress is occurring rapidly, and new and improved tests are continuously becoming available. The contents are based on experience to date and indicate the feasibility of a number of current approaches. Readers contemplating new programmes are encouraged to contact epidemiological and laboratory-based researchers to identify the ever more appropriate technologies being developed.

Background

The STIs and reproductive tract infections that are most amenable to inclusion in survey-based research and which will be discussed in this chapter are:

- *Neisseria gonorrhoeae*, the causal agent of gonorrhoea, can result in male urethral and female cervical infections, genital discharge, infertility, pelvic inflammatory disease and, if transmitted to the infant during birth, ocular infection which can cause blindness. Between two-thirds and three-quarters of initial infections are asymptomatic in both men and women (Gray et al., 1999; Grosskurth et al., 1996; Paxton et al., 1998).
- *Chlamydia trachomatis*, which, like gonorrhoea, results in urethral and cervical infections, can lead to fallopian tubal damage and infertility in women, and transient ocular infection in infants infected at the time of delivery. Over 80 per cent

of cases in men and women are asymptomatic (Gray et al., 1999; Grosskurth et al., 1996; Paxton et al., 1998).

- *Treponema pallidum*, the causal agent of syphilis, can have protean long-term effects in both men and women, including cardiovascular and neurological sequelae. In women with early untreated syphilis during pregnancy, adverse effects are observed in over two-thirds of births, and include spontaneous abortion, congenital infection and malformations in the newborn.
- *Trichomonas vaginalis*, a vaginal infection, is associated with vaginal discharge and, as suggested by some data, low birth weight and increased susceptibility to HIV infection.
- Bacterial vaginosis is a condition in which the vaginal ecology is disrupted. Lactobacillus species normally predominate in a healthy vagina and produce lactic acid and hydrogen peroxide, which inhibit other organisms (including gonorrhoea, gardnerella and mobiluncus). Bacterial vaginosis is characterized by a depletion of lactobacilli and an overgrowth of largely Gram-negative organisms. This condition is not a classical STI: while sexual intercourse is associated with a higher prevalence of bacterial vaginosis, the condition also occurs among sexually inexperienced women. Although the precise reason for its deleterious effects is not understood, bacterial vaginosis is associated with pelvic inflammatory disease and poor birth outcomes, including premature rupture of the membranes, low birth weight and postpartum upper genital tract infection (Glantz, 1997; Hillier et al., 1995). A number of studies also suggest that bacterial vaginosis increases the risk of acquiring HIV infection (Cohen et al., 1995; Sewankambo et al., 1997). Although bacterial vaginosis can be associated with symptoms (vaginal discharge, fishy amine vaginal odour), many cases do not result in recognized symptoms.
- Herpes simplex type 2 (HSV-2) is a viral, genital, ulcerative condition that can result in sepsis in infants infected during birth. In adults, HSV-2 infection generally persists indefinitely, and results in recurrent, progressively less symptomatic ulcerative episodes.
- HPV, which causes genital warts in both men and women, is now recognized as the primary etiologic agent of cervical cancer.
- HIV is transmitted sexually (via heterosexual and homosexual contact), through infected blood products and in utero from mother to child. In developing country settings, in the absence of expensive anti-retroviral medications and therapies for many opportunistic infections, median survival from infection to death is estimated at approximately 8 years.

In addition to their direct health effects, many STIs and reproductive tract infections mentioned earlier have been associated with increased risk of HIV transmission and acquisition. Thus, given their importance for health and reproduction, their demographic effects (Gray et al., 1999; Sewankambo et al., 1994) and their inextricable link to behaviours, studies that combine the social sciences and epidemiology represent a priority.

In a research setting, identification of some or all the forementioned conditions may be desirable. Selecting the conditions to be tested will depend on a number of considerations.

First, research goals need to be defined. Goals should include:

- Descriptive research to determine levels of prevalent and/or new incident infection (in the entire population or in key subgroups) in relation to reported behaviours and sociodemographic characteristics. This will help to determine behavioural and biological risk factors for infection and morbidity, assess the demographic effects of selected conditions, develop national projections of infection and morbidity, set priorities, and plan preventive and treatment programmes.
- Programme monitoring to assess whether the incidence or prevalence of selected conditions diminishes over time.[1]
- Validation of behavioural research data (for example, are declines in STI rates consistent with reported behavioural change).

A second consideration in selecting target conditions is the research setting itself. Home-based specimen collection necessarily imposes limits on sampling methods, since pelvic examinations cannot be conducted and specimens collected must be stable in field conditions, pending their transport to the laboratory.

The training and experience of the research team will influence the selection of samples to be collected. Interviewers with no prior experience can readily be taught to collect urine and finger stick blood specimens, and to instruct participants in the collection of self-administered vaginal swabs. However, the collection of venous blood specimens would be difficult for such interviewers and would require substantial practice with the procedure prior to study implementation.

Finally, the resources available, including financial resources, access to a laboratory and the capacity to transport samples for testing, will determine which combination of tests is appropriate in a given setting.

Ideally, a diagnostic test should include:

- Samples that are easily collected, through non-invasive procedures that are culturally acceptable.

---

[1] Incidence is the rate of new infections (or other conditions) in a defined population or subgroup occurring during a specified period of time. Incidence is generally expressed as the number of new cases per 100 person years of observation. In order to determine incidence rate, it is usually necessary to follow a population over time. Prevalence is the proportion of persons having the given infection or condition in a defined population at a point in time.

- Samples that are stable in field conditions and do not necessitate complex handling or processing.
- The test should provide immediate results.
- It should be technically simple to perform in the field or a small field laboratory.
- It should have high sensitivity and specificity in order to correctly identify all participants with or without the condition or infection.[2]
- It should differentiate between current infection and previous exposure.

Unfortunately, the tests currently available do not meet all these conditions. The advantages and disadvantages of different tests are described in detail below. In general, however, the potential for comprehensive testing in community-based research settings has improved substantially in the 1990s, such that the advantages of combining behavioural and biological data collection can far outweigh the extra complexity of such an endeavour. Recent improvements include the ability to identify HIV from saliva, urine and finger stick samples; diagnose gonorrhoea, chlamydia, trichomonas, HPV and bacterial vaginosis from self-administered vaginal swabs; and detect gonorrhoea and chlamydia from urine samples. Although some of the tests performed on these samples are still expensive, sample collection itself has been sufficiently simplified to permit the design of comprehensive population-based STI, reproductive tract infection and HIV surveys.

In the following section, we describe a number of feasible testing procedures. Many of the experiences are drawn from the Rakai STD Control for AIDS Prevention Project (1994–99), a randomized community-based trial to determine the effects of intensive STI control on HIV transmission and acquisition. The project has been described in detail (Hayes et al., 1997; Wawer et al., 1998, 1999). Briefly, all adults aged 15–59 years, resident in 56 rural Ugandan villages, were visited in the home every 10 months for survey and biological sample collection. The study enrolled and followed over 12 000 subjects, and thus acquired substantial experience with biological sampling in home-based survey research. Specimens were collected under challenging circumstances, in dispersed rural villages, which included many single-room homes with no electricity or running water. Samples were then processed and/or tested in a simple, two-room field laboratory, of which the main components were a generator for electrical backup, a backup water tank, a refrigerator, a freezer (operating at $-20\,^{\circ}$C), a microscope, a centrifuge, a plate rocker and an incubator – equipment which is either available or can readily be made available in most district-level hospitals in the developing world. The Rakai experiences can thus be adapted to other settings.

---

[2] Sensitivity refers to a test's ability to correctly identify true cases of a given condition or infection. A highly sensitive test produces a low proportion of false-negative results (i.e. results in which a person who has the target infection is incorrectly classified as being uninfected).

Specific diagnostic tests

Specific diagnostic tests will be described based on the type of specimen collected.

Tests based on self-administered vaginal swabs

Home-based, self-administered vaginal swab collection has proved to be highly feasible and well accepted in populations as diverse as rural Rakai district, Uganda (Gray et al., 1998a; Serwadda et al., 1999; Wawer et al., 1995), Ethiopia (C. Stanton, 1997, pers. comm.) and among Latina women living in New York City (Cushman, Kalmuss and Wawer, 1998). In these settings, over 90 per cent of study participants agreed to provide multiple vaginal swabs (up to four swabs in Rakai) in a single home visit, and reported the procedure to be easy and acceptable. In both Rakai and New York, over 98 per cent of women who self-collected vaginal swabs provided samples of good quality (determined by the presence of vaginal epithelium and vaginal organisms, detected on Gram-stained slides) (see section on Bacterial vaginosis).

To collect the swabs, women are given Dacron or cotton swabs (a 20-cm stick length is ideal). They are instructed to squat and gently insert the swab (one at a time) high into the vagina and rotate the swab in the vaginal vault as high as the swab will comfortably go. The swabs are immediately given to the survey worker. Swabs can be used for the identification of trichomonas, bacterial vaginosis, chlamydia, gonorrhoea and HPV.

Collection and testing of vaginal cells and fluid can also be performed with self-administered tampons (Haughie, Ames and Madsen, 1975) in cultures where women are accustomed to their use. However, the per unit cost of swabs is considerably less than that of tampons, and the latter may be less acceptable in populations with no prior exposure to tampons.

The following tests were performed during the Rakai Project with self-administered swabs.

Trichomonas culture

The InPouch TV™ culture kit (Biomed Diagnostic, San Jose, CA, USA) provides a feasible means of detecting trichomonas in survey settings (Wawer et al., 1995). After the woman has prepared the swab, as described above, she is asked to hand it immediately to the interviewer, who then inserts the tip of the swab into the InPouch, breaks off the remaining stick and keeps the InPouch at ambient temperature until the sample is brought to the laboratory. The InPouch kit is incubated at 37°C for 24–72 hours, where it is then read every 12 hours for 2 or 3 days. The pouch is viewed under a low power (100×) microscope and motile trichomonads are readily observed. Even personnel without prior laboratory experience can be easily trained to interpret InPouch results. This test is well established with high sensitivity and specificity (Borchardt and Smith, 1991; Draper et al., 1993). Only current infections are detected.

Requirements for specimen reading are simple: a small incubator (the Latina women's project in New York used a simple agricultural egg incubator costing $60) and an inexpensive microscope, such that reading can be conducted even in a non-laboratory setting.

The cost of each InPouch kit is approximately US$2. Since trichomonasis is highly prevalent in many populations (prevalence rates of 15–25 per cent have been reported among women in rural Africa (Grosskurth et al., 1995; Wawer et al., 1998)), and is also highly transmissible, culture provides a simple means of assessing the extent of high-risk sexual behaviour, and can be used for programme monitoring and validation of reported behaviours. For example, decline in trichomonas prevalence suggests reduction in high-risk behaviour and/or improved treatment and treatment seeking, any of which may be key study outcomes. If, on the other hand, rates remain unchanged despite reported behavioural change, the data suggest that such change has been inadequate or inconsistent.

The prior discussion refers solely to trichomonas culture from female vaginal swabs. The InPouch has also been successfully used to assess trichomonas in male urine samples in clinic-based settings: the samples are centrifuged at low speed and the sediment is cultured in the InPouch (Borchardt et al., 1995). However, in the Rakai field setting, trichomonas culture from male urine resulted in poor yields, possibly because of the long lag time (up to 8 hours) between urine collection in the field, and centrifugation and incubation in the field laboratory. (The project was not equipped to centrifuge urine at the village level.) New urinary polymerase chain reaction (PCR) tests, which can be conducted on male and female urine, are being developed but are substantially more expensive and complex than the InPouch TV culture.

Bacterial vaginosis

The conventional clinical diagnosis of bacterial vaginosis requires testing fresh vaginal fluid and is difficult to conduct in a field setting. However, new diagnostic methods are based on slides prepared from self-administered vaginal swabs, and slides can readily be prepared in the field. The self-administered vaginal swab is immediately rolled onto a glass slide, which is then air-dried. The slide can be stored at room temperature in a slide box for up to several months. In order to diagnose bacterial vaginosis, the slide is Gram-stained in the laboratory. The Gram-stained slide is examined under a high power oil immersion lens (1000×) and bacterial vaginosis is diagnosed using the quantitative morphological method, which scores the vaginal flora from 0 to 10, depending on the relative predominance or absence of lactobacilli and other Gram-negative bacteria (Hillier, 1993; Morse, Moreland and Holmes, 1996). Scores of 7–10 indicate bacterial vaginosis; scores of 9–10 are considered to be severe bacterial vaginosis (total absence of lactobacilli and major overgrowth of Gram-negative organisms). The test detects current bacterial vaginosis status.

Bacterial vaginosis slides can serve as a quality control check for other swabs. A correctly collected specimen will have many epithelial cells and bacteria; the lack of either will give an indication that the specimen was incorrectly collected and test results on other swabs collected by the same participant should be considered questionable.

The cost of preparing a Gram-stained slide is under $0.30 a specimen (including the swab, slides and reagents). Slides are easy to prepare: over 35 000 such slides were prepared in the field and read in the Rakai Project field laboratory during the STD Control for AIDS Prevention project. Since slides are stable for long periods after staining, they can be reread for quality control. (The Rakai Project sent approximately 10 per cent of its slides to Johns Hopkins University and Pittsburgh University in the US for the purpose of quality control.) A disadvantage of the Gram-stain technique is the requirement that the technicians reading the slides be well trained and acquire substantial experience (based on the supervised reading of several hundred slides) in order to ensure reliability in score assignment. Periodic refresher courses are advisable.

Since bacterial vaginosis is not a classical STI and recurs following treatment, monitoring of this condition does not provide direct evidence of behavioural change. The utility of bacterial vaginosis for programme evaluation or validation of reported behaviours is thus limited.

Gonorrhoea and chlamydia

Gonorrhoea and chlamydia can both be detected from self-administered vaginal swabs using a number of technologies, including amplification methods such as PCR (Roche Molecular Systems, Alameda, CA, USA), ligase chain reaction (LCR) (Abbott Laboratories, Abbott Part, IL, USA) or DNA probe methods such as the Digene Hybrid Capture microtitre assay (Digene, Silver Spring, MD, USA) (Gray et al., 1999).

For each of these tests, self-administered swabs are collected as described earlier, and are immediately stored in the field in a pre-packaged transport vial containing an appropriate medium (PCR buffer, LCR buffer or Digene specimen transport medium). The cost per vial is approximately US$1 for the PCR and LCR medium, and US$2 for the Digene Hybrid Capture transport medium. Samples are kept in a cool box with ice packs in the field, and frozen at $-200\,°C$ once they reach the laboratory at the end of the day.

Testing the samples requires high-tech equipment and trained technicians. Although PCR, and to a lesser extent LCR, are becoming available in tertiary care research laboratories in developing countries, hybrid capture is generally not yet available outside Western countries. Thus, samples need to be shipped to appropriate laboratories, potentially to another country. Air shipment requires the use of IATA-approved insulated biological specimen boxes: specimens can be shipped on wet ice, ideally pre-frozen to $-700\,°C$. Costs per test vary from approximately US$15–30 per PCR or LCR (depending on the laboratory used). An advantage of the hybrid capture (which costs approximately US$6–10 depending on the laboratory) is that the sample is tested simultaneously for both organisms, and only those specimens that are positive require additional testing to determine which infection is actually present. This substantially reduces costs, particularly if the prevalence of gonorrhoea and chlamydia is relatively low. PCR, LCR and hybrid capture detect current infections only. Off-site testing increases the time between sample collection and testing (sometimes up to several months), limiting project capacity to provide care or referral based on results. Thus, in many developing countries, the tests are more useful for research purposes than for clinical management.

PCR, LCR and hybrid capture greatly simplify specimen collection and handling in the field, permitting population-based assessment of the prevalence of gonorrhoea and chlamydia. The need for high-tech laboratory facilities and the costs of the tests, however, restrict this approach to fairly intensive epidemiological research, or potentially to a single-shot survey to ascertain the prevalence of these infections for modelling, projections and programme planning.

As an alternative to the tests mentioned, a chlamydia antigen capture enzyme immunoassay (IDEIA, NovoNordisk Diagnostics, Cambridge, UK) is less expensive and can more readily be implemented in laboratories in developing countries. However, the test, which is less sensitive than amplification techniques, has not been tested using self-administered swabs and does not identify gonorrhoea.

Human papillomavirus

HPV causes cervical cancer. New developments in HPV detection, such as the Pap smear, show promise as a research and screening tool for the identification of women at high risk of cervical cancer. One test, the Digene Hybrid Capture II (HCII) microtitre assay (Digene, Silver Springs, MD, USA), uses molecular diagnostic methods (HPV RNA probes) linked to immunoassay, to detect 11 carcinogenic HPV viruses and to quantify virus shedding (Lorincz, 1996). The Rakai experience with this assay in 1000 women has shown that samples can be obtained by self-administered vaginal swabs in a home setting (Serwadda et al., 1999). The prevalence of HPV infection in the rural Rakai population was 18 per cent, with very high prevalence (>25 per cent) in younger women under 25 years. (It should be noted that the majority of young women with HPV do not have discernible cervical precancerous or cancerous lesions.)[3] HPV prevalence and shedding were also much greater in HIV infected women (Serwadda et al., 1999). Since HPV is prevalent among adolescent and young women in many populations, the virus can serve as an epidemiological marker of sexual debut and high-risk sexual activity.

Self-administered vaginal swabs for hybrid capture analysis are collected as described earlier, and are immediately inserted into a transport vial containing Digene specimen transport medium. Specimens can be maintained in cold boxes (coolers with ice packs) for approximately a day, at which time they should be frozen at −20°C. Sample collection is thus easy, and the cost of each Digene specimen transport medium vial is approximately US$2. However, testing the specimens requires complex technology and is not readily feasible in most developing country settings. The Rakai Project shipped frozen samples (packed on wet ice in IATA-approved specimen transport boxes) to the US for testing. The costs per test are approximately US$ 6–10, depending on the laboratory used. HPV can also be detected from self-administered swabs by PCR. However, PCR does not obviate the need to ship samples to a specialized laboratory, and the cost of the test itself is substantially more than that of hybrid capture. Both hybrid capture and PCR only detect current infections.

Given that samples need to be shipped to the US or Europe for testing and the cost of the test, the detection of HPV is most suited to epidemiological research projects.

Tests based on urine samples

Urinary tract inflammation

The leucocyte esterase dehydrogenase (LED) urine dipstick test identifies white blood cell markers of urinary tract infection from fresh urine samples. Although the test does not distinguish between inflammation caused by bacteria (including *Neisseria gonorrhoeae* and *Chlamydia trachomatis*), parasites such as urinary tract schistosomiasis or other causes, it can be a useful screening test to identify individuals requiring additional sample collection. This approach was used in the Mwanza STI control for AIDS prevention trial in Tanzania (Grosskurth et al., 1995, 1996; Hayes et al., 1997). Because of poor specificity in women, the LED is generally reserved for testing in men. A LED dipstick is inserted into a fresh urine specimen, and in the presence of leucocytes, undergoes a colour change which is compared to a standard colour reference chart. The test is thus very easy to conduct. It is also inexpensive, costing approximately US$0.05 per sample.

---

[3] If a woman continues to shed HPV into her 30s and 40s, her risk of having a lesion is substantially higher.

Chlamydia and gonorrhoea

In the presence of cervical or urethral infections with chlamydia or gonorrhoea, urine, preferably a first catch sample, contains sufficient cells for the detection of these organisms using sensitive DNA amplification methods. Urine sampling is particularly useful in assessing the prevalence of infection in males since male urine collection is simple and substantially more acceptable than urethral swab collection. Samples are collected in plastic cups with screw-top lids. There is no need to wipe or otherwise clean the perineum or urethral meatus prior to collection. Urine volumes of 15 ml or more are suitable for testing. For transport, the urine is placed in a cold box.

Urine tests for chlamydia and gonorrhoea are largely based on DNA amplification techniques such as LCR. The Rakai Project used the Abbott LCR, which can be conducted on fresh or frozen urine collected from both men and women. Specimens can be kept in a domestic refrigerator (2–8 °C) for up to 4 days or can be frozen for several weeks at −20 °C prior to processing. The latter procedure can be carried out in a simple field laboratory, and consists of boiling, centrifugation and buffering to produce a pellet for long-term storage (at −20 °C) for shipment and for testing.

Processed pellets are shipped frozen on wet ice to a laboratory with the required specialized equipment. In the literature, the urinary LCR assay for gonorrhoea and chlamydia has been reported to have a sensitivity and specificity of over 95 per cent (Ching et al., 1995; Gaydos and Quinn, 1995; Koumans et al., 1998; Lee et al., 1995) in both men and women. In the Rakai Project field setting, urinary LCR performed with high sensitivity and specificity for the identification of chlamydia in women, when compared with amplification methods performed on self-administered vaginal swabs. However, sensitivity was lower for the identification of gonorrhoea in female urine samples (approximately 70 per cent compared to results from vaginal swabs tested by LCR, PCR and/or Digene Hybrid Capture): the relatively lower yield may have been due to the delay (up to 10 hours) between urine sample collection and processing in Rakai field conditions.

LCR and PCR only detect current infections. Costs per LCR or PCR test are approximately US $15–30, depending on the laboratory. As discussed in the section on vaginal swab testing for gonorrhoea and chlamydia, PCR and LCR greatly simplify specimen collection and handling in the field, permitting population-based assessment of the prevalence of gonorrhoea and chlamydia. The need for high-tech laboratory facilities and the costs of the tests, however, restrict this approach to fairly intensive epidemiological research, or potentially to a single-shot survey to ascertain the prevalence of infection.

HIV

HIV can be assessed from venous blood samples. However, assessment in surveys has been greatly facilitated with the introduction of urine-based and saliva-based tests, and with use of finger stick blood samples collected on filter paper. In this section, the urine-based assay is discussed.

The Calypte enzyme immunoassay (EIA) for HIV-1 antibodies in the urine was recently approved by the US Food and Drug Administration (Calypte, Berkley, CA, USA). A fresh 15-ml urine sample placed in a polypropylene tube containing a Stabilur tablet can be stored in a domestic refrigerator for up to a year prior to assay. The EIA can be run in any laboratory that routinely conducts HIV EIA testing, and can thus be readily performed in many developing country settings. The cost per single test is approximately US$2.50, slightly higher than the US$1.50 for a standard serum-based EIA test. However, the urinary EIA produces more false-positive results than EIA testing based on serum. It is thus advisable to repeat the urine EIA at least twice, and to confirm positive results with urinary Western blot. With Western blot confirmation, urinary HIV testing is over 99 per cent sensitive and specific (Berrios et al., 1995; Meehan et al., 1999). Urinary HIV testing is thus more expensive than that based on serum but nonetheless offers advantages in programmes where logistical considerations or cultural factors preclude the collection of blood samples. The Rakai Project conducted urinary HIV testing on subjects who declined to provide a serological sample but who consented to a urine specimen (approximately 10 per cent of all participants).

Pregnancy tests

Urine can also be used to test for pregnancy using human chorionic gonadotrophin (hCG) test kits. The Rakai Project screened all women in the home for early pregnancy using this procedure. This allows more complete ascertainment of pregnancies and subsequent pregnancy loss than that based solely on participant reporting. The Rakai Project observed a 19.3 per cent prevalence of pregnancy in women aged 15–49 years, and a fifth of these pregnancies were detected by hCG. The cost per hCG test varies from US$1.00 to US$2.50, depending on the sensitivity of the test used.

Tests based on blood samples

The following tests can be conducted on 5–10 ml of blood collected in a serum vaccutainer tube (commonly referred to as a red top tube). Tubes are labelled and placed in a cold box for transport to a basic laboratory, where samples are centrifuged and divided into separate 1 ml serum aliquots for testing and archival purposes. Although samples can be stored at $-20°C$, freezing to $-700°C$ is recommended if samples are to be stored for more than several months.

HIV

The following summary focuses on HIV-1, which is the predominant HIV virus. HIV tests are performed on serum using EIAs, among other types of tests. EIAs detect antibodies to HIV, and generally become positive within 2 months after initial HIV infection (i.e. after a window period). In a limited proportion of cases, however, the window period can extend for a longer time.

Commercial EIA kits are 99.0–99.6 per cent sensitive and 99.2–99.8 per cent specific. Generally, HIV diagnosis and reporting of results is based on more than one EIA test. The most efficient and cost-effective strategy is to conduct two separate EIAs (using EIA kits produced by two different manufacturers) and to retest all samples in which the two EIAs produce discordant results. If resources are adequate, a Western blot, which is highly specific, can be done on all EIA- positive samples as a confirmatory test (Holmes et al., 1990; Morse et al., 1996). In West Africa where HIV-2 is prevalent, separate EIAs for this virus are required. The cost of a standard EIA is approximately US$1.25–1.50 depending on the exact test used, and thus double EIA testing costs add up to approximately US$2.50–3.00 per subject. Each Western blot costs between US$10–15. EIA and Western blot testing is routinely conducted in developing country settings. Transport of samples from the research site to the laboratory can be done in one of two ways: red top tubes can be delivered in cool boxes to the laboratory on the day of collection, or if resources permit, the samples can be centrifuged in a field laboratory, the serum frozen at −200°C and the samples brought to the laboratory at a later date.

In some research circumstances, early infections during the window period (i.e. before the EIA is positive) can be diagnosed by PCR or the detuned p24 antigen assay (Brookmeyer and Quinn, 1995; Brookmeyer et al., 1995). Such testing permits estimation of HIV incidence rates from a single cross-sectional survey. However, these methods are expensive, require testing of large numbers of HIV-negative specimens, and in the case of the p24 assay, have not yet been validated on all HIV subtypes. Thus such research is of limited application in many field settings.

HIV testing can also be carried out on finger stick blood samples stored on filter paper. The survey worker makes a small puncture on the subject's finger using a standard lancet, and gently squeezes a few drops of blood onto special filter paper. The filter paper is then air-dried in the field and stored refrigerated or frozen in the laboratory until testing, which can be conducted months after collection. The advantages of this approach are ease of sample collection (obviating the need for venipuncture) and low cost, since special collection devices (as in the case of saliva sampling; see section Saliva-based testing) are not required. Standard serum HIV EIA can be performed (at a cost of approximately US$1.25–1.50 a test). A disadvantage is the necessity of the additional laboratory step required for elution of the filter paper, but with training, technicians in laboratories that routinely perform EIAs master this step with no difficulty.

Finally, rapid HIV EIA tests, including the Capillus HIV-1/HIV-2 (Cambridge Diagnostics Ireland Limited, Galway, Ireland), the SeroCard HIV (Trinity Biotech, Dublin, Ireland), the Multispot HIV-1/HIV-2 (Sanofi Pasteur, Paris, France) and the Determine (Abbott Laboratories, Abbott Park, IL, USA) are now available. The tests can be conducted on blood collected via venipuncture or, more conveniently, via a finger stick specimen collected in a capillary tube. In both cases, the specimen needs to be centrifuged to separate out the serum for testing, but the procedure is amenable to implementation in the field. Algorithms that combine different rapid tests to maximize sensitivity and specificity have been developed and tested (Downing et al., 1998). However, the use of rapid tests in the field raises issues related to participant confidentiality and the provision of results. Rapid testing would be inappropriate in a field setting if the subject's results cannot be maintained in strict confidence, or where appropriate counselling is not immediately available.

Syphilis

Serological testing for syphilis is inexpensive and can readily be conducted in a small field laboratory. None the less, testing is somewhat complex because interpretation of results varies with the stage of infection. In addition, two tests are required for diagnosis – a screening test and a specific treponemal confirmatory test.

Screening tests are indirect or nontreponemal tests, and include the Rapid Plasma Reagin (RPR) test or the Toluidine Red Unheated Serum Test (TRUST). Both are card tests performed on serum, and do not require a microscope (Parham et al., 1984; Pettiti and Larsen, 1983). The tests can be conducted in a simple field laboratory, or in the field itself if the latter is equipped with a centrifuge for serum separation. The cost of a TRUST test is approximately US$0.15 per titre; generally, three titres are run on each person at a total cost of US$0.45. Samples can be frozen indefinitely.

In a laboratory, the serum can be diluted to estimate the titre, or the strength of any positive reactions, and this can be used as a test of cure since successful treatment is followed by falling titres. The specific treponemal tests can only be performed in a laboratory and are used as confirmatory tests. The most commonly used are the Fluorescent Treponema Antibody Absorption (FTA-ABS) test and the Micro Hemagglutination Assay for Antibodies to *Treponema pallidum* (MHA-TP), the *T. pallidum* Hemagglutination test (TPHA) (Holmes et al., 1990; Morse, Moreland and Holmes, 1996) and the *T. pallidum* Particle Agglutination test (TPPA). The cost of a TPHA or TPPA is approximately $0.50.

Algorithms to determine whether a given syphilis infection is new or old are somewhat complex. New infections are associated with very high rates of poor pregnancy outcomes (including stillbirth and congenital infection), whereas old infections can result in severe neurological and cardiovascular sequelae.

Syphilis testing generally requires a venipuncture blood draw. However, the Centers for Disease Control, Atlanta, GA, USA (Dr. J. Lewis) have successfully conducted syphilis RPR and TPHA testing on finger stick samples collected on filter paper.

Herpes simplex virus-2 (HSV-2)

HSV-2 is the causal agent of genital herpes infections. Serological tests for HSV-2 include the MRL Diagnostics dual EIA system to detect type specific antibodies and differentiate between HSV-1 (which generally causes oral herpes but can also be found in genital lesions) and HSV-2 (classical genital herpes) (Prince, Ernst and Hogrefe, 2000). Serological tests for HSV-2 do not differentiate between previous exposure to the virus and currently active infections, and once exposed, the individual is generally seropositive for life. HSV-2 is highly prevalent in many populations, with very high rates of incidence of new infection occurring among adolescents and young adults (Obasi et al., 1999). HSV-2 thus represents an excellent epidemiological tool to examine high-risk behaviours and the effects of behavioural prevention programmes: decline in the incidence of HSV-2 in the young is a good indicator of success.

Saliva-based testing

HIV

HIV antibodies can be detected in saliva samples. Specimen collection methods include the OraSureR HIV Oral Collection device used in the Rakai Project. The OraSure collection device uses a treated cotton-fibre pad attached to a handle. The pad is placed in the subject's mouth between the lower cheek and gum, rubbed gently until moist, held in place for 2 minutes, then inserted into the manufacturer's transport vial. The sample can be held at room temperature (approximately 23 °C) for a week. After elution and centrifugation of the stored specimen, sample testing is conducted using standard HIV EIA tests and protocols, such as the Vironostika HIV-1 Microelisa System (Organon Teknika Corp, Research Triangle Park, NC, USA). The cost of the collection device is US$2, and the cost of the subsequent standard EIA is approximately US$1.25–1.50 per test.

Genital ulcer swab testing

A number of assays are available to determine the etiology of a reported or observed genital ulcer, including the Multiplex PCR, which differentiates between syphilis, chancroid and genital herpes (HSV-2). Genital ulcers are gently debrided and swabbed, swabs are stored in vials of PCR buffer and the specimens are then transported frozen on wet ice to the testing laboratory. Because sample collection requires genital examination by the survey worker, it is generally less feasible in non-clinical research settings, although the Rakai Project collected such samples in the home from men reporting an ulcer. The Multiplex PCR is not available commercially, but is being conducted in an increasing number of laboratories (including the Centers for Disease Control and Prevention in Atlanta, GA, USA) for research purposes.

The HERPCHEK Direct Herpes Simplex Virus Antigen Test (El Dupont De Numours and Co. Medical Products, Charlotte, NC, USA) identifies herpes in genital lesions: both HSV-2 and HSV-1 (generally considered to be the oral herpes virus but is also found in genital lesions) are both detected by the test. The test is conducted on swabs collected in the same manner as those for the Multiplex PCR. Swabs are stored in the HerpTran transport medium prior to testing in the laboratory.

Placental pathology

Examination of the placenta can provide important information on the presence of a number of conditions, including malaria and placental membrane inflammation (chorioamnionitis and funisitis). Inflammation, which can be caused by organisms such as those associated with bacterial vaginosis, causes low birth weight and premature delivery, and predisposes to maternal postpartum upper genital tract infections. In the Rakai Project, where most deliveries occur in the home, mothers were provided with covered plastic buckets containing 10 per cent formalin and the mother or her attendant (such as the traditional midwife) asked to place the placenta in the container after delivery. The formalin-fixed placentas can be kept for prolonged periods prior to processing in the pathology laboratory. The processed tissue, in the form of paraffin blocks or slide-mounted sections, can be kept indefinitely. The Rakai Project obtained over 78 per cent compliance with placenta collection, and the prevalence of chorioamnionitis in the samples tested to date has been approximately 20 per cent.

Summary

Combined biological and behavioural data provide a wealth of information on reproductive health. New sample collection techniques and tests greatly facilitate such integrated research.

For an evaluation of the laboratory methods see also Table 10.1.

Table 10.1. Evaluation of laboratory methods for diagnosis of reproductive tract infections

Test	Price (USD)	Sensitivity	Specificity	Equipment	Special training required
Gram stain for bacterial vaginosis	1	97%	79–100%	Microscope	Yes
TRUST	0.16				
TPHA	0.28				None
Trichomonas InPouch	2	96%	100%	Microscope	No
Organon HIV EIA test	1.5	100%	99.9%	Plate washer	Yes
Serum Western blot	20.37	100%	100%	Vacuum aspirator	Yes
Urine Western blot	26.5	99.1–100%	96.3–99.4%	Rocker	Yes
Chemstrip LET	4.72	97.2%	90.1%	None	No
Urine EIA (Calypte)	2	98%	81%	See other EIA	Yes
Multiplex PCR GUD	30			Thermocycler	Yes
Syphilis		91%	99.2%		
HSV		100%	100%		
Haemophilus ducreyi		98.4%	99.6%		

Specimen collection and applicability to different research settings

New sample collection methods based on urine, self-administered vaginal swabs, saliva and finger stick blood collection make it possible to collect samples in the home (or in virtually any setting) for assessing HIV, gonorrhoea, chlamydia, trichomonas, bacterial vaginosis, HPV and pregnancy. Over time, an ever greater number of tests will be adapted to noninvasive sample collection. In addition, there is experience with home-based collection of male genital ulcer swabs and placentas, suggesting that with adequate preparation of the population and motivation of subjects, there are few insurmountable barriers to the acceptability of many reproductive health-related research activities.

As discussed earlier, however, ease of specimen collection is not necessarily linked to inexpensive and technologically simple sample testing. Many of the tests described (LCR, PCR, hybrid capture) are revolutionizing our understanding of the epidemiology, transmission and behavioural risk factors for key infections in the general population, but require shipping to specialized laboratories for expensive testing.

A possible approach to the integration of laboratory testing and behavioural and survey research projects could include the following considerations. In projects where it is important to acquire an understanding of disease prevalence, a baseline survey may incorporate both high-tech and low-tech testing. Thus, some combination of sample collection for LCR, PCR or hybrid capture for gonorrhoea, chlamydia and HPV may be selected, in addition to moderately low-tech testing for HIV and syphilis, and very low-tech testing for trichomonas. Follow-up surveys may only require testing for selected conditions, such as HIV and trichomonas, as a means of monitoring rates of new infection. A study with very limited resources may elect to only conduct trichomonas culture using the InPouch TVTM culture system as a means of validating reported behaviour and following changes in prevalence over time. Only clinical studies or highly specialized field research sites are likely to include genital ulcer swab collation or placental collection.

Experience in Africa and the US suggests that adding biological sample collection to a survey does not inhibit subject participation: over 90 per cent of eligible residents in Rakai participated in the study, and of these persons, over 94 per cent provided biological samples (Wawer et al., 1999). Similarly, in the New York study, more than 90 per cent of women who consented to respond to the questionnaire also consented to provide samples (Cushman et al., 1998). In both studies, subjects were clearly informed that they could elect to provide samples but were not obliged to do so.

Similarly, it is possible to collect very detailed behavioural information to enhance the interpretation of data on disease prevalence/incidence. The Rakai Project routinely initiates a home visit with a 30–45 minute questionnaire on socio-demographic characteristics, such as travel and migration. Details are sought on pregnancy history, health status including potential STI symptoms, circumcision, sexual behaviours and networks (as well as detailed data on the last four sexual partners, their place of residence, relationship to the respondent, sexual activities undertaken with these partners, use of condoms and other contraception, use of alcohol with partners and violent/non-consensual sex). Data are also collected on vaginal practices (such as douching) and male and female genital hygiene. Over 90 per cent of subjects responded to the full questionnaire, and the data have been invaluable in identifying behavioural and demographic risk factors for observed patterns of infection.

Personnel issues

In deciding which tests to perform, consideration must be given to personnel needs, including the number of staff available, their training and experience. Where well trained, qualified laboratory personnel are difficult to locate, testing should be limited to those methods that do not require complex sample processing, and are easy-to-run and interpret. Diploma-level laboratory technicians can readily be trained to read the InPouch TVTM culture, run EIAs and conduct syphilis serology.

The more involved tests, such as PCR and LCR, are labour-intensive and require highly trained laboratory staff.

Ethical considerations

Projects that plan to identify reproductive health problems need to consider research ethics. Participants must be informed of the conditions or infections being assessed by the project. Both interview and biological data must be safeguarded to ensure participant confidentiality. In addition, researchers need to carefully consider their obligation to persons who report STI symptoms or are found to be positive on laboratory testing. For example, in the control arm of the Rakai Project, persons who reported symptoms were referred for free treatment to Rakai Project clinics, and subjects with serious and treatable infections identified in Uganda (such as syphilis) were also referred for free treatment. However, the project did not routinely inform women who had bacterial vaginosis, or provide them with treatment if they were neither symptomatic nor pregnant, since data suggest very low utility of routine treatment for this condition. Results of potentially serious infections (such as chlamydia and gonorrhoea) diagnosed in external laboratories were often not available for 6–12 months because of batch shipment and testing procedures. The Rakai Project provided mass treatment to all participants at the end of the STD Control for AIDS Prevention Project to cover any such potential infections. Since this approach will not be possible in many settings, researchers should discuss treatment issues with the government and local leaders in order to arrive at feasible and ethically acceptable approaches to the provision of care. At the very least, research projects should ensure that subjects have access to the prevailing standard of care, through mechanisms such as referral to government clinics which the project may help stock with selected drugs if necessary.

HIV testing raises issues related to the provision of serological results and counselling services. In Uganda, Ministry of Health policy indicates that research subjects are free to know their results, but cannot be coerced to do so, and that results may not be passed on to a third party without written consent from the subject. The Rakai Project makes results available in a voluntary and confidential manner to all subjects who choose to receive them, and strongly encourages participants to avail of their results and counselling. The project has trained a team of counsellors who travel to different communities to provide these confidential services. Projects that do not have the capacity to provide counselling may elect to establish a system of referral to other programmes that offer the service. Anonymous testing – in which no identifiers are collected – obviates the necessity of providing results and counselling, but has disadvantages and may not be acceptable to the host country or study population.

REFERENCES

Berrios D, Andrew LA, Haynes-Sanstad K et al. (1995) Screening for Human Immundeficiency Virus antibody in urine. *Archives of pathology and laboratory medicine*, **119**: 139–141.

Borchardt KA, Smith RF (1991) An evaluation of an InPouch™ TV culture method for diagnosing *Trichomonas vaginalis* infection. *Genitourinary medicine*, **67**: 149–152.

Borchardt KA, al-Haraci S, Maida N (1995) Prevalence of *Trichomonas vaginalis* in a male sexually transmitted disease clinic population by interview, wet mount microscopy and the InPouch TV test. *Genitourinary medicine*, **71**: 405–406.

Brookmeyer R, Quinn TC (1995) Estimation of current Human Immunodeficiency Virus incidence from a cross-sectional survey using early diagnostic tests. *American journal of epidemiology*, **141**: 166–172.

Brookmeyer R, Quinn T, Shepherd M et al. (1995) The AIDS epidemic in India: A new method for estimating current Human Immunodeficiency Virus (HIV) rates. *American journal of epidemiology*, **142**: 709–713.

Ching S, Lee H, Hook III et al. (1995) Ligase chain reaction for detection of *Neisseria gonorrhoeae*. *Journal of clinical microbiology*, **33**: 3111–3114.

Cohen CR, Duerr A, Pruithithada N et al.(1995) Bacterial vaginosis and HIV seroprevalence among female commercial sex workers in Chiang Mai, Thailand. *AIDS*, **9**: 1093–1097.

Cushman L, Kalmuss D, Wawer M (1998) Home-based STD screening of women in Washington Heights: a feasibility study. Abstract B7, National STD Prevention Conference, Dallas, Texas, 6–9 December.

Dallabetta GA, Gerbase AC, Holmes KK (1998) Problems, solutions and challenges in syndromic management of sexually transmitted diseases. *Sexually transmitted infections*, **74**(Suppl. 1): S1–11.

Downing RG, Otten RA, Marum E et al. (1998) Optimizing the delivery of HIV counseling and testing services: The Uganda experience using rapid HIV antibody test algorithms. *Journal of AIDS and human retrovirology*, **18**: 384–388.

Draper D, Parker R, Patterson E et al. (1993) Detection of *Trichomonas vaginalis* in pregnant women with the InPouch TV Culture System. *Journal of clinical microbiology*, **31**: 1016–1018.

Gaydos CQ, Quinn TC (1995) DNA amplification assays: a new standard for diagnosis of *Chlamydia trachomatis* infections. *Venerology*, **8**: 234–239.

Glantz JC (1997) Screening and treatment of bacterial vaginosis during pregnancy: a model for determining benefit. *American journal of perinatology*, **14**(8): 487–490.

Gray RH, Wawer MJ, Girdner J et al. (1998a) Use of self-collected vaginal swabs for detection of *Chlamydia trachomatis*. Letter. *Sexually transmitted diseases*, **8**: 450.

Gray RH, Wawer MJ, Sewankambo NK et al. (1998b) Population-based study of fertility in women with HIV-1 infection in Uganda. *Lancet*, **351**: 98–103.

Gray RH, Wawer MJ, Sewankambo NK et al. (1999) Relative risk and population attributable fraction of incident HIV associated with symptoms of STDs and treatable STDs in Rakai, Uganda. *AIDS*, **13**: 2113–2123.

Grosskurth H, Mosha F, Todd J et al. (1995) Impact of improved treatment of sexually transmitted diseases on HIV infection in rural Tanzania: randomised controlled trial. *Lancet*, **346**: 53–56.

Grosskurth H, Mayaud P, Mosha F et al. (1996) Asymptomatic gonorrhoea and chlamydia infection in rural Tanzanian men. *British journal of medicine*, **312**: 277–280.

Haughie GE, Ames WR, Madsen EF (1975) The use of tampons for identifying asymptomatic *N. gonorrhoea* infections. *Journal of American Venereal Disease Association*, **2**(2): 26–28.

Hayes R, Wawer MJ, Gray RH et al. (1997) Randomized trials of STD control for HIV prevention: report of an international workshop. *Genitourinary medicine*, **73**: 432–443.

Hiller S (1993) Diagnostic microbiology of bacterial vaginosis. *American journal of obstetrics and gynecology*, **169**: 455–459.

Hillier SL, Nugent RP, Eschenbach DA et al. (1995) Association between bacterial vaginosis and preterm delivery of low-birth-weight infants. *New England journal of medicine*, **333**(26): 1737–1742.

Holmes KK, Mardh P-a, Sparling PF et al. (1990) *Sexually transmitted diseases.* New York, McGraw-Hill, Inc.

Kapiga SH, Vuylsteke B, Lyamuya EF et al. (1998) Evaluation of sexually transmitted diseases diagnostic algorithms among family planning clients in Dar Es Salaam, Tanzania. *Sexually transmitted infections*, **74**(Suppl. 1): S132–138.

Koumans EH, Johnson RE, Knapp JS et al. (1998) Laboratory testing for *Neisseria gonorrhoeae* by recently introduced nonculture tests: a performance review with clinical and public health considerations. *Clinical infectious disease*, **27**: 1171–1180.

Lee HH, Max A, Chernesky JS et al. (1995) Diagnosis of *Chlamydia trachomatis* genitourinary infection in women by ligase chain reaction assay of urine. *Lancet*, **345**: 213– 216.

Lorincz A (1996) Hybrid capture TM method for detection of human papillomavirus DNA in clinical specimens. *Papillomavirus report*, **7**: 1–6.

Meehan MP, Sewankambo N, Wawer M et al. (1999) Sensitivity and specificity of HIV-1 testing of urine compared with serum specimens: Rakai, Uganda. *Sexually transmitted diseases*, **13**: 37–39.

Morse S, Moreland AA, Holmes KK (1996) *Sexually transmitted diseases and AIDS.* Barcelona, Mosby-Wolfe.

Obasi A, Mosha F, Quigley M et al. (1999) Antibody to herpes simplex virus type 2 as a marker of sexual risk behavior in rural Tanzania. *Journal of infectious disease*, **179**: 16–24.

Parham CE, Peittiti DE, Larsen A et al. (1984) Interlaboratory comparison of the toluidine red unheated serum test antigen preparation. *Journal of clinical microbiology*, **20**: 434–437.

Paxton LA, Sewankambo N, Gray R et al. (1998) Asymptomatic non-ulcerative genital tract infections in a rural Ugandan population. *Sexually transmitted infections*, **74**: 421–425.

Pettiti DE, Larsen SA (1983) Harbec PSea: toluidine red unheated serum test, a nontreponemal test for syphilis. *Journal of clinical microbiology*, **18**: 1141–1145.

Prince HE, Ernst CE, Hogrefe WR (2000) Evaluation of an enzyme immunoassay system of measuring herpes simplex virus (HSV) type 1-specific and HSV type 2-specific IgG antibodies. *Journal of clinical laboratory analysis*, **14**: 13–16.

Serwadda D, Wawer MJ, Shah K et al. (1999) Use of a hybrid capture assay of self-collected vaginal swabs in Uganda for detection of HPV. *Journal of infectious diseases*, **180**: 1316–1319.

Sewankambo NK, Wawer MJ, Gray RH et al. (1994) Demographic impact of HIV infection in rural Rakai District, Uganda. *AIDS*, **8**: 1707–1713.

Sewankambo NK, Gray RH, Wawer MJ et al. (1997) Human immunodeficiency virus type-1 infection associated with abnormal vaginal flora morphology and bacterial vaginosis. *Lancet*, **350**: 546–550.

Wawer MJ, McNairn D, Wabwire-Mangen F et al. (1995) Self-administered vaginal swabs for population-based assessment of *Trichomonas vaginalis* infection. Letter. *Lancet*, **345**: 131–132.

Wawer MJ, Gray RH, Sewankambo NK et al. (1998) A randomized, community trial of intensive STD control for AIDS prevention, Rakai, Uganda. *AIDS*, **12**: 1211–1225.

Wawer MJ, Sewankambo NK, Serwadda D et al. (1999) Control of sexually transmitted diseases for AIDS prevention in Uganda: a randomized community trial. *Lancet*, **353**:525–535.

11

The value of the imperfect: the contribution of interview surveys to the study of gynaecological ill health

John Cleland[1] and Siobán Harlow[2]

[1] Centre for Population Studies, London School of Hygiene and Tropical Medicine, London, UK; [2] University of Michigan, Ann Arbor, USA

There are three main ways of measuring gynaecological morbidity: clinical examinations by trained medical practitioners, laboratory tests on biological specimens such as blood and urine, and questioning individuals or groups about their perceptions and experiences of illness. Clinical and laboratory approaches have been addressed in Chapters 8, 9 and 10. The central purpose of Chapters 11, 12 and 13 is to assess the role of the third approach to the measurement of gynaecological morbidity, its causes and consequences. The focus of this chapter is on structured interview surveys.

Interview surveys on health have been a familiar form of enquiry for decades. Many lessons have been learnt about their utility and limitations, and about measurement issues. Much of this experience is relevant to the design of surveys on gynaecological morbidity in low-income countries. Accordingly, this chapter starts with a summary of these lessons and the application of the survey method to two important dimensions of gynaecological morbidity – reproductive tract infections and menstrual dysfunction. These two morbidities have been chosen because they are the most prevalent gynaecological problems that women of reproductive age face, if not the most serious. As will become apparent, menstrual dysfunction lends itself well to investigation by the survey method and there is a growing body of experience upon which to draw. Conversely, the study of reproductive tract infections by surveys is relatively recent and has encountered serious problems.

General lessons from health interview surveys

Lack of correspondence between self-reported morbidity and results of clinical examinations or laboratory tests

The fact that self-reported ill health (or perceived morbidity) may have only a tenuous relationship with diagnoses based on clinical examination or laboratory tests (often called observed morbidity) has been known for a long time. Some of the reasons for these discrepancies are obvious. Infections may be completely asymptomatic, sometimes for long periods of time, as in the case of many intestinal parasites and, of course, HIV. Conversely, some pathologies are only too apparent to the individual, such as backache or menorrhagia, but may exhibit no signs detectable by the clinician. Conditions regarded by subjects as a normal part of life may be defined by medical practitioners as pathological (e.g. anaemia) or vice versa.

However, the lack of correspondence between perceived and observed morbidity is too striking to be entirely explained by such obvious factors, and has led many medical anthropologists such as Arthur Kleinman (1980) to propose a fundamental distinction between disease and illness. Disease is defined as a malfunction in a biological or psychological sense. Illness is the social meaning attached to perceived disorders by the sufferer. This social meaning includes notions of cause, appropriate behaviour for the individual and appropriate treatment. There may be disease without illness, as when an observable morbidity or condition remains socially unacknowledged or unrecognized. And there may be illness without disease.

Kleinman's distinction has important implications for a correct understanding of the role of interview surveys in the study of ill health. Self-reported morbidity corresponds largely to the concept of illness. Laboratory tests are entirely disease-oriented, while clinical diagnosis often occupies an intermediate position because it is usually based partly on an examination and partly on the patient's verbal account of the illness. The fundamental dilemma for the self-reported approach to the measurement of ill health is to recognize when to accept that disease and illness are two very different dimensions that cannot and should not be reconciled, and when to attempt to narrow the gap between these two approaches by skilful questioning (e.g. verbal algorithms).

The lack of correspondence between results obtained from different measurement approaches applies with particular force to gynaecological morbidity. As already mentioned, HIV infection is asymptomatic for long periods, and the same may be true, particularly in women, of classical sexually transmitted infections (STIs). Thus, women may be infected with serious, even fatal, diseases without any awareness of the abnormality. The reverse is also true. Women presenting at health facilities with symptoms of reproductive tract infections (e.g. vaginal discharge, lower abdominal pain) are often found to be free of any biomedically detectable infection or pathology (e.g. Hawkes et al., 1999; Wilkinson et al., 1999). Similarly, reported symptoms gathered in community-based surveys of reproductive tract infections correlate poorly with the results of clinical examination or laboratory testing (e.g. Bulut et al., 1997; Sadana, 2000; Zurayk et al., 1995). Another consequence of the subjective nature of perceived morbidity is that comparisons of the nature or overall burden of morbidity between populations are extremely difficult to interpret. Murray and Chen (1992) point out that the self-reported burden of morbidity is higher in the US than in India despite the fact that life expectancy is nearly 20 years longer in North America. In India, the self-reported burden is highest in Kerala (the state with the lowest mortality). Similarly, within the same population, self-reported morbidity often rises with household income or educational status. To conclude that perceived morbidity always rises as the risks of death fall would be an exaggeration, but, clearly, feelings of ill health and/or willingness to express them bear little relation to more 'objective' measures, such as life expectancy, nutritional status, parasitic load or extent of functional disability.

The proposed reasons for these counter-intuitive relationships are speculative but presumably reflect a rise in expectations regarding health in parallel with improvements in living standards, education and availability of effective health care. Conditions once regarded as a normal part of life are no longer tolerated and awareness grows that remedies are available. Ailments previously regarded as trivial and therefore ignored invoke treatment seeking responses. Rising incomes make possible greater use of services. Shifts in beliefs about aetiology – from spiritual to biological explanations – may also act to alter perceptions of morbidity.

The paucity of comparable cross-national data prevents any firm conclusions regarding the link between educational and living standards in a population and the burden of self-reported gynaecological illness. However, the available evidence suggests that the subjective meanings given to gynaecological symptoms vary between cultures, and that these variations have a major influence on the importance attached to symptoms and the propensity to report them. For instance, in South Asia, vaginal discharge appears to cause much greater concern than in other regions because it is thought to lead to progressive weakness. Reporting of discharge may reflect a general feeling of ill health or anxiety rather than the existence of a specific reproductive tract infection per se (Trollope-Kumar, 1999). Consequently, both ethnographical studies and surveys in South Asia tend to yield high estimates of self-reported symptoms (Bang and Bang, 1994; Koenig et al., 1998) that may well exceed the level of underlying biomedical infection (Hawkes et al., 1999).

The value of information on consequences and severity

The preceding section addresses one of the major weaknesses of health interview surveys, namely their limited ability to generate reliable information on the incidence or prevalence of biomedical diseases. However, the value of surveys that are merely restricted to the enumeration of the presence or absence of symptoms is limited because data are so difficult to interpret. The greatest contribution of the interview approach is to explore the subjective dimension of ill health. Such exploration requires information on the consequences of the reported symptoms or illness for the individual, which may include impairment, disability and handicap, and the effect on social or psychological sense of well being.

Some definitions may be clarified at this juncture. In WHO terminology (World Health Organization, 1999), impairment (of bodily function and structure) is a departure from some norm in an individual's biomedical status, disability (or activity limitation) refers to the loss of an ability to perform normal activities, and handicap (or participation restrictions) refers to the social or economic consequences of impairments or disabilities. For instance, excessive vaginal discharge is an impairment. A consequent disability might include a reluctance to engage in sexual intercourse, and this in turn leads to a serious handicap, namely the inability to perform a full conjugal role. The point to stress here is that the reported impairment may or may not correspond to some biomedically verifiable pathology, but the consequences – the disability and handicap – are important realities in their own right, both from the individual's viewpoint and from the perspective of providing a comprehensive assessment of the burden of illness and setting health priorities.

A huge amount of literature exists on the measurement of physical impairment, disability and handicap, as well as on scales that assess generic health-related quality of life and psychological well-being (for useful reviews see Bowling, 1995, 1997). For instance, Bowling (1995) lists no less than 135 protocols or scales. The focus of these instruments is broad, covering variously a general sense of good health, physical disability (e.g. inability to dress, work, walk), psychological dimensions (e.g. depression, anxiety), handicap (e.g. inability to work), social support, satisfaction with therapeutic regimes and adjustment to illness.

Some of the more specialized scales reviewed by Bowling have possible direct relevance to investigations of gynaecological morbidity, particularly the McGill instrument to measure the intensity and nature of pain (Melzack, 1987) and the Lasry sexual functioning scale (Lasry, 1991). Some have been adapted for the study of specific gynaecological conditions such as breast cancer, postpartum ill health and menopause. However, most are designed for specific non-gynaecological diseases (e.g. asthma, stroke) or are specifically adapted to the study of ill health among the aged, and nearly all are more appropriate for use in industrialized countries than low-income settings. This body of literature provides useful experience of the conceptual issues of measuring ill health and its consequences in population-based surveys, but rather little by way of scales or sets of questions that can be directly incorporated in studies of gynaecological morbidity in low-income countries.

The consequences of gynaecological ill health are often mediated by local beliefs and practices. For instance, the consequences of menstrual dysfunction depend

Table 11.1. Examples of questions to elicit consequences and severity of reported gynaecological illness

	Not at all	Only a little	Some	A lot
How much did SYMPTOM usually prevent you from carrying out housework and other daily activities?	0	1	2	3
How much did SYMPTOM usually affect your ability to leave the house for any reason?	0	1	2	3
How much did SYMPTOM usually affect your sexual life?	0	1	2	3
How much did SYMPTOM usually affect your social life?	0	1	2	3
To what extent has SYMPTOM affected your overall sense of contentment?	0	1	2	3
How serious a threat to your overall health is SYMPTOM?	0	1	2	3

critically on the type of menstrual hygiene used and on beliefs about impurity that, in some populations, severely curtail the activities of menstruating women. Accordingly, the development of questionnaires requires detailed knowledge of the local culture and/or prior ethnographic work. Another general consideration is that gynaecological morbidity may affect several spheres of life (e.g. work, domestic duties, social activities, sexual conduct). A comprehensive documentation of consequences may require separate questions on each sphere (see examples in Table 11.1).

The systematic measurement of consequences, both in terms of disability and handicap, will capture the most important dimension of severity, namely the extent to which the reported illness results in curtailment of activities and roles that are considered normal, given the respondent's age, sex and social setting. Details of health-seeking behaviour and costs (see next section) may provide further insights into severity, though, of course, considerations of access and affordability may be equally important determinants of health seeking behaviour as is perceived severity of illness.

Some forms of gynaecological morbidity, such as excessive menstrual bleeding or vaginal discharge, require specific questions on direct consequences such as staining of clothes, bed linen or furniture and the need to use extra protection to minimize soiling. Women's perceptions of 'normality' with regard to menstrual bleeding and discharge are subjective, and it is therefore useful to obtain more objective, albeit indirect, measures of the volume of flow and the inconvenience caused, as will be discussed in greater detail (see also Table 11.7).

Severity also has an entirely subjective dimension (i.e. perceived severity) that

Table 11.2. Selected facets of World Health Organization's quality of life assessment

Overall quality of life

How would you rate your quality of life?

How satisfied are you with your quality of life?

In general, how satisfied are you with your life?

How satisfied are you with your health?

Pain and discomfort

How often do you suffer physical pain?

Do you worry about your pain or discomfort?

How difficult is it for you to handle any pain or discomfort?

To what extent do you feel that physical pain prevents you from doing what you need to do?

Activities of daily living

To what extent are you able to carry out your daily activities?

To what extent do you have difficulty performing your routine activities?

How satisfied are you with your ability to perform your daily activities?

How much are you bothered by any limitations in performing your everyday activities?

Sexual activity

How would you rate your sex life?

How well are your sexual needs fulfilled?

How satisfied are you with your sex life?

Are you bothered by any difficulties in your sex life?

Source: WHOQOL Group (1998).

does not necessarily correlate highly with more objective measures of disability, handicap and health seeking. Beliefs about aetiology, or long-term prognosis, are likely to influence an individual's rating of the severity of the illness. While interview surveys are not well suited to a full investigation of beliefs about causation, they should attempt to obtain an indication of perceived severity.

Generic measures of health and well being

Reproductive health has been defined as a 'state of complete physical, mental and social well-being and not merely the absence of disease or infirmity in all matters relating to the reproductive system and to its functions and processes' (United Nations, 1994). This holistic concept has considerable rhetorical appeal but we are unaware of any successful attempts to derive a battery of indicators that could be measured in interview surveys. Indeed, it is probably impossible to separate reproductive well being from general health status, particularly for women, because the two are so intertwined. For instance, problems of a reproductive or sexual nature may lead to generalized depression or vice versa, anaemia is a risk feature for poor obstetric outcomes and repeated pregnancies may cause or exacerbate anaemia.

Because of this difficulty of disentangling reproductive from general health, researchers should consider the option of including one of the many instruments that have been developed to measure overall health-related quality of life. The inclusion of such an instrument in surveys of gynaecological morbidity should sharpen the focus on consequences, by establishing, for instance, to what extent women suffering from symptoms of gynaecological morbidity have a lower quality of life than non-sufferers. One of the general instruments that has been developed and tested for cross-cultural use is WHO's quality of life assessment (WHOQOL Group, 1998). This covers 25 aspects or facets of health-related quality of life, each of which is measured by four questions (the most relevant are listed in Table 11.2).

The obvious overlap or redundancy in these groups of questions reflects a fundamental tenet of psychometric measurement, namely that a characteristic can be better measured by combining responses to a set of questions rather than by relying on answers to a single question. In the WHO instrument, answers to all questions are recorded as five-point Likert scales (i.e. ordered sequences of words or phrases such as never, occasionally, sometimes, usually, always). Answers are assigned numerical values (i.e. 1 to 5) and statistical analysis is performed to choose questions the score of which correlates highly with the aggregate score of other questions in the same set or battery. This procedure ensures that the final set of questions indeed measures the same characteristic or facet.

Because it has been tested in a variety of low and high income populations (albeit with literate or semi-literate subjects), the WHO quality of life assessment provides a good starting point for investigators who wish to study the consequences of gynaecological morbidity in developing countries.

Treatment seeking and costs

Another strength of interview surveys on illness is the information that can be gathered on treatment seeking and associated costs. Unlike issues of impairment, disability and handicap, the huge literature on treatment seeking and costs from industrialized societies is complemented by a rich body of experience from developing countries, particularly with regard to the treatment of childhood illnesses. The value of such data is multifaceted. They can provide overall measures of potential demand for specific types of health service; establish the relative contributions of self-treatment; resort to indigenous or traditional practitioners or to allopathic practitioners in therapeutic strategies; identify the contributions of private and public sector health provision; estimate the financial or economic consequences of ill health; and disclose barriers to quick and effective treatment. The advantages of the community-based survey approach over other methods of obtaining information about responses to illness and service utilization apply particularly to the study of gynaecological problems in low-income countries. The available evidence suggests that women in some societies may be reluctant to seek professional advice or treatment for gynaecological complaints because of embarrassment or shame, or the perception that the condition is normal (Antrobus, Germain and Nowrojee, 1994). For instance, Bang et al. (1989) found a high level of gynaecological problems in their Indian study population that went largely untreated. Their clear demonstration of the unmet need for gynaecological services had a considerable policy impact, as did the well-known Giza study (Younis et al., 1993) which demonstrated a large burden of gynaecological problems. Enquiries restricted to clinical populations would have captured only a small unrepresentative fraction of women suffering from reproductive ill health.

As documented in Chapter 2, response to illness may take the form of a complex web of consultations and behaviour in which different types of treatment may be pursued simultaneously or in sequence. In many countries, the partial blending of different medical systems adds to the difficulty of identifying a clear therapeutic strategy (Durkin-Langley, 1984; Nichter, 1980). Interview surveys can be used to gather two types of information about response to illnesses and health-care seeking: general information and episode-specific information. General information may include questions on knowledge and beliefs about ways to treat particular illnesses, knowledge of alternative sources of treatment and advice, evaluation of these alternatives in terms of access, cost, perceived quality and effectiveness, and past use. Such general data, however, can also be gathered more cheaply and in greater depth by non-survey methods (e.g. free listing, pile sorting and focus group discussions). The real strength of structured surveys lies in the documentation of individual therapy seeking behaviour in connection with recent illness episodes. Decisions to seek expert help depend partly on perceived aetiology of the illness and its perceived consequences. The views of other family members may carry as much weight as the woman's own views. To do justice to this complexity may require repeated semi-structured interviewing. In a structured interview survey, some of the detail, elucidation of the nature of social interactions and explanatory depth has to be sacrificed. Nevertheless, skilfully designed questionnaires are able to yield information of great value.

In designing questionnaires, the following considerations should be borne in mind:

- Self-treatment, including diet modifications, requires specific probing. Otherwise, it may remain unreported.
- Because of social desirability bias, respondents may be more likely to report allopathic treatment in the formal health service than traditional, spiritual or

informal health care seeking. Specific prompts or probes on non-allopathic therapies are required to collect comprehensive information.

- More than one practitioner may be consulted, particularly for more serious or prolonged illness episodes. Accordingly, the questionnaire should make provision for at least two and perhaps three types of consultations.
- A consultation with the same practitioner may involve more than one visit, and the questionnaire may need to take this into account.
- Accurate health expenditure data require separate questions on cost of travel, consultation, fee and cost of drugs. Indirect or opportunity costs (e.g. lost wages or lost output) are more difficult to measure but should be considered.
- Community-based surveys are not ideally suited to the collection of information on the diagnostic and therapeutic procedures of practitioners, particularly in uneducated populations. More accurate data will be obtained from facility-based studies using observation, practitioner interviews and exit interviews with clients, similar to the situation analysis methodology developed by the Population Council (Miller et al., 1997).
- Prospective surveys are more suitable for gathering high quality data on treatment seeking than single-round studies (this point is discussed in detail later).

An interesting example of the application of some of these guidelines is provided by a study of primary infertility in Andhra Pradesh, India (Unisa, 1999). As infertility is defined as a prolonged time without conceiving, a long reference period was necessarily employed and ample provision had to be made for multiple treatment seeking sequences. The section of the questionnaire concerning treatment seeking started with an enumeration (first spontaneous, then probed) of all the types of treatment that the couple had sought (see Table 11.3). The chronological order of each course of treatment was then ascertained. For each type of treatment, a sequence of 11 questions was administered. These included timing of start of treatment, duration of treatment, number of visits and cost. The results showed that, while the majority of infertile couples had experienced less than three courses of treatment, a few had tried six or more courses, at an average total cost of over Rs 22,000 (about US$490 at 1999 exchange rate).

General versus illness-specific enquiries

Surveys on ill health may attempt to measure a generic sense of health-related quality of life, the entire range of illnesses, a particular subset of illnesses or a single type of illness. Examples abound for each of these measures. Most large household surveys in developing countries attempt to cover the entire range of chronic and acute morbidities. Typically, introductory questions are asked about chronic conditions, and these are followed by items requesting information on illnesses of each

Table 11.3. Example of questions on types of health seeking

		Spontaneous	Probed	Order
Couples visit many different kinds of people for help to become pregnant. They visit doctors and hospitals, as well as traditional doctors, herbalists, vaids and hakims. I would be interested in hearing about all the people you might have consulted. Have you seen anyone for advice or treatment for this problem?	Allopathy			
	Primary health centre	1	2	[ ]
	Private hospital	2	2	[ ]
	Government hospital	3	3	[ ]
	Private doctor/clinic	4	4	[ ]
	Pharmacy	5	5	[ ]
	Ayurvedic	6	6	[ ]
	Homeopathy	7	7	[ ]
	Unani	8	8	[ ]
	Herbalist	9	9	[ ]
	Dai	10	10	[ ]
	Traditional practitioners	11	11	[ ]
	Home remedies (elders)	12	12	[ ]
	Religious/superstitious practice	13	13	[ ]
	Don't remember/don't know	14	14	
	Not consulted	99	99	

Note: Let the respondent answer and code all treatment and advice without any probing. For each type of treatment not mentioned spontaneously, probe and circle positive responses in the second column. In the third column, write the order in which treatments were sought.

Source: Adapted from Unisa (1999).

household member in the preceding two or four weeks. This broad approach is ill-suited to the study of gynaecological problems. Interviewers and the main respondent, the household head, are often men. Such proxy reporting is disastrous. Even when an adult female is the respondent, embarrassment and shyness inhibit reporting of gynaecological problems, unless specific probes are used. As a result, gynaecological problems are conspicuous only by their absence in the published results from general health enquiries.

Surveys on gynaecological morbidity require the use of female interviewers and female respondents and a reasonable degree of privacy for the interview. Two main options for structuring such surveys can be considered. A restricted option would focus solely on gynaecological conditions. A more general option would enquire about all illnesses of the woman, with a checklist to ensure that the more sensitive gynaecological issues are not overlooked. The relative merit of these two approaches depends, of course, on the aims of the study. For many purposes, a narrower focus on gynaecological problems will be the preferred option as it permits detailed questioning on symptoms, consequences and treatment seeking. However, when a more comprehensive account of women's ill health is required or when an estimate of the contribution of gynaecological morbidity to the overall burden of ill health is needed, a broader approach will be necessary.

A recent example of the broad approach comes from the work of Bhatia and Cleland (1999) in Karnataka, India. In this study, reproductive ill health (mainly of a gynaecological nature) accounted for about half of all days of reported illness and for 31 per cent of health expenditure in a sample of young married women. Among the 12 major diagnostic categories of the World Health Organization's International Classification of Diseases (ICD-10; World Health Organization, 1992), genitourinary symptoms were by far the most commonly reported.

Longitudinal versus cross-sectional surveys

The vast majority of health interview surveys, particularly those with national coverage, are single-round, cross-sectional enquiries. In such designs, most questions about illnesses are restricted to a recall period of two or four weeks. This type of study is attractive because it can provide useful summary snapshots of the health status of a population at a relatively low cost. Cross-sectional surveys are particularly well suited to the measurement of common acute conditions such as respiratory infections and diarrhoeal diseases. Results may be presented in terms of point prevalence (the percentage ill at the time of interview), period prevalence (the percentage reported ill at any time during the recall period), the percentage of days of illness in the recall period and the incidence (the number of new episodes of illness that started in the recall period per 1000 persons).

One of the great disadvantages of the cross-sectional approach is that the inevitably short recall period cuts across episodes of illness in an arbitrary manner. Thus, episodes may have started before the recall boundary and may not have ended by the time of interview. This element of arbitrary censoring greatly complicates the collection of useful information on consequences, treatment seeking and costs, which ideally should be collected for completed episodes of illness. The longer the duration of illness episodes, the less satisfactory the cross-sectional approach.

These considerations have direct implications for community-based surveys of gynaecological morbidity. Episodes of the latter tend to be longer in duration than episodes of acute respiratory or gastrointestinal morbidity. For instance, Bhatia and Cleland (2000a) found in south India that the median duration of episodes of a genitourinary nature was 46.7 days: 67 per cent of such episodes exceeded 28 days in duration and 38 per cent exceeded 60 days. These figures contrast with a median duration of only 12.4 days for all illness episodes reported by young married women, of which only 16 per cent exceeded 60 days in duration.

The prolonged nature of many gynaecological disorders (e.g. menstrual problems, excessive vaginal discharge) reduces the utility of the cross-sectional approach. Within a 4-week reference period, very few gynaecological episodes will both start and finish. Extension of the reference period to 6 months or even one year is a possible solution but this tactic increases problems related to accuracy of recall and the consequent likelihood of a decline in the quality of data. Women are likely to forget less severe episodes that ended several months prior to the interview, and may have difficulty in remembering details of health care seeking. One superficially attractive alternative is to first identify current or recent episodes, establish their duration and finally attempt to reconstruct the consequences and related health-seeking patterns since the initial onset of symptoms. For chronic and severe conditions such as infertility and prolapse, this approach has considerable merits but its great defect is the selectivity of the episodes that are included. Specifically, episodes that are relatively short, self-limiting or successfully treated will be omitted, leading to a biased picture.

A more satisfactory alternative is to employ a prospective or longitudinal study design in which women are interviewed at regular intervals (e.g. every four weeks) over a period of one or two years, as this approach solves many of the methodological problems inherent in a cross-sectional design. The onset and end of most episodes can be clearly identified and a comprehensive account can be obtained of consequences, health seeking and costs per completed episode. This method also permits the collection of more detailed information than a cross-sectional approach, and may facilitate the development of close rapport between the interviewer and subject over time that in turn may lead to better reporting.

It is generally accepted that prospective studies are superior to cross-sectional enquiries in the study of ill health and its consequences. The disadvantages are largely of a practical nature. Costs are high per subject and thus sample sizes tend to be small. Given the logistical problems of repeated observations on the same subjects, most such studies are restricted to a small geographical area where adequate supervision, transport and so on can be assured. Data management issues can be daunting because of the sheer volume of data and the need to link information from successive rounds. Sample attrition may be a drawback, particularly in more mobile urban populations. Finally, ethical issues must also be addressed, such as how to handle cases in which women present with severe conditions as well as the more general requirement of avoiding possible exploitation.

While it is clear that successful execution of a prospective study demands an experienced and skilful research team, these problems are not insurmountable. In our view, small prospective studies will usually be more rewarding in terms of new knowledge on gynaecological morbidity than larger cross-sectional surveys.

Measurement lessons

Many general reviews of health interview surveys have been published (e.g. Kroeger, 1983; Murray et al., 1992; Ross and Vaughan, 1986; Timaeus et al., 1998; Van Ginneken, 1993). The purpose of this section is to distil the key measurement lessons that have relevance to gynaecological studies in low-income populations.

Use of appropriate vocabulary

Questionnaire construction should be preceded by ethnographic research to establish the appropriate words for specific symptoms or illnesses. The same general symptom may be represented in local languages by several different words or phrases, each of which may convey subtle variations in meaning. For instance, in many countries there are several different words for diarrhoea (Yoder, 1991) and, similarly, different types of fever are distinguished in the Gambia (Hill and David, 1990). The same complex taxonomy of illness may apply to gynaecological morbidities. Bang and Bang (1994) identified no less than 12 different terms for vaginal discharge in a community in central India. The characteristics of the discharge, its perceived cause and severity were among the principles underlying this classification (see Table 11.4). Use of appropriate local vocabulary is likely to result in more precise and interpretable data than would otherwise be the case.

Formal allopathic disease classifications should be avoided. Instead, a widely understood term in the local language should be used if an appropriate one exists. In the absence of such a term, a symptom or group of symptoms should be used. For instance, in the Giza study, uterine prolapse was described as 'a feeling of heaviness down below'. Similarly, Graham et al. (1995) recommended the following questions to identify fistulae: 'Sometimes, after childbirth, women are not able to

Table 11.4. Local classification of vaginal discharge (central India)

Khalai (or kharai)	The mildest and most common variety, manifested as thin white discharge with minimal smell and staining of underclothes. The women believe that it generally occurs due to weakness
Pandhara pani ('*white discharge*')	Whitish in colour but greater in amount. It wets underclothing and the white stain that it leaves remains even after washing
Pandhara pani	May be thin, like rice water (hence also called *dhupani* or *dhuwani* meaning 'rice water'). When the underclothes are washed, the wash water comes out like white 'rice water'. Otherwise, it may be thick like curds or sticky white like nasal discharge
Dhattu (or dhat)	The white discharge passed with urine in men. Some said that *dhat* is also seen in women's urine
Poo parma (or wasi parma or dhatu parm)	A more severe variety, where the discharge is yellowish, smells foul like pus and stains underclothing. Sores in the vulval region are accompanied by burning and itching, and a burning sensation while urinating often characterize this condition
Pair (or pair parma or ragat parma)	The most severe variety, with a reddish discharge and foul smell. Women feel that death is almost certain as all the blood in the body is being drained off

Source: Bang and Bang (1994).

control the leaking of faeces or urine. Has this ever happened to you?' *If yes,* 'Is this leaking continuous or does it happen when you cough, laugh or lift heavy objects?'

In this example, the purpose of the second question is to distinguish stress incontinence from fistulae. This is a simple example of what is commonly called a verbal algorithm: a carefully constructed sequence of questions to measure a combination of symptoms with the intention of bringing about a closer correspondence between self-reports and biomedical diagnosis. Such verbal algorithms have been widely applied in the study of childhood illnesses and cause of death (e.g. neonatal tetanus, dysentery, measles and acute respiratory infections). Because the main purpose is to narrow the gap between self-reported symptoms and biomedical conditions, verbal algorithms ideally require validation against biomedical diagnosis.

Use of symptom checklists

Though many health surveys have used open-ended questions to enquire about recent illnesses, there is a near-consensus among researchers that such an approach leads to selective under-reporting of low-level chronic conditions and less acute ill-nesses and, no doubt, more sensitive or embarrassing symptoms. Reporting is improved by the use of a checklist of symptoms, or illnesses in the local language, which is read out to the respondent. In their review of Indian studies, Koenig et al. (1998) adduce evidence that explicit probing with a symptom checklist substantially increases positive reporting of gynaecological problems compared with open-ended questioning. The most marked increase was observed for dyspareunia, suggesting that symptoms directly linked to sexual intercourse may be particularly vulnerable to under-reporting. Careful preparation of this checklist is one of the keys to good questionnaire design.

While combinations of symptoms, clinical signs and behavioural reports form the essence of clinical management of many gynaecological morbidities, their relevance to interview surveys is not well established. There are several possibilities (e.g. a combination of vaginal discharge and genital itching in the diagnosis of lower reproductive tract infections or lower abdominal pain plus fever in the diagnosis of pelvic inflammatory disease). However, we are unaware of any evidence that such combinations result in significant improvements in the diagnostic accuracy of self-reported symptoms when gauged against the results of clinical examinations or laboratory tests.

Recall periods

Wide agreement exists that accurate recall of brief common illnesses, such as respiratory infections, can only be attempted over a short recall period. Two weeks is often the preferred option, though there is some evidence that even this may be too extended for some purposes. As already mentioned, the use of such short recall periods is unsuitable for the study of gynaecological illnesses because of their relatively long duration. A variety of alternative approaches have been used. Some studies (e.g. Bhatia and Cleland, 1995; Kaufman et al., 1999) have restricted attention to current episodes and thus yield estimates of point prevalence only. This approach has the advantage of simplicity, but the disadvantage that no valid estimates of durations of episodes can be derived, that self-limiting or successfully treated episodes are excluded and that symptoms characterized by intervals of remission followed by reappearance may be missed.

For these reasons, application of the 'current status' approach to the measurement of gynaecological problems in cross-sectional surveys is far from ideal. In most studies it may be preferable to use a longer reference or recall period. The most commonly used recall time frame is three months; this was used in the classic WHO multi-site study of gynaecological morbidity (Omran and Standley, 1976, 1981) and in the Istanbul and Giza studies (Bulut et al., 1997; Younis et al., 1993). A 12-month span for the measurement of symptoms of STIs (Ferry, 1995) was used in the series of surveys coordinated by the Global Programme on AIDS, while others have used an even longer reference period (Jain et al., 1996).

In view of the variety of endpoints in gynaecological surveys, the variability of reference periods currently employed and the lack of methodological studies in this area, emphatic recommendations are not justified. However, for most purposes a recall period of 3 or 6 months is appropriate for the study of many gynaecological conditions, though 12 months may be preferred in the case of menstrual dysfunction. Care should be taken to distinguish episodes that started before the reference period from those that started within it, so as to allow correct estimation of episode length and incidence, if required. It is also important to establish which episodes are still continuing at the time of interview to allow point prevalence estimates.

Complexities in the measurement of chronic conditions with an episodic nature

In most of the literature on health surveys, the simplifying assumption is implicitly made that morbidities fall into two broad categories. The first comprises chronic conditions or disabilities that are typically irreversible, though the effects of some can be controlled by medication (e.g. diabetes, hypertension). The second category consists of acute conditions, usually resulting from infections. It is assumed that these tend to be short, with a recognizable onset and end of symptoms, and that the cessation of symptoms signifies the end of the infection. Measurement of chronic conditions requires a current status question, supplemented perhaps by enquiry into the approximate date of onset. No reference period is needed. Adequate measurement of acute conditions, on the other hand, demands a precise recall period.

Complexities of measurement arise when illnesses do not fall neatly into either category as is often the case with reproductive ill health. Some problems of reproductive health can be regarded as chronic conditions, for example, prolapse and fistulae. Though these conditions are, in principle, curable by surgery or other means, it is reasonable to assume that most cases in low-income countries will not be effectively treated. Other problems fall clearly into the acute category, such as post-abortion septicaemia. However, there are many other illnesses that do not fit neatly into either category. For instance, some menstrual dysfunctions, such as heavy bleeding or severe pain, may be experienced periodically but not every month. Similarly, symptoms of reproductive tract infection may be intermittent, with intervals of remission. In such instances, short separate episodes can easily be confused with episodic manifestations of the same long-term underlying condition. Categorizing infertility, or episodes of sub-fertility, can be even more complex. Probably the best strategy at the moment is to allow the respondent to make the distinction, but practical difficulties of identifying a clear onset and clear end can be anticipated.

The interview context

There is convincing evidence that the identity of the interviewer, the location of the interview and the perceived link to health services may influence the propensity of women to report symptoms of ill health. One major factor has already been noted – the sex of the interviewer. For obvious reasons, women are less likely to report intimate details to a man than to a woman. Experience also suggests that symptoms are more readily reported to medical practitioners than to lay persons (Koenig et al., 1998). Even the expectation of future treatment may result in increased reporting. In an Indian study, higher estimates of illness were recorded by the interviewers when subjects were questioned on the day before a clinical examination than when interviewed on previous occasions (Bhatia and Cleland, 2000b). The degree of rapport or familiarity between investigator and subject may also influence women's responses. Some evidence from India suggests that women are readier to report illness in later than in earlier rounds of longitudinal studies (Bhatia and Cleland, 2000b; Koenig et al., 1998). These considerations have profound implications for the comparability of results obtained from different studies. Those with a clinical component cannot be compared with those that lack such a component and, similarly, results from prospective designs involving repeated contact cannot easily be compared with those from cross-sectional surveys.

In the next two sections of this chapter, we discuss in detail the application of the interview survey approach to the study of reproductive tract infections and menstrual dysfunction. As mentioned earlier, these two dimensions of gynaecological morbidity have been chosen because they are the most common problems faced by women in low-income countries.

Application to the study of reproductive tract infections

Symptomatology

Together with menstrual dysfunctions, reproductive tract infections are the most common category of gynaecological problems found in most populations. A classification of reproductive tract infections is presented in Chapter 2 and risk factors and consequences are discussed in Chapter 3. It remains here to outline the symptoms that may be associated with different types of reproductive tract infections (see Table 11.5). The symptoms of vaginal or cervical infection include abnormal vaginal discharge, dyspareunia, dysuria, itching, blisters and sores. Upper reproductive tract infections or pelvic inflammatory disease may be associated with lower abdominal pain (typically bilateral and sub-acute) and high fever.

The details shown in Table 11.5 illustrate the fact that symptoms of specific infections often overlap. Moreover, many infections are entirely asymptomatic or

Table 11.5. Symptoms associated with common reproductive tract infections

Biomedical condition/infection	Possible symptoms
Candidiasis	White, lumpy discharge Pain during intercourse (dyspareunia) Vaginal soreness/irritation/itchiness Burning feeling when urinating (dysuria)
Bacterial vaginosis	White discharge with fishy smell Mild vaginal itching
Trichomonas vaginalis	Grey or yellow discharge with bad smell Vaginal itching
Gonorrhoea/chlamydia	Yellow or green discharge Pain/burning feeling when urinating (dysuria) Pain/bleeding during intercourse (dyspareunia) Lower abdominal pain Fever
Genital herpes	Genital itching/pain Small blisters that burst and form open genital sores
Chancroid	Painful genital sores that bleed easily High fever Feeling of weakness Discharge Pain/bleeding during intercourse (dyspareunia)
Pelvic inflammatory disease	Lower abdominal pain High fever Feeling of weakness Discharge Pain/bleeding during intercourse (dyspareunia)

produce clinical signs that remain unnoticed by the sufferer. For these reasons, clinical diagnoses (based on reported symptoms and genital examination) tend to be inaccurate when judged by the results of laboratory tests. It is thus hardly surprising that self-reported symptoms alone correspond very poorly with laboratory tests (Bulut et al., 1997; Kaufman et al., 1999; Zurayk et al., 1995).

This lack of correspondence between self-reported symptoms of reproductive tract infections and biomedical diagnosis has radical implications. It implies that interview surveys cannot be used to distinguish the prevalence of more serious infections (e.g. gonorrhoea and chlamydia) from those with less serious health consequences (e.g. candidiasis and trichomonas vaginalis). It also implies that assessment of causes or risk factors will be inadequate. While most of the conditions listed in Table 11.5 are sexually transmitted, the most common ones are not primarily transmitted in this way (candidiasis, bacterial vaginosis). Because self-reports cannot be used to separate aetiologically distinct categories, a severe problem of what epidemiologists term 'case mis-specification' arises, thereby undermining attempts to measure statistical associations between possible risk factors and specific outcomes. Of course, interview methods can be used in tandem with community-based collection of specimens for laboratory analysis and such designs permit proper investigation of behavioural, iatrogenic and other types of determinant or risk factors (e.g. sexual behaviour, hygiene, antibiotic use, recent history of intrusive medical procedures). However, until cheaper and less intrusive diagnostic techniques are developed, community-based studies of reproductive tract infections with a laboratory component will remain expensive, complex and may encounter serious problems of compliance (see Chapters 6 and 7 for further discussion).

Much has been learnt about the role of community-based interview surveys in the investigation of reproductive tract infections in the last 10 years. Prior to 1990, there were very few enquiries based on reasonable representative samples. The single most significant exception is WHO's pioneering multi-country study (Omran and Standley, 1976, 1981). This showed a high prevalence of self-reported symptoms of reproductive tract infection in a wide variety of populations. The 3-month period prevalence of symptoms of vaginal discharge ranged from 17 to 56 per cent and of genital itching from 11 to 34 per cent among married women of reproductive age. These data were almost totally ignored, perhaps because gynaecological morbidity was a low international priority at the time and no doubt also because the WHO study collected no information on the severity and consequences of reported symptoms.

With the more recent results from the Giza study, and similar studies that have used multiple methods to assess gynaecological morbidity in a community setting, it is an appropriate time to attempt a radical appraisal of the aims and content of future interview surveys. Two key points are already clear from the earlier discussion. Surveys without a biomedical component cannot be used to assess disease prevalence and are inappropriate for the proper investigation of biomedical risk factors. These are serious limitations. By contrast, the interview survey approach has a uniquely valuable role to play in documenting the consequences of reproductive tract infection symptoms for women, including details of therapy seeking behaviour. As already discussed, these subjective dimensions of illness are important for any comprehensive assessment of the burden of illness, and for setting priorities in health information campaigns and in the design of improved health services.

Table 11.6. Possible structure of a questionnaire on the prevalence and consequences of symptoms of reproductive tract infections

---

Section 1 *Socio-economic and demographic characteristics*
           Education, employment, age, marital status, childbearing history, characteristics of husband, etc.

Section 2 *General assessment of health-related quality of life*
           Overall health self-assessment, degree of interference with daily activities, pain, sexual activity, etc.

Section 3 *Symptoms of illness, including reproductive tract infections, in the last three months*
           Symptom checklist, measurement of episode lengths

Section 4 *Consequences and severity of specific illnesses*
           Disability and handicap in relevant spheres of life. Subjective measures of severity

Section 5 *Therapy seeking behaviour in relation to reported symptoms in the last three months*
           Resort to home remedies, use of expert advice/treatment, cost of treatments, etc.

Questionnaire content

We have already argued that longitudinal studies represent a better option than cross-sectional surveys. Nevertheless, for practical reasons, cross-sectional surveys will no doubt continue to be the dominant design. Accordingly, in this section, suggestions regarding the content of future surveys are discussed with the cross-sectional model in mind, though much will also be relevant to future longitudinal studies.

A possible structure for a survey questionnaire with the major aim of documenting the prevalence of reproductive tract infection symptoms, their consequences and health seeking responses is presented in Table 11.6. This structure is equally relevant to enquiries on menstrual dysfunction (see next section) and studies with a broader focus on all types of gynaecological morbidity. It is a sound tactic to start any interview with a set of relatively straightforward questions that serve to put the respondent at ease and to allow time for rapport to be established. The amount of demographic and socio-economic detail to be collected will depend on the characteristics of the study population, and it is unnecessary to discuss this further.

The purpose of Section 2 is to measure overall health-related quality of life, which could be based on an adapted version of WHO's instrument (see Table 11.2). The questions should be asked of everyone in the sample, regardless of whether or not they have experienced any recent illnesses. This strategy will permit a comparison of women with and without specific recent symptoms of reproductive tract infections or other illnesses in terms of their perceived quality of life. Such comparisons are essential for a rigorous assessment of the possible consequences of reproductive tract infections for women's lives, yet we are unaware of any community-based study that has attempted such analysis. As usual with cross-sectional studies, such data will not allow a clear-cut disentangling of cause, concomitant or consequence. For instance, a statistical analysis may show that women with recent symptoms of reproductive tract infection report a significantly lower health-related quality of particular facets or dimensions of their life. This association may be indicative of a causal relationship: reproductive tract infection symptoms reduce the quality of life. But it is equally possible that self-reported reproductive tract infection symptoms are primarily an indication of some underlying psychological state (depression, anxiety, marital unhappiness), in which case the causal link is in the opposite direction. Despite this interpretative ambiguity, strong statistical associations would further justify more intensive enquiries while the absence of any association would constitute convincing evidence that the consequences of reproductive tract infections for women's lives were of little importance in that particular study population (though the biomedical consequences might be severe).

In the third section of the questionnaire, symptoms of morbidity, their characteristics, timing and duration are covered. As discussed earlier, investigators can choose to cover all types of morbidity or restrict attention to gynaecological symptoms, or some subset of these, such as reproductive tract infections. On balance, we would advocate a broad-ranging approach to the measurement of illness because this will allow estimation of the contribution of gynaecological symptoms to the overall burden of illness, and this is a considerable advantage if the study is principally designed to provide an assessment of health needs. In this chapter, however, only the measurement of reproductive tract infections is discussed.

A suggested sequence of questions for the third section is presented in Appendix 11.1, though it should be emphasized that vocabulary and classification should be based on preliminary ethnographic work. The following features of the recommended approach should be noted:

- All the main symptoms of reproductive tract infections (see Table 11.5) should be included in the checklist; however, because by itself fever is not specifically gynaecological, the occurrence of this symptom should only be ascertained if other symptoms are reported.
- Positive reporting of abnormal vaginal discharge should be followed up with additional questions on colour, odour and persistence.
- Multiple symptoms should be classified as the same illness or different illnesses according to the perspective of the woman.
- The approximate date of onset and date of end (where applicable) of symptoms and current status should be established.

- The perceived cause of illness should be ascertained using pre-coded categories (based on prior ethnographic work). These data may be useful in the analysis of therapy seeking.

The fourth section addresses the consequences and severity of specific illnesses/symptoms (see Table 11.1 for illustrative questions). The last section of the illustrative questionnaire addresses therapy seeking actions and uses of treatment. We shall not repeat the main considerations to be borne in mind as they were discussed earlier in the chapter. It may be noted, however, that reasons for non-treatment and reasons for choice of a specific type of therapy or practitioner are not recommended for inclusion because such in-depth data on motivations are more appropriately gathered with qualitative approaches.

Applications to the study of menstrual dysfunction

Menstrual morbidities lend themselves well to measurement in the context of health surveys. In contrast to other gynaecological morbidities such as reproductive tract infections, clinical diagnosis of menstrual dysfunction is itself highly dependent on a woman's self-reported clinical history. Although evaluation of the aetiology of a specific complaint may require clinical examination, ultrasound imaging and/or laboratory evaluations, clinical assessment relies heavily on self-reports of menstrual characteristics and symptoms. As the classification of menstrual morbidity has not been addressed elsewhere in this volume, this section first considers the problem of classification and then addresses general measurement issues. A suggested sequence of questions for specific morbidities is provided in Appendix 11.2.

Perhaps the major issue in the measurement of the prevalence or severity of menstrual disorders is clarification of the type of menstrual dysfunction. Data on levels and determinants of menstrual dysfunction in low-income and middle-income countries are scarce and extant studies often lump together diverse and aetiologically distinct complaints into a single category of 'any menstrual complaint'. Such questions are not generally useful since distinct menstrual disorders differ in their aetiologies, health consequences and treatment.

Classification of menstrual morbidity

Menstrual dysfunction may be defined primarily in terms of disruptions in bleeding patterns (e.g. menorrhagia or heavy or prolonged bleeding), polymenorrhoea (frequent menstruation), oligomenorrhoea (infrequent menstruation) and amenorrhoea (cessation of menses). These definitions encompass problems related both to abnormal uterine bleeding, where the amount, duration or frequency of vaginal bleeding per se is the focus of concern, as well as to disruptions in the timing of menstrual cycling. A second, entirely separate, construct of menstrual dysfunction stems from a consideration of pain (dysmenorrhoea) and other symptomatology (premenstrual syndrome) associated with the onset of menses. A third menstrual dysfunction may be defined by disturbance of ovarian function (e.g. anovulation and luteal deficiency), which may or may not manifest as alterations in bleeding patterns. As identification of functional disturbances requires the measurement of hormones and/or daily monitoring (e.g. of basal body temperature), health interview surveys are limited to measurement of disruptions in bleeding pattern, including cycle length disorders and bleeding disorders, menstrual symptomatology, and the consequences of these menstrual disorders on women's quality of life and social functioning.

Cycle length disorders

Amenorrhoea is defined as the cessation of menses. Primary amenorrhoea refers to failure to achieve menarche by age 16, and secondary amenorrhoea refers to cessation of menses after menarche. Although the clinical criterion for amenorrhoea is absence of menses for 6 months or for three times the length of the previous menstrual cycle (Speroff, Glass and Kase, 1994), in research a definition of no menses for 90 days is most commonly used. Oligomenorrhoea is defined as the absence of menses for shorter intervals or as unevenly spaced menses, and is generally operationalized as menstrual cycles of 35–90 days in length. Polymenorrhoea is defined as frequent menses, generally operationalized as menstrual cycles shorter than 21 days.

Although health professionals and the lay public often use the term 'irregular' to describe menstrual cycle disorders, the term is imprecise and has no commonly understood meaning. Some women whose cycles vary by a few days consider their cycles to be irregular precisely because they vary. Other women, whose cycles vary by several days but are consistently one length or the other, consider their cycles to be regular because there is a consistent pattern. Qualitative studies in Bangladesh (Intermediate Technology Bangladesh, 1992) indicate that women use the term to refer both to oligomenorrhoea and having short periods. The lack of utility of questions about irregular bleeding is clearly illustrated by the wide range of prevalences reported for irregular bleeding in the WHO multi-country study of gynaecological morbidity (8–83 per cent) (Omran and Standley, 1976, 1981). Health interview surveys should therefore approach the measurement of cycle length disorders either by obtaining specific information on the range of cycle lengths experienced by a woman during the reference period, or by inquiring whether or not she has had any cycle of lengths consistent with the definitions of oligomenorrhoea, amenorrhoea or polymenorrhoea.

Women have difficulty responding to questions about cycle length primarily for two reasons. First, the language used is often not adequate to distinguish the concept of menstrual periods (i.e. consecutive days of bleeding) from the concept of menstrual cycles (i.e. the time from the start of one menstrual period to the start of the next menstrual period). Thus terms such as cycle length and menstrual period need to be explicitly defined. Furthermore, attention to these two distinct constructs of bleeding episodes and menstrual cycling varies across cultures. Some cultures place little focus on the precise length of intervals between bleeding episodes; thus, asking questions about the relative frequency of bleeding episodes will be more productive than efforts to obtain a precise estimate of length. Second, questions about usual cycle length can be difficult to answer when women have variable cycles. Additional questions on the shortest and longest cycles over the reference period should be included to improve the reliability and validity of the survey instrument (see Appendix 11.2).

Several studies of the quality of interview data have examined women's ability to report characteristics of their previous or usual menstrual cycle (Bean et al., 1979; WHO, 1981). These studies have found that women have difficulty remembering the date of their last menstrual bleed, demonstrate strong digit preference for 28-day and 30-day cycles and, as discussed earlier, have difficulty reporting an average or usual cycle length when their cycles tend to vary in length. The recall of duration of bleeding was found to be more accurate than recall of cycle length. Because many women have difficulty recalling specific details about their menstrual history, prospective recording of bleeding experience using menstrual calendars or diaries is preferable to obtain more precise and valid data on menstrual patterns.

Bleeding disorders

A range of terms are used to describe excessive, prolonged or too frequent bleeding, depending upon the amount of information available on the actual bleeding pattern, the underlying ovarian function and the presence of organic pathology. In the absence of precise information on one or more of these parameters, the term abnormal uterine bleeding is commonly used to describe bleeding complaints. Definitions based on specific bleeding patterns include menorrhagia (regular, normal intervals, excessive flow and duration), metrorrhagia (irregular intervals, excessive flow and duration) and polymenorrhoea (intervals less than 21 days) (Speroff et al., 1994).

In health interview surveys, differential diagnoses based on ovarian function or organic pathology are generally not possible; thus only abnormal uterine bleeding, or particular conditions such as menorrhagia, which are defined by specific alterations in menstrual bleeding patterns, can be measured. Excessive blood loss is defined as blood loss of more than 80 ml per menses (Hallberg et al., 1966), while prolonged menstruation is often defined as bleeding for more than seven or eight

Table 11.7. Example of an approach to quantifying amount of blood flow in a survey format

Light bleeding (change protection 1–3 times per day)

Moderate bleeding (change protection every 3–4 hours)

Heavy bleeding (change protection every 2 hours, or change every hour for less than a 4-hour period)

Very heavy bleeding (change protection every hour or sooner, for more than a 4-hour period)

days. However, a cutpoint of 10 days is thought to distinguish better between abnormal and normal bleeding.

Measuring the amount of menstrual flow using structured interview surveys is more problematic than measuring length of menstruation. Hence interview questions should include criteria to help women define the amount of flow, and should focus on the time elapsed between changes of menstrual protection or on level of interference with their daily routine. Counting the number of pads/tampons used per day is not recommended as women may use sanitary protection for reasons other than bleeding (e.g. for incontinence) and focus group research suggests that women construct their experience of bleeding in terms of elapsed time between changes. An example of such definitions is provided in Table 11.7 (see also Appendix 11.2).

Two recently developed instruments – a pictorial blood loss assessment scale (Higham, Obrien and Shaw, 1990) which can be filled out over the course of one bleeding episode and a 13-item screening questionnaire (Ruta et al., 1995) – have been shown to be sensitive and specific for the diagnosis of menorraghia and to gauge its severity, respectively. These should be easily adaptable to low-income and middle-income country settings.

Studies have shown that many women who experience considerable blood loss do not report excessive bleeding (low sensitivity); however, mean blood loss for women who do report heavy bleeding is greater than mean loss for women who report light or moderate bleeding (Fraser et al., 1984; Hallberg et al., 1966). In a study of Turkish women, 13 per cent reported experiencing long bleeding episodes (>8 days), frequent periods and/or inter-menstrual spotting, while 16 per cent were diagnosed with abnormal uterine bleeding upon clinical examination. The sensitivity and specificity for a complaint of heavy bleeding in this study was 45 per cent and 93 per cent, respectively (Filippi et al., 1997). In another study, where 56 per cent of women complaining of heavy bleeding were found to have blood loss >80 ml, the sensitivity and specificity for a complaint of heavy bleeding was 74 per cent and 74 per cent, respectively. The addition of a subjective assessment of the volume based on a pictorial chart increased the predictive value from 56 per cent to 86 per cent (Janssen, Scholten and Heintz, 1995). Data from one study of post-partum women suggest that self-reports can describe individual changes fairly accurately and that reports of lighter than normal bleeds accurately predict anovu-lation (Campbell and Gray, 1993).

Dysmenorrhoea

Although the term dysmenorrhoea is sometimes used to refer to a broad panorama of symptomatology, it is appropriately defined as abdominal pain, cramping or backache associated with menstrual bleeding. Related gastrointestinal symptoma-tology, such as nausea or diarrhoea, may also occur. Dysmenorrhoea results from secondary effects of the production of prostaglandins during menstruation, or may be secondary to other conditions such as chronic pelvic infections, fibroids or endometriosis.

As few quantitative measures of pain exist, questions about menstrual cramps or backache generally include a subjective rating of pain and questions about dura-tion of pain, its impact on functioning and the use of palliative treatments or medi-cation to control pain (see Appendix 11.2 for examples).

General measurement issues

Widely divergent estimates of the prevalence of menstrual disorders will result if careful attention is not given to the difference between eliciting information on the occurrence of symptoms, perception of illness and care-seeking behaviour. For example, the likelihood of a woman reporting abnormal uterine bleeding in the past 6 months will depend upon whether she is asked if she has *experienced* any epi-sodes of unusually heavy bleeding, whether she has *had a problem* with unusually heavy bleeding or whether she has *sought care* for unusually heavy bleeding. The likelihood of women defining a given characteristic to be a problem depends on the objective severity of the condition, the extent to which the condition interferes with a woman's daily life, her ability to develop effective coping strategies, and her knowledge and perception of normality.

Evaluations of disruption of daily life vary considerably between women, and also are likely to vary across cultures. First, a woman's perception of dysfunction may depend upon her own life stage. In general, women have little knowledge about normal changes in menstrual function over the reproductive life span, making it difficult for them to distinguish normal age-related changes in bleeding patterns from menstrual morbidity. During life stages characterized by change in menstrual patterns, such as the menopausal transition, women may be more likely to report menstrual dysfunction simply because their periods or cycles have changed. In a similar vein, menstrual symptoms may be considered a problem only when they are associated with another concern, such as fertility or cancer.

Other influences on women's perception of dysfunction include social factors such as cultural restrictions on activity during periods of bleeding, a woman's ability to adjust her occupational or social commitments to menstrual hygiene needs, a woman's or society's level of social discomfort with bleeding accidents, the availability of effective menstrual hygiene products, and the availability of simple and effective treatment. For example, a woman who works outside the home may indicate she has had a problem with heavy bleeding in the past 6 months if she is unable to change her menstrual protection every hour and if any bleeding accident would be unduly embarrassing, while a woman who works at home may report no bleeding problem in the past 6 months if, despite the discomfort of the symptom, she can easily cope with the hygiene demands of the excessive flow. Affordable, disposable hygiene products may make it easier to cope with excessive bleeding, and availability of non-steroidal anti-inflammatory medications may also increase women's ability to cope with pain or heavy bleeding, thus reducing the possibility that women will translate these symptoms into a complaint.

Previous research has suggested that any given menstrual morbidity may differentially affect distinct social spheres, and specific questions are needed to assess the impact of menstrual symptoms on work, home, social/leisure and sexual activity. As perception of dysfunction may be influenced by menstrual hygiene options, in many countries survey questions about menstrual hygiene practices may need to be included.

Specification of precise and consistent reference periods is particularly important for measuring the prevalence of menstrual dysfunction. Given the variable nature of menstrual function and the often episodic nature of menstrual disturbances, questionnaires that focus on the last cycle or the last month are likely to underestimate the prevalence of menstrual dysfunction. Conversely, questionnaires that use an extended recall period may overestimate dysfunction. Although more work is needed to define optimal time frames, reference periods of the past 6 months or the past year are generally appropriate.

As menstrual periods are repeated events, one must also consider the distinction between usual experiences and episodic occurrences of particular symptoms. Asking questions about a woman's usual experience will elicit information about her normative experience but will miss dysfunction, which presents intermittently. Women who report excessive bleeding, disabling pain or having cycles longer than three months as their usual or average experience will represent one subgroup of severely affected women. However, many more women may experience one episode of symptoms in a six-month reference period. As the level of pain tends to vary from menstrual period to menstrual period (Harlow and Park, 1996), an important subgroup of women may usually have mild to moderate pain but experience disabling pain every third or fourth bleeding episode. Thus investigators must carefully consider which subgroups of affected women they wish to identify with their survey instrument. Finally, menstrual cycle characteristics may be altered by contraception, and amenorrhoea may be attributable to a recent pregnancy or lactation. Interview surveys therefore must include screening questions to ensure that the subgroup of menstruating women can be identified for analysis.

REFERENCES

Antrobus P, Germain A, Nowrojee S (1994) *Challenging the culture of silence: building alliances to end reproductive tract infections.* New York, International Women's Health Coalition.

Bang R, Bang A (1994) Women's perceptions of white vaginal discharge: ethnographic data from rural Maharashtia. In: Gittelsohn J. ed. *Listening to women talk about their health,* pp. 79–94. New Delhi, Har-Amand Publications.

Bang RA, Bang AT, Baitule M et al. (1989) High prevalence of gynaecological diseases in rural Indian women. *Lancet,* 1(8629): 85–88.

Bean JA, Leper JD, Wallace RB et al. (1979) Variation in the reporting of menstrual histories. *American journal of epidemiology,* 109(2): 181–185.

Bhatia JC, Cleland J (1995) Self-reported symptoms of gynaecological morbidity and their treatment in south India. *Studies in family planning,* 26(4): 203–216.

Bhatia JC, Cleland J (1999) Health-seeking behaviour of women and costs incurred: an analysis of prospective data. In: Pachauri S, Subramanian S, eds. *Implementing a reproductive health agenda in India: the beginning,* pp. 207–232. New Delhi, The Population Council.

Bhatia JC, Cleland J (2000a) Perceived gynaecological morbidity, health-seeking behaviour and expenditure in Karnataka, India. Paper presented at the meeting on Reproductive Health in India: New Evidence and Issues, Pune, 28 February–1 March.

Bhatia JC, Cleland J (2000b) Methodological issues in community-based studies of gynaecological morbidity. *Studies in family planning,* 31(4): 267–273.

Bowling A (1995) Measuring disease: a review of disease-specific quality of life measurement scales. Buckingham, Open University Press.

Bowling A (1997) *Measuring health: a review of quality of life measurement scales.* Buckingham, Open University Press.

Bulut A, Filippi V, Marshall T et al. (1997) Contraceptive choice and reproductive morbidity in Istanbul. *Studies in family planning,* 28(1): 35–43.

Campbell OMR, Gray RH (1993) Characteristics and determinants of postpartum ovarian function in women in the United States. *American journal of obstetrics and gynecology,* 169: 55–60.

Durkin-Langley M (1984) Multiple therapeutic strategies in urban Nepal. *Social science and medicine,* 19(8): 867–872.

Ferry B (1995) Risk factors related to HIV transmission: sexually transmitted infections, alcohol consumption and medically-related infections. In: Cleland J and Ferry B, eds. *Sexual behaviour and AIDS in the developing world*, pp. 193–207. London, Taylor and Francis.

Filippi V, Marshall T, Bulut A et al. (1997) Asking questions about women's reproductive health: validity and reliability of survey findings from Istanbul. *Tropical medicine and international health*, 2(1): 47–56.

Fraser IS, McCarron G, Markham R et al. (1984) A preliminary study of factors influencing perception of menstrual blood loss volume. *American journal of obstetrics and gynecology*, 149: 788–793.

Graham W, Ronsmans C, Filippi V et al. (1995) *Asking questions about women's health in community-based surveys: guidelines on scope and content.* London, London School of Hygiene and Tropical Medicine, Maternal and Child Epidemiology Unit.

Hallberg L, Hogdahl AM, Nilsson L et al. (1966). Menstrual blood loss – a population study. Variation at different ages and attempts to define normality. *Acta Obstet Gynecol Scan*, 45: 320–351.

Harlow SD, Park M (1996) A longitudinal study of risk factors for the occurrence, duration and severity of menstrual cramps in a cohort of college women. *British journal of obstetrics and gynaecology*, 103: 1134–1142.

Hawkes SL, Morison L, Foster S et al. (1999) Reproductive tract infections in women in low-income, low-prevalence settings: assessment of syndromic management in Matlab, Bangladesh. *Lancet*, 354: 1776–1781.

Higham JM, Obrien PMS, Shaw RW (1990) Assessment of menstrual blood loss using a pictorial chart. *Obstetrics and Gynaecology*, 97: 734–739.

Hill A, David P (1990) *An experimental survey on childhood mortality and cause of death conducted in the Central Gambia.* Report to the Diarrhoeal Disease Programme, WHO. London, London School of Hygiene and Tropical Medicine.

Intermediate Technology Bangladesh (1992) *Investigation into the sanitary protection needs of poor women in Bangladesh.* Dhaka.

Jain AK, Slein K, Arends-Koenning M et al. (1996) *Measuring reproductive morbidity with a sample survey in Peru.* Programs Division Working Paper Number 9. New York, The Population Council.

Janssen CAH, Scholten PC, Heintz APM (1995) A simple visual assessment technique to discriminate between menorrhagia and normal menstrual blood loss. *Obstetrics and Gynaecology*, 85: 977–982.

Kaufman J, Liqin Y, Tongyin W et al. (1999) A study of field-based methods for diagnosing reproductive tract infections in rural Yunnan Province, China. *Studies in family planning*, 39(2): 112–119.

Kleinman A (1980) *Patients and healers in the context of culture.* Berkley and Los Angeles, University of California Press.

Koenig M, Jejeebhoy S, Singh S et al. (1998) Investigating gynaecological morbidity in India: not just another KAP survey. *Reproductive health matters*, 6(11): 84–97.

Kroeger A (1983) Health interview surveys in developing countries: a review of the methods and results. *International journal of epidemiology*, 12(4): 465–481.

Lasry JC (1991) Women's sexuality following breast cancer. In: Osoba D, ed. *Effect of cancer on quality of life*, pp. 215–228. Boston, CRC Press.

Melzack R (1987) The short-form McGill Pain Questionnaire. *Pain*, **30**: 191–197.

Miller R, Tisher A, Miller K et al. (1997) *The situation analysis approach to assessing family planning and reproductive health services: a handbook*. New York, The Population Council.

Murray CJL, Feachem RG, Phillips MA et al. (1992) Adult morbidity: limited data and methodological uncertainty. In: Feachem RG et al., eds. *The health of adults in the developing world*, pp. 113–160. New York, Oxford University Press.

Murray CJL, Chen LC (1992) Understanding morbidity change. *Population and development review*, **18**(3): 481–506.

Nichter M (1980) The lay person's perception of medicine as perspective into the utilisation of multiple therapy systems in the Indian context. *Social science and medicine*, **14**(4): 225–233.

Omran AR, Standley CC (1976) *Family formation patterns and health*. Geneva, World Health Organization.

Omran AR, Standley CC (1981) *Family formation patterns and health: further studies*. Geneva, World Health Organization.

Ross DA, Vaughan JP (1986) Health interview surveys in developing countries: a methodological review. *Studies in family planning*, **17**(2): 78–94.

Ruta DA, Garratt AM, Chadha YC et al. (1995) Assessment of patients with menorraghia: how valid is a structured clinical history as a measure of health status? *Quality of life research*, **4**: 33–40.

Sadana R (2000) Measuring reproductive health and well-being: review of community-based approaches to assessing morbidity. *Bulletin of the World Health Organization*, **78**(5): 640–654.

Speroff L, Glass RH, Kase NG (1994) *Clinical gynecologic endocrinology and infertility*, 5th edn. Baltimore, Williams and Wilkins.

Timaeus I, Harpham T, Price M et al. (1998) Health surveys in developing countries: the objectives and designs of an international programme. *Social science and medicine*, **27**(4): 359–368.

Trollope-Kumar K (1999) Symptoms of reproductive tract infection: not all are like they seem to be. *Lancet*, **354**: 1745–1746.

Unisa S (1999) Childlessness in Andhra Pradesh, India: treatment seeking and consequences. *Reproductive health matters*, **7**(13): 54–64.

United Nations (1994) Programme of Action of the 1994 International Conference on Population and Development. New York.

Van Ginneken J (1993) Measurement of morbidity and disability with cross-sectional surveys in developing countries. In *International Population Conference, Montreal*, vol. 1, pp. 483–499. Liege, International Union for the Scientific Study of Population.

Wilkinson D, Karim A, Harrison A et al. (1999) Unrecognised sexually transmitted infections in rural South African women: a hidden epidemic. *Bulletin of the World Health Organization*, **77**(1): 22–28.

World Health Organization (1992) *The International Statistical Classification of Diseases and Realted Health Problems*, 10th revision. Geneva, World Health Organization.

World Health Organization (1999) *International Classification of Impairments, Disability and Handicap*. Geneva.

World Health Organization Quality of Life Assessment (WHOQOL Group) (1998) Development and general psychometric prospects. *Social science and medicine*, **46**(12): 1569–1585.

World Health Organization Task Force on Psychosocial Research in Family Planning, Special Programme of Research, Development and Research Training in Human Reproduction (1981) Women's bleeding patterns: ability to recall and predict menstrual events. *Studies in family planning*, **12**: 17–27.

Yoder PS (1991) Cultural conceptions of illness and the measurement of change in morbidity. In: Cleland J and Hill A, eds. *The health transition: methods and measures*, pp. 43–60. Canberra, Australian National University, Health Transition Centre.

Younis N, Khattab H, Zurayk H et al. (1993) A community study of gynaecological and related morbidities in rural Egypt. *Studies in family planning*, **24**(3): 175–186.

Zurayk H, Khattab H, Younis N et al. (1995) Comparing women's reports with medical diagnosis of reproductive morbidity conditions in rural Egypt. *Studies in family planning*, **26**(1): 14–21.

Appendix 11.1

Measurement of symptoms of reproductive tract infections using a reference period of three months

	1	2	3	4	5	6
	At any time in the last three months have you experienced?	How long ago did you first notice (SYMPTOM)?	Is it continuing or has it stopped?	IF STOPPED How long did it last?	(During the illness), did you have the symptoms all the time or sometimes?	Did you also experience fever while you were suffering from (SYMPTOM)?
A. Discharge from your vagina that was abnormal in amount, in colour or in smell	YES 1 NO 2	→ WEEKS ☐☐ OR MONTHS ☐☐	STOPPED 1 CONTINUED 2	WEEKS ☐☐ OR MONTHS ☐☐	ALL 1 SOMETIMES 2	YES 1 NO 2
B. Sores or blisters in the genital area	YES 1 NO 2	→ WEEKS ☐☐ OR MONTHS ☐☐	STOPPED 1 CONTINUED 2	WEEKS ☐☐ OR MONTHS ☐☐	ALL 1 SOMETIMES 2	YES 1 NO 2
C. Pain in your lower abdomen	YES 1 NO 2	→ WEEKS ☐☐ OR MONTHS ☐☐	STOPPED 1 CONTINUED 2	WEEKS ☐☐ OR MONTHS ☐☐	ALL 1 SOMETIMES 2	YES 1 NO 2
D. Pain or burning sensation when urinating	YES 1 NO 2	→ WEEKS ☐☐ OR MONTHS ☐☐	STOPPED 1 CONTINUED 2	WEEKS ☐☐ OR MONTHS ☐☐	ALL 1 SOMETIMES 2	YES 1 NO 2
E. Pain or bleeding during intercourse	YES 1 NO 2	→ WEEKS ☐☐ OR MONTHS ☐☐	STOPPED 1 CONTINUED 2	WEEKS ☐☐ OR MONTHS ☐☐	ALL 1 SOMETIMES 2	YES 1 NO 2

7. INTERVIEWER: TICK ONE BOX

MORE THAN ONE SYMPTOM REPORTED ☐ ▼	ONE SYMPTOM REPORTED ☐ ▼	NO SYMPTOMS REPORTED ☐ ▼
	GO TO Q.10	GO TO NEXT SECTION

8. You mentioned (SYMPTOMS). Do you think that they are part of the same illness/condition or are they separate illnesses?

SAME ILLNESS	1
SEPARATE ILLNESSES	2

9. IF SEPARATE ILLNESSES. Which do you think is the more (most) serious symptom?

A. DISCHARGE	1
B. SORE/BLISTERS	2
C. PAIN IN LOWER ABDOMEN	3
D. PAIN DURING URINATION	4
E. PAIN DURING INTERCOURSE	5

10. ASK FOLLOWING QUESTIONS ABOUT MOST SERIOUS SYMPTOM. What do you think is the cause of this illness?

_____

_____

_____

_____

_____

(N.B. use pre-coded answer categories, based on prior ethnographic work)

11. Did your husband (partner) experience similar symptoms?

YES	1
NO	2
D.K.	3

ADDITIONAL QUESTIONS FOR THOSE REPORTING VAGINAL DISCHARGE

12. What was the colour of the discharge?

WHITE	1
YELLOW	2
GREEN	3
GREY	4
OTHER	5

13. Did it have an unpleasant smell?

YES	1
NO	2

14. Did you experience the discharge all the time or only on certain days of the month?	ALL THE TIME	1
	CERTAIN DAYS	2
15. Did you use special protection, such as a sanitary towel, while you were having the discharge?	YES	1
	NO	2
16. Did you have to change your undergarments more than once a day while you were having the discharge? IF YES How many times a day?	NO	1
	ONCE	2
	TWICE	3
	THREE + TIMES	4

Appendix 11.2

Measurement of menstrual dysfunction using a reference period of 12 months

Condition	Questions	Comments
Primary amenorrhoea *(Restricted to women aged 16 or more years)*	Have you ever had a menstrual period? IF YES: At what age did you have your first menstrual period?	If 'no' to both questions, the woman may be considered to have primary amenorrhoea.
	Have you ever been pregnant? IF YES: At what age did you first become pregnant?	If a girl became pregnant with her first ovulation, menses may not have presented.
Menstrual cycle length and cycle length disorders *(Restricted to menstruating women who are not pregnant, lactating or using hormonal methods of contraception)*	Thinking about the last 12 months, on an average, how many days are there from the first day of one menstrual period until the first day of your next period?	Information on usual cycle length, longest and shortest cycle length can be used to identify women with amenorrhoea (>90 day cycles), oligomenorrhoea (35–90 day cycles), and polymenorrhoea (cycles <21 days).
	Over the past 12 months, has the number of days from one menstrual period to the start of the next changed or varied?	Alternative cutpoints for short and long cycles may also be of interest.

Condition	Questions	Comments
	IF YES: What was the longest number of days from the start of one period to the next?	'On average' may be defined as more than half the time.
	IF YES: What was the shortest number of days from the start of one period to the next?	
	Approximately how many menstrual periods have you had in the past 12 months (1–3, 4–9, 10–15, 16 or more)?	1–3 cycles per year is consistent with amenorrhoea, 4–9 cycles are consistent with oligomenorrhoea/amenorrhoea, 16 or more may be consistent with polymenorrhoea
	In comparison with your experience over the previous year, in the past 12 months have your periods become farther apart, closer together, more variable, less variable or stayed the same?	Question 4 is useful to assess change in menstrual function and entry into perimenopause.
Secondary amenorrhoea	In the past year, have you gone without a menstrual period for longer than 90 days? OR In the past year, have you ever gone without a menstrual period for 3 months or longer?	
Oligomenorrhoea	In the past year, have you ever had a menstrual cycle that lasted 35–90 days? OR In the past year, have you ever not had a period for one or two months?	

Condition	Questions	Comments
Polymenorrhoea	In the past year, have you ever had a menstrual cycle that was shorter than 21 days? OR In the past year, have you ever had a menstrual period two or more times in the same month?	
Amount and duration of menstrual flow and bleeding disorders *(Restricted to menstruating women who are not pregnant, lactating or using hormonal methods of contraception)*	Thinking of the past 12 months, on average how many days do you bleed when you have your menstrual period? (Count from the day bleeding or spotting starts to the day it completely stops) In the past 12 months, has the number of days that you bled when you had your menstrual period sometimes changed or varied? IF YES: How many days was the LONGEST period of bleeding and/or spotting that you experienced in the last 12 months? IF YES: How many days was the SHORTEST period of bleeding and/or spotting that you experienced in the last 12 months?	'On average' may be defined as more than half the time. Women with intrauterine devices should be evaluated separately taking into account type of device (i.e. containing progesterone or not)

Condition	Questions	Comments
	Thinking about the past 12 months, on average do you consider the amount you bleed on the heaviest day of your menstrual period to be light, moderate, heavy or very heavy?	
	IF HEAVY OR VERY HEAVY: How many days does heavy bleeding last?	
	In comparison with your experience over the previous year, in the past 12 months have your periods become heavier, lighter, more variable, less variable or stayed the same?	These questions may help detect age-related changes in menstrual function, entry into perimenopause or onset of menstrual dysfunction.
	In comparison with your experience over the previous year, in the past 12 months have your periods become longer, shorter, more variable less variable or stayed the same?	
Prolonged flow	During the past 12 months, did you ever have a menstrual period where you bled or spotted for more than 10 days without stopping ?	
Excessive flow	During the last 12 months, have you had any episodes of unusually heavy bleeding where you had to change your sanitary protection every 20 minutes to one hour?	Heavy bleeding, which lasts for more than 24 hours, distinguishes women who are most likely to seek treatment for their bleeding and be diagnosed with abnormal uterine bleeding.

Condition	Questions	Comments
	IF YES: For how many hours did this heavy bleeding last?	
Dysmenorrhoea (menstrual cramps, backache, or pain with menstruation) *(Restricted to menstruating women who are not pregnant, lactating or using hormonal methods of contraception)*	Do you usually experience menstrual cramps, abdominal pain or backache when you have your menstrual period? IF YES: Is the pain usually mild, moderate or severe? IF YES: Do you usually take medication to relieve the pain? IF YES: Do you usually need to rest, lie down or stop your normal activities because of the pain? IF YES: For how long (part of the day, the whole day, more than one day)?	

12

Qualitative methods in gynaecological morbidity research

Nandini Oomman[1] and Joel Gittelsohn[2]

[1] Bethesda, USA; [2] Johns Hopkins University, Baltimore, USA

Initial community-based studies in the late 1980s and early 1990s that explored the issue of gynaecological morbidity focused mainly on the clinical assessment of prevalence (Bang et al., 1989; Younis, Khattab and Zurayk, 1993). These early studies faced several methodological challenges in assessing valid prevalence figures due to the sensitive nature of gynaecological morbidity (Koenig et al., 1998; Population Council, 1996). A few studies tested the predictive value of symptoms, such as vaginal discharge, for reproductive tract infections (Bulut et al., 1995; Zurayk and Khattab, 1995). Others tested algorithms as a tool for the diagnosis and management of reproductive tract infections (e.g. Vuylsteke et al., 1993). Still others moved beyond prevalence studies and used qualitative methodological approaches to explore women's perceptions of reproductive tract infections. These methods enabled researchers to explore women's perceptions of the gynaecological problems they encounter in terms of etiology, symptoms, and to some degree the severity of illnesses and health seeking behaviours (Gittelsohn et al., 1994; Oomman, 1996). In spite of a decade of research in the field, several dimensions of gynaecological morbidity remain relatively unexplored and could be more comprehensively investigated using a qualitative research approach. The social, behavioural and biomedical determinants, including sexual and reproductive health-related behaviours and men's roles in women's health, require further elucidation. Similarly, the consequences of gynaecological morbidity, including health seeking behaviour and the impact of morbidity on women's physical and mental health, have not been well described. Skilfully-used information gathered using qualitative methods could complement quantitative information more fully to investigate the different dimensions of gynaecological morbidity.

This chapter serves as a preliminary guide to field researchers, policy makers and programmers who would like to use qualitative methods in gynaecological morbidity studies. It provides an introduction to the concept of a qualitative approach, its basic elements, a list of selected qualitative methods, and a brief review of available gynaecological morbidity studies with examples of the use of qualitative methods. The chapter also lists guidelines for the use of two models of qualitative research for gynaecological morbidity research; guidelines for the use of qualitative methods for specific dimensions of gynaecological morbidity; and a practical guide to steps in the implementation of a qualitative study. A list of qualitative research manuals that could be useful to researchers interested in gynaecological morbidity research is presented in Appendix 12.1.

A qualitative research approach

Qualitative methods can be viewed both as an approach and as a set of techniques for data collection. As an approach, they enable researchers to investigate perceptions and behaviours from the informant's perspective. As data collection techniques, they can facilitate an inquiry of sensitive issues like abortion, extramarital or premarital sex, sexual behaviour and violence, which are often difficult to investigate through survey methods. These methods can also be used to generate hypotheses by exploring new and sensitive issues and to confirm or challenge existing hypotheses.

A qualitative research approach has four basic elements – triangulation, iteration, flexibility and contextualization (Gittelsohn et al., 1994). There are three basic types of triangulation. Data triangulation compares different data sources (primary and secondary sources), investigator triangulation compares data from different investigators since many qualitative studies have several investigators, and methodological triangulation uses multiple methods to study the same social phenomenon. Researchers are often encouraged to use several methods for data collection on the same topic to gain access to the 'truth' about a certain social phenomenon. The assumption that different methods will necessarily lead to a convergence of findings and hence greater validity of data is erroneous (Mathison, 1988). Rather, as Mathison suggests, the 'value of triangulation lies in providing evidence – whether convergent, inconsistent or contradictory – such that the researcher can construct good explanations of the social phenomena from which they rise' (Mathison, 1988: 15). Regardless of whether the process of triangulation leads to convergent, inconsistent or contradictory outcomes, each of these need to be interpreted from the data itself, from the immediate and historic context, and from a general understanding of the larger social world in which the phenomenon under investigation is being studied. Multiple data sources, investigators and methods provide the opportunity to understand better beliefs and behaviours.

Iteration is a cumulative process that allows earlier steps of data collection and analysis to inform later stages of data collection. The process is not necessarily linear; researchers are encouraged to reflect back on data collected at different stages. Iteration also helps researchers follow up on new ideas, facilitating a process that can be focused and expansionary at the same time. Qualitative research can be iterative between methods of data collection, between stages of data collection and between rounds of interviews with the same informant. For example, Oomman (1996) used data from one round of data collection to inform the next steps. Initial focus groups, key informant interviews and observations were used to identify the domain of 'women's illnesses' rather than reproductive or gynaecological health problems. These data were used to construct primary and secondary questions for free listing, checklisting, body mapping and illness narratives. Similarly, follow-up interviews with key informants were conducted to ensure expansion of issues that emerged in the first interview. Immediate analysis of the first interview enabled an interviewer to return to the key informant to further probe particular topics.

Flexibility refers to the researcher's ability to substantially modify data collection plans during data collection. If a particular method is found to be ineffective in generating the expected type of data, new methods should be adopted and/or developed for data collection. There are different reasons why a particular method may not generate the appropriate data. For instance, a topic may be too sensitive and the respondent unwilling to make such information public; respondents may feel that they are being tested rather than interviewed, especially when they are instructed to do a task like pile sorting; respondents may not understand specific methods and cannot complete an interview task correctly; and respondents may provide hypotheticals instead of narratives of themselves. Free listing, for instance, was found to be a somewhat unsuccessful technique when women in two studies in India were asked to list 'women's illnesses' as they were unable or unwilling to list women's illnesses (Jaswal and Harpham, 1997; Oomman, 1996). To overcome this obstacle, free listing was modified to a 'checklist' of illnesses in the Oomman (1996) study. A checklist was created from open-ended interviews and used for further data collection to question women on whether they had heard of a specific illness, its causes, symptoms and treatment. In the study by Jaswal and Harpham (1998), prompting was useful in assisting women to list illnesses, such as dyspareunia, that are considered 'dirty'.

Contextualization describes an emphasis on understanding the broader set of social, cultural and economic factors that affect perceptions and behaviours around health. This aspect is critical when one is exploring sensitive issues like sexuality, and sexual and reproductive behaviours. The delineation of the context of gynaecological morbidity is critical to the success of any study as it provides clues to the further study of the determinants and consequences of gynaecological morbidity. Lane and Meleis (1991) are exemplary in their attempt to delineate the context of women's health perceptions and health resources. This study describes women's health needs as a reflection of their multiple roles and responsibilities in rural

Table 12.1. Selected qualitative methods: interview and observation

Interview methods	Observation methods
Less structured	*Direct observation*
Key informant interviews	Continuous monitoring
In-depth interviews	Time allocation
Semi-structured interviews	Spot checks
Focus group discussions	
Natural group discussion	*Participant observation*
Body mapping	
Community mapping	
Structured or systematic	
Free lists	
Pile sorts	
Triads	
Ranking, e.g., severity ranking	
Paired comparisons	
Structured matrices	

Egypt. The researchers used participant observation to observe women's work and their daily lives, structured observation to observe household activities and in-depth interviews to elicit descriptions of the daily lives of women and the activities expected of them as wives, mothers, homemakers and farmers.

Qualitative methods

Qualitative research methods are not defined and described in this chapter. Instead we provide a list of selected qualitative methods to which we will refer (Table 12.1). Specific methods in qualitative research are detailed in several sources (Bernard, 1988; also see Appendix 12.1 on manuals). Interview methods form a continuum of methods, from less structured methods to systematic or structured methods. Less structured methods like key informant interviews, focus groups and in-depth interviews generate textual data that can be analyzed for thematic patterns on topics of interest. Systematic methods like free listing, pile sorting, ranking and triads generate textual data that can be quantified for analysis. Observation methods involve direct observation of a situation while participant observation necessitates that the observer participates in a particular situation while conducting the observation. Rapid assessment procedures (RAP) for women's health are also available to conduct a short, quick assessment (see Appendix 12.1).

A review of available studies using qualitative methods in gynaecological morbidity research

This section presents a methodological review of 21 studies that specifically used qualitative methods for gynaecological morbidity and related research (see Table 12.2).[1] About half these studies are entirely qualitative while other studies use both qualitative and quantitative methods. The studies are discussed with respect to the use of the qualitative approach, choice of method, sampling and research topics.

Use of the qualitative approach

It is difficult to learn from the studies listed in Table 12.2 the extent to which investigators may have directly used different elements of the qualitative approach. Since the research protocol is not described in detail in these papers, one cannot comment on the extent to which iteration and flexibility were important aspects, except for studies where this is explicitly stated. Similarly, only three studies (see earlier section) discuss the context of women's illnesses (Khattab, 1995; Lane and Meleis, 1991; Oomman, 1996). Alternatively, one can comment on the extent to which methodological triangulation was followed in these studies as this is more apparent. Specific details of the combinations of methods and triangulation are discussed later in this section. Here we cite one example of a study in which investigators were able to triangulate and one where they did not. Ross et al. (1998) employ a combination of open-ended techniques (in-depth interviews and semi-structured matrix interviews) and more systematic methods (free listing, pile sorting and severity ratings) to determine women's health priorities in Bangladesh. As a result, they were able to draw on data from different methods to gain several perspectives on the same topic. In contrast, Palabrica-Costello et al. (1997) depended solely on focus group discussions to determine beliefs and practices about reproductive tract infections in the Philippines. While a series of focus group discussions yield plentiful data on reproductive tract infections, the approach is problematic; it is difficult to draw conclusions about individual-level perceptions and actual practices around reproductive tract infections from group discussion data. Focus group discussions as a group method may only yield a normative perspective, and not necessarily the most valid one. People may respond differently when they participate in individual interviews and group discussions, especially with regard to sensitive issues like sexual behaviour. Relying on a single method, such as focus groups, allows an investigator to draw conclusions based only on a singular perspective, and limits the range and depth of information collected.

---

[1] The list was compiled from a computer search of the Popline database using different combinations of keywords such as reproductive health, gynaecological morbidity, reproductive tract infections, family planning and qualitative methods. The authors also accessed available unpublished papers and reports.

Table 12.2. Studies using qualitative methods for gynaecological morbidity research

Study and author	Location	Method used	Sampling frame	Sampling	Topics of research
Women's health priorities: cultural perspectives on illness in rural Bangladesh Ross JL, Laston SL, Nahar K et al. (1998)	Rural Bangladesh: a community residing near the Dhonagoda river	Only qualitative 1. In-depth interviews to explore the domain of 'women's illnesses', gather examples of illness episodes and delineate explanatory models. 2. Free listing of every general illness and ailment they could think of 3. Pile sorting to obtain more systematic information on the domain of 'women's illnesses' 4. Severity ratings to explore the degree of seriousness of women's illnesses and other characteristics 5. Structured matrix interviews to examine women's choice of health care providers	Married women of reproductive age. All were Muslim, most were illiterate	Methods 1–4: Women were selected from *baris* (groups of households sharing the same courtyard). Those who agreed to participate were interviewed Method 5: 43 women were selected from the community	Focus is on exploring the perceptions of reproductive health-related problems. Women believe RTIs are important problems that merit attention and treatment Also examines women's health seeking behaviour, particularly what women do to treat RTIs (through structured matrix or community mapping interviews)
Application of rapid assessment procedures in the context of women's morbidity: experiences of a non-government organization in India	Vadodara, India: two low-income slum communities. Muslim families in slum A and Hindu families in slum B	Only qualitative. 1. Focus group discussions (19) to build rapport with women and obtain a general framework of women's morbidity (types, etiology, treatment) 2. Free listing and pile sorting (*n* = 60) to elicit information on the range of women's illnesses, including local terms used to describe each illness and its symptoms, and to understand	Methods 1–4 conducted with married women (20–50 years) with at least one child Method 5 conducted with health service	1. FGDs naturally formed as curious women joined discussions 2–3. Subjects were contacted in their house and asked to participate	Mainly an assessment of women's perceptions of RTIs, but includes a discussion of how women and health practitioners view treatment seeking for RTIs Includes some information

Table 12.2 (cont.)

Study and author	Location	Method used	Sampling frame	Sampling	Topics of research
Kanani SJ (1992)		how women categorize different illnesses 3. Ethnographic interviews ($n=50$) to obtain socio-economic and political information, information on women's perceptions/beliefs and on health-seeking behaviour 4. Narratives ($n=50$) to obtain illness episodes and provide a range of health-seeking behaviours 5. Key informant interviews ($n=6$) to generate information on women's morbidity and health-seeking behaviour	providers (TBAs and indigenous medical practitioners)	4. Identified through health records, matched by illness disorder and contacted 5. Health practitioners identified through observation, then contacted	on treatment patterns

Listening to women talk about their health: issues and evidence from India
Gittelsohn J, Bentley ME, Pelto PJ et al., eds. (1994)

Study and author	Location	Method used	Sampling frame	Sampling	Topics of research
A. Chapter 3 *Illness beliefs and health-seeking behaviour of the Bhil women of Panchamahal district, Gujarat state* Patel P (1994), pp. 55–66	Ahmedabad, Gujarat: two villages (Kathala and Sahada) in Dahod, Panchamahal district. Both are 10 km from Ahmedabad	Qualitative and quantitative methods 1. FGDs (2) on decision making, control of money, health and marriage 2. Free listing (41) of women's illnesses 3. Severity ranking (26): 10 most commonly mentioned women's illnesses 4. Pile sorting (26): 10 most commonly mentioned women's illnesses 5. In-depth interviews (2) on white discharge and treatment	Local women	Local women were asked to gather for informal discussions	Focus on perceptions of health problems, but there is discussion on what women do for illness. Women discuss what they do for RTIs during in-depth interviews and group discussions Prioritization of RTIs through severity ranking and pile sorting

B. Chapter 4 *Some experience in the rapid assessment of women's perceptions of illness in rural and urban areas in Tamil Nadu* Narayan KA, Srinivasa DK (1994), pp. 67–78	Pondicherry, Tamil Nadu: Jawaharlal Institute urban and rural health centres. The urban centre is in an urban slum, divided into two areas – Kuruchikuppam and Vazhakulam. The rural centre is in Ramanathapuram Gadchiroli,	Only qualitative 1. Free listing of 'illnesses that women suffer from in the area' 2. Pile sorting of 19–25 of the most commonly mentioned conditions in the free listing exercise	40 women: 26 in the rural centre and 14 in the urban slum	Women selected by two social scientists and asked to participate	Focus on perceptions of health problems
C. Chapter 5 *Women's perceptions of white vaginal discharge: ethnographic data from rural Maharashtra* Bang R, Bang A (1994), pp. 79–94	Maharashtra: a remote district in central India	Qualitative and quantitative methods This study had two phases Phase 1 (quantitative): Structured surveys to record rural women's perceptions of white discharge Phase 2 (qualitative): 1. Focus groups discussions 2. In-depth interviews 3. Open-ended structured interviews	Women and men from the village and the SEARCH clinic. Method 1: with women and TBAs. Method 2: with TBAs and couples where the wife had white discharge. Method 3: conducted with women	No details on actual sampling procedures	Focus on perceptions of white vaginal discharge. No ranking of RTIs, but classification of white discharge During group and individual interviews, respondents reported treatment-seeking behaviours for white discharge

Table 12.2 (cont.)

Study and author	Location	Method used	Sampling frame	Sampling	Topics of research
D. Chapter 7 *Application of qualitative methodologies to investigate perceptions of women and health practitioners regarding women's health disorders in Baroda slums* Kanani S, Latha K, Shah M (1994), pp. 116–130	Baroda, Gujarat: two slum communities – Akhrot and Gothi	Only qualitative 1. Focus groups for an overview of women's illnesses 2. Key informant interviews for more specialized information on women's illnesses 3. In-depth interviews for detailed information on specific women's illnesses 4. Free listing to generate lists of women's illnesses and illness categories 5. Pile sorting of women's illnesses and illness categories mentioned in the free lists. 6. Illness narratives for episode-specific descriptions of selected illnesses 7. Illness scenarios for desired and actual health seeking behaviours of women, according to health practitioners	Methods 1, 3, 4, 5, 6: slum women Methods 2 and 7: indigenous health practitioners, TBAs Method 2: informal leaders (women) in the community	From health centre records, women who had sought treatment for symptoms of any one disorder (white discharge, menstrual problems or weakness) during the past 3 months	Main focus on beliefs and behaviours. Ranking of illnesses by women through free listing and pile sorting Treatment seeking behaviour (as reported by women) for health problems elicited through in-depth interviews with women. Behaviour as seen by health practitioners reported through illness scenarios
E. Chapter 8 *Listening to women talk about their reproductive health problems in the urban slums and rural areas of Baroda* Patel BC, Barge S, Kolhe R et al. (1994), pp. 131–144	Baroda, Gujarat: 4 villages and 3 slums (Sawad, Kalali Fatak, Jayaram Nagar) on the outskirts of Baroda	Only qualitative 1. In-depth interviews, with or without prompting, to explore local health situations and women's general health problems 2. Free listing of gynaecological illnesses 3. Focus groups on women's health problems	In-depth interviews with young women, elderly women and TBAs. Free listing with women. FGDs with low and high caste women	No information on sampling	Perceptions of symptoms, causes of illnesses and ranking of women's views on gynaecological problems assessed through free listing, interviews and FGDs Treatment-seeking behaviour also discussed in interviews and FGDs

Study / Author	Location	Methods	Sample	Focus
Poverty and pathology: comparing rural Rajasthani women's ethnomedical models of reproductive morbidity: implications for women's health in India Oomman NM (1996)	Bikaner district, Rajasthan, India	Qualitative and quantitative Quantitative: survey and clinical, conducted after qualitative phase 1. Village mapping for context 2. Key informant interviews: illnesses, causes, treatment, women's work, childbirth, menstruation, sexual behaviour, food and nutrition 3. Focus groups: as above 4. Body mapping: ethnoanatomy and physiology, women's illnesses 5. Direct observation: local treatments, caste, housing, wealth 6. Participant observation: women's work, local treatments, childbirth, sterilization operations 7. Free list/checklist: women's illnesses 8. Illness narratives: causes, progression, treatment sought, confidants 9. Semi-structured interviews: treatments	1. Men and women 2. TBAs, local healer, older women in the community, health centre staff 3. Village women's groups 4. Village women and TBAs 5. Local healers, men and women 6. Women's work, medicine shops, sterilization camps 7–8. Village women 9. Local health service providers Purposive sampling strategy from each for a particular method	Mainly women's perceptions of: Their bodies – ethnoanatomy and ethnophysiology. Women's illnesses – causes and progression of RTIs and other gynaecological morbidities such as menstrual disorders and prolapse. Treatments for the above. Some discussion of reported health-seeking behaviour from women during illness narratives and from local health service providers
Getting sensitive information on sensitive issues: gynaecological morbidity Jaswal S, Harpham, T (1997)	Mumbai, India	Only qualitative Part of a larger study of women's gynaecological and mental health. The following techniques were used during in-depth interviews with women: Free listing of women's illnesses Rank ordering of severity of women's illnesses	Low-income urban women Purposive sampling of women who were identified as key informants	Focus on women's perceptions of gynaecological morbidity: seriousness of illnesses, knowledge about their bodies as related to body functions and reported illness, causes of illness

Table 12.2 (cont.)

Study and author	Location	Method used	Sampling frame	Sampling	Topics of research
		Body mapping perceptions of the body and illnesses			Minimal reporting of results of health seeking behaviour
Iron deficiency anaemia in women of South Asian descent: a qualitative study Chapple, A (1998)	Northwest England: women of Indian and Pakistani descent	Only qualitative Semi-structured (in-depth) interviews to explore reasons for the relatively high level of iron deficiency anaemia among South Asian women in Britain	Women suffering from menorrhagia	Theoretical or purposive sample (not selected from medical records)	Focus on perceptions of RTIs. RTIs were ranked using information from women's discussion of their beliefs about heavy menstrual flow Main focus on the problems women encounter in obtaining satisfactory treatment for menorrhagia
Social factors associated with abortion-related morbidity in the Philippines Ford NJ, Manlagnit AB (1994)	Manila, the Philippines (rural)	Qualitative and quantitative methods Quantitative methods: schedule-structured survey Qualitative methods: 1. In-depth interviews 2. Focus groups To obtain information on the main types of abortion, the processes women go through to obtain illegal termination, and community attitudes to, and the political context of, abortion	1. In-depth interviews with policy-makers, doctors, TBAs and community leaders 2. FGDs with women who were abortion cases; hospital and community controls	Participants were selected from those receiving care from two main hospitals in Manila	Focus on perceptions and behaviours related to abortion

Study	Setting	Methods	Sample	Sampling	Focus
Community-based research and advocacy on health among poor women in Davao City, Philippines Sanchez RD, Juarez MP (1995)	Philippines: two 'squatter' settlements' of more than 1000 households each near Davao City	Qualitative and quantitative methods. Quantitative methods: survey, physical and laboratory examinations. Qualitative methods: Focus groups with adolescents to explore perceptions of menstruation, premarital sex, family planning and abortion. Discussions with women to examine changes in sexual feelings/responses, family relationships and financial situations	1256 women participated. Three groups: 1. Single or never married (15–19 years) 2. Ever married of reproductive age 3. Ever married, past menopause	No information on sampling	Focus on perceptions of menstruation and a minor focus on women's perceptions of RTIs
Beliefs and practices about reproductive tract infections: findings from a series of Philippine FGDs, Philippines Palabrica-Costello M, Chaves CM, Echavez C et al. (1997)	The Philippines: Three study communities: The Urban National Capital Region (Barangay Kamuning, Quezon City, Metro Manila). A lower-class neighbourhood (Barangay Lapasan) in the medium-sized city of Cagayan de Oro. A rural community of Jasaan, Misamis Oriental	Only qualitative. FGDs (4) were held in each of the study communities to discuss: 1. Concepts of health and illness 2. Knowledge and beliefs about RTIs 3. Social dimensions of RTIs 4. Preventive and curative practices	FGD 1: Women in their 20s and early 30s FGD 2: Women in their late 30s and older FGD 3: Men in their 20s and early 30s FGD 4: Men in their late 30s and older	Selection of participants was based on the following criteria: community of residence, age, sex, social class	Focus on beliefs/ perceptions. 50% of the participants were women, and about half their discussion(s) revolved around their views on RTIs. No information on what women do to treat RTIs

Table 12.2 (cont.)

Study and author	Location	Method used	Sampling frame	Sampling	Topics of research
The meaning of RTI in Vietnam: a qualitative study of illness representation: collaboration or self-regulation? Gorbach PM, Hoa DTK, Eng E et al. (1997)	Two communes in the northern provinces of Vietnam: Hai Hung (urban) and Ha Bac (rural)	Qualitative and quantitative methods Quantitative methods: self-administered surveys Qualitative methods: 1. Ethnographic interviews to explore general health, marital history, childbearing, family planning practice, IUDs, menstrual experiences, RTIs 2. Structured interviews to expand on issues raised in ethnographic interviews	32 women, 16 from each commune (no further information provided)	Participants selected on the basis of history of IUD-use and other criteria (ethnic group, hamlet in rural commune and employment in urban commune)	Focuses on the relationship between perceptions and behaviour – how women interpret reproductive problems and how they subsequently decide upon and seek treatment During initial interviews, women denied feeling anything about RTI symptoms. Later interviews were successful in eliciting their views about RTIs
In search of truth: comparing alternative sources of information on reproductive tract infection Bulut A, Yolsal N, Filippi V et al. (1995)	Yenibosna, Istanbul: an area of rapid urbanization	Qualitative and quantitative methods Quantitative methods: clinical and lab examinations Qualitative methods: 1. Focus groups for input on designing a survey on self-reported symptoms that might be signs of an RTI 2. Structured interviews with open-ended questions on reproductive health problems to gather demographic and socioeconomic details, and reproductive and contraceptive history	Married women (15–44 years) using contraception, have had an induced abortion and reside in the catchment area (via the maternal and child health and family planning centre)	FGDs drawn from a systematic sample of 1204 women taken from the previous year's records of the maternal and child health and family planning centre	Focuses on the differences between women's perceptions and the clinical diagnoses of their reproductive problems. Although there was minimal mention of how this relates to women's treatment choices, health seeking behaviour was a minor aspect of the study

Study	Setting	Methods	Sample	Sampling	Focus/Findings
Reproductive tract infections among women in Ado-Ekiti, Nigeria: symptoms recognition, perceived causes and treatment choices Erwin JO (1993)	Ado-Ekiti, Nigeria: an urban centre in south-west Nigeria with a population of 150000	Qualitative and quantitative methods. Quantitative methods: clinical investigations and household survey. Qualitative methods: 1. In-depth interviews to assess local knowledge and etiological concepts that give meaning to illness episodes and determine the health-seeking and sexual behaviours of women suffering from RTIs. 2. Focus groups to discuss symptoms, causes, possible long-term effects, management, treatment and the prevention of various reproductive health-related illnesses	In-depth interviews (2) with a herbalist and a diviner. FGDs with women of various ages, educational levels and marital status (10 groups were formed and 40 FGDs held)	No information provided on sampling	Focus mainly on beliefs. Findings indicate that women associate the symptoms of RTIs with negative effects to their health and the ability to bear children. This is assessed through FGDs in which women connect symptoms with outcomes and associated feelings/beliefs. It is not assessed through women's demonstration of a biomedical understanding of RTIs. Some information given pertaining to the health-seeking and sexual behaviours of women suffering from RTIs. Provides information on what women in the study reported doing when suffering from an RTI
Perceptions of reproductive tract morbidity among	Lagos, Nigeria: Yoruba in Shomolu and	Only qualitative. 1. Focus groups to develop an understanding of men's and women's perceptions of	FGDs (10): 1. Sexually active adolescent girls	No information provided on sampling	About two-thirds of the study focuses on beliefs and one-third on health seeking

Table 12.2 (*cont.*)

Study and author	Location	Method used	Sampling frame	Sampling	Topics of research
Nigerian women and men Olukoya AA, Elias C (1996)	Mushin, low socio-economic status communities of peri-urban Lagos	reproductive tract symptoms, the way people acquire, prevent or deal with such conditions, and the perceived accessibility and quality of family planning and other reproductive health services 2. In-depth interviews with herb sellers in the market who are commonly consulted by women seeking remedies for RTIs	(15–19 years) 2. Non-sexually active adolescent girls 3. Women of reproductive age (20–45 years) attending the clinic 4. Women of reproductive age (20–45 years) not attending the clinic 5. Pregnant women 6. Postpartum women 7. Menopausal women 8. Sexually active single men 9. Sexually active married men 10. Male traditional healers In-depth interviews conducted with 10 women selling herbs in the local market		behaviour. The main emphasis is on women's views of RTIs Study also provided information on what women do to treat RTIs by discussing the topic during about 25% of the FGDs and through in-depth interviews with women herbalists

| Synopsis of a report on a qualitative research study on knowledge, attitude and practice related to female genital mutilation in the northern province of Sierra Leone Greene, PAS (1996) | Northern province of Sierra Leone | Only qualitative 1. Focus groups (20) 2. In-depth interviews ($n = 50$) | Women of reproductive age (21–45 years) male and female youth (15–21 years), both in and out of school, adult men (both literate and illiterate opinion leaders), practitioners of female genital mutilation (TBAs, traditional healers, society heads) | No information on sampling | Objective of the research was to collect information on FGM and build an information base; identify reasons for the strong opposition to eradicating this practice; identify sociocultural factors related to female genital mutilation that would inform an IEC campaign; and sensitize and change attitudes of men and women The study highlighted perceptions of FGM. Not much information on women's opinions of RTIs but does include information on attitudes toward FGM and knowledge that the practice is associated with health problems (loss of babies during delivery, anaemia, difficult urination and defecation) |

Table 12.2 (*cont.*)

Study and author	Location	Method used	Sampling frame	Sampling	Topics of research
Female circumcision: a report on focus group discussions from Embu, Nyeri and Machakos districts of Kenya Zimmerman M, Radeny S, Abwao S (1996)	Kenya: Embu, Nyeri and Machakos districts	Only qualitative. Focus groups were conducted to determine why female circumcision has been abandoned in some communities and not in others. FGDs (16) were held in two divisions of each of the three districts	FGDs held with mothers and fathers, teachers and students (boys and girls). All participants were identified by the study's research assistants who resided in the districts and worked in these communities	Students were selected with the help of teachers	Focus on perceptions of female genital mutilation
Roles, work, health perceptions and health resources of women: a study in an Egyptian delta hamlet Lane SD, Meleis AI (1991)	Gamileya, northern Egypt: a small farming community	Only qualitative. 1. Participant observation to observe women's work, and women's and children's daily lives. 2. In-depth interviews on women's daily lives and the activities expected of them in their roles as mothers, wives, homemakers and farm workers. 3. Structured observation of household activities	Method 1: village women. Method 2: village women, female leaders, female traditional healers. Method 3: randomly selected households	Researchers obtained permission to observe women in structured observations a day prior to activity. No other sampling information given	Women's perceptions of roles, health and work, with the main focus on observing behaviour. Includes a discussion of gynaecological morbidity associated with circumcision and health issues related to menstruation

The silent endurance: social conditions of women's reproductive health in rural Egypt Khattab HAS (1995)	Egypt: two villages in Giza district (adjacent to Cairo)	Qualitative and quantitative methods Quantitative methods: medical information surveys, clinical examinations Qualitative methods: 1. Participant observation to record the response of women and their families to learning of health problems 2. In-depth interviews to gain a deeper understanding of the sociocultural and economic conditions contributing to ill health	Ever married women residing in one of the two villages	Households were visited in the selected areas and eligible women were invited to participate once they were informed of all phases of the research Participant observation was undertaken on cases referred for follow-up at the university hospital	Some discussion of behaviour, but focuses on women's perceptions of illnesses, problems with treatment, and relationships with healthcare providers Although findings indicate a high prevalence of RTIs, in many cases RTIs were dismissed by women as being unimportant Personal accounts cover treatment seeking related to RTIs in detail Women talk about health resources and what they do for illnesses when detected and if they persist or get worse

Notes:

FGD, focus group discussion; FGM, female genital mutilation; IUD, intrauterine contraceptive device; RTI, reproductive tract infection; TBA, traditional birth attendant.

Methods

The most frequently used qualitative methods are focus groups (82 per cent) and in-depth interviews (76 per cent) (see Table 12.2, col. 3). A small proportion of researchers (29 per cent) used semi-structured interview methods with open-ended questions on women's reproductive health problems, and close-ended questions on demographics, socio-economic status, and reproductive and contraceptive history. Studies that used systematic methods (such as free listing and pile sorting) are mainly those in the group of Indian organizations (under a joint Ford Foundation/Johns Hopkins research training project) who were specifically trained to use a range of qualitative methods (Bentley et al., 1992; Gittelsohn et al., 1994). Other useful and well-developed qualitative methods, such as key informant interviewing, observation, case studies and severity ranking, have been minimally employed in these studies. Only a few studies have been creative in trying more innovative methods to explore women's health issues. Kanani et al. (1994) and Oomman (1996) used illness narratives to obtain episode-specific information. Both studies also used body mapping as a tool to understand women's perceptions of their bodies and illness. Ross et al. (1998) used a structured matrix interview to examine women's choices of health care providers for reproductive tract infections. Khattab's (1995) use of participant observations and in-depth interviews to develop a series of case studies of women with reproductive tract infections is innovative.

A review of the combination of methods suggests that five of the 21 research teams used only focus groups and in-depth interviews, three used these two methods in combination with one other method, three used only focus groups, and one used only semi-structured in-depth interviews. In our experience of training and working with researchers, we find that they have been exposed mainly to focus group and in-depth interview methods, and therefore use them frequently. There is perhaps a widespread belief that these methods are 'easy to do' and that researchers often use them without any training; in fact, these methods are not easy to use. Both these methods require highly trained and experienced interviewers and data analysts, and are not necessarily the best methods to use just because one knows about them. Instead, the choice and combination of methods for gynaecological morbidity research should be based on specific criteria that we outline in a later section.

Sampling

Most studies focus on low income, semi-literate married women of reproductive age from urban and rural areas (90.5 per cent) (Table 12.2, col. 4). There are a few exceptions. Bang et al. (1994) and Palabrica-Costello et al. (1997) also interviewed men; others interviewed local/indigenous health practitioners and traditional birth attendants (Erwin, 1993; Ford and Manlagnit, 1994; Kanani, Latha and Shah, 1994; Oomman, 1996; Patel et al., 1994). Some researchers interviewed community leaders and policy makers (Ford and Manlagnit, 1994; Kanani, Latha and Shah, 1994). A few studies also included youth and adolescents in their sampling frame (Greene, 1996; Olukoya and Elias, 1996; Zimmerman, Radeny and Abwao, 1996).

Given that women and adolescents have been the focus of research in the 1990s, researchers should turn their attention to other subgroups. Additional studies on men's roles and their impact on women's reproductive lives are also needed. Similarly, research on male and female youth would reflect their sexuality and reproductive health status more accurately in the context of their fast-changing lives. The gynaecological health of older women has also been more or less neglected due to global attention on adolescent girls and women in childbearing years.

Of the papers that describe their sampling strategy (15 studies), purposive sampling is the most frequently used (60 per cent). Others have sampled women who volunteered to speak (27 per cent) and a few identified women from health records (13 per cent). Purposive sampling is defined as a strategy by which researchers intentionally seek out and select informants for their specific cultural knowledge of a topic under inquiry. For instance, researchers interested in studying women's health in rural India would approach traditional birth attendants for their specialized knowledge about pregnancy and childbirth in the community, and create a purposive sample. However, purposive selection of a sample can result in data collection that is not useful, as some informants are not necessarily cultural experts on the topic under investigation. Purposive and/or random samples may be selected when structured methods such as free listing, pile sorting or semi-structured interviews are being used to gather more confirmatory data. Opportunistic samples may also be used in qualitative research; Oomman (1996) used existing *mahila mandals* (village women's groups) to conduct focus group discussions and body mapping sessions on women's health problems.

Sampling strategies in qualitative research can vary depending on the method and the stage of the study. Some general guidelines for the selection of study subjects are outlined later in the chapter.

Research topics

Qualitative research interest in gynaecological morbidity has mainly focused on women's perceptions of illness and, to some extent, health-seeking behaviour (Table 12.2, col. 6). Women's perceptions of illnesses (symptoms, local terminology) were addressed by most studies (76 per cent). Fewer than half the studies had a minor health-seeking behaviour component (48 per cent), and only two studies focused on health-seeking behaviour (10 per cent). Examples of specific topics in these studies include ranking of illnesses using severity ranking/ratings (Kanani, Latha and Shah, 1994; Ross et al., 1998) and how illnesses relate to each other using an analytical technique called multidimensional scaling (Ross et al., 1998). Zimmerman et al. (1996) and Greene (1996) explore female genital mutilation and associated issues, including mutilation-related morbidity. Ford and Manlagnit (1994) focus on abortion-related morbidity in the Philippines, using mainly in-depth interviews and focus groups to obtain their data. Lane and Meleis (1991) use exclusively qualitative methods to examine the links between women's roles, their work, women's health perceptions and health resources while Oomman (1996) looks at the links between poverty and gynaecological illness as described by women.

Clearly, several topics related to gynaecological morbidity remain unexplored. Researchers should consider focusing research on health-seeking behaviours, determinants and consequences of gynaecological morbidity. Determinants of reproductive tract infections, especially those related to iatrogenic procedures such as sterilization and abortion, female genital mutilation, psychosocial distress and sexual behaviour, need further investigation. In addition, several aspects of sexuality and sexual behaviour other than the type and frequency of sexual acts need to be described in greater detail. Women's and men's desires, the circumstances under which protected or risky sexual encounters occur and the relational aspects of sexual encounters require greater attention. The consequences of gynaecological morbidity, such as decision-making around health-seeking behaviour, actual health-seeking behaviour, mental and emotional health consequences, and physical health consequences (such as infertility), remain poorly described in the literature and warrant attention. These topics may be suitably researched using qualitative methods, since many of them are sensitive issues and are rarely covered accurately in one-time survey interviews.

There is also a need for researchers to begin testing effective service delivery models for the diagnosis and treatment of gynaecological morbidity. Qualitative methods are particularly useful to develop reproductive tract infection case management protocols and to observe and describe patient–provider interactions. The RAP approach is extremely useful for programme-related research: it facilitates a quick assessment of health beliefs and health-seeking behaviour for the prevention and cure of gynaecological health problems (Kanani, 1992).

Two models for qualitative methods in gynaecological morbidity research

Based on a review of the available literature and our experience with qualitative research, we present two models for qualitative methods in gynaecological morbidity research. The decision to use a particular combination and number of qualitative methods should be based on objectives of the study, capacity for qualitative research (i.e. presence of seasoned qualitative researchers on the study team), time period, budget and the linkage of the study to a quantitative component. The two models we outline here are stand-alone qualitative research, and interlinked qualitative and quantitative research.

Stand-alone qualitative research

Stand-alone qualitative research involves qualitative methods exclusively. Researchers may combine a variety of qualitative methods to investigate gynaecological morbidity and its related issues.

Guidelines

Researchers who conduct stand-alone qualitative studies are often tempted to use a variety of different methods to provide evidence (whether convergent, divergent or contradictory) on the phenomena that they are studying. However, this approach has limitations. An experienced qualitative researcher (generally an anthropologist who has extensive training in using different qualitative methods and is able to analyse vast amounts of textual and systematic data meaningfully) would be a necessary member of the study team. The researcher would train data collectors specifically in these methods and would need to work closely with them through the entire course of the study. Hence, we do not advise quantitative researchers who are interested in doing qualitative research to use this approach, unless they themselves have been through intensive training in qualitative research methods. Additionally, an in-depth, stand-alone, qualitative study will generally require a long study period for a thorough training of interviewers and to establish rapport with the community, and at least 12–18 months to conduct repeated interviews and observations to document perceptions and behaviour patterns, and to analyze data. Examples of such studies include Ross et al. (1998) and Kanani et al. (1994).

Alternatively, seasoned researchers may use a few qualitative methods to conduct a stand-alone qualitative study. The study by Lane and Meleis (1991) is a good example of how researchers carefully selected three methods to yield data that would allow them to draw conclusions about women's work, their roles and their perceptions. One of the authors lived in the Egyptian hamlet on and off for about 5 months and used participant observation to study women's daily lives at home and at work. The data from these observations formed the basis for more in-depth interviews with women. Key informant interviews were conducted with women leaders and traditional healers. Finally, households were randomly selected for structured observations. The researchers specifically state that they used this combination of methods to cross-check whether women's reports from interviews

matched the observation data. The authors do not report any divergence or contra-
diction in the data drawn from alternative sources. A combination of interviews
and observation methods served these researchers well; they wisely restricted themselves to a few methods that would yield large amounts of data from different perspectives to describe the relationships between women's work, their social roles,
their health perceptions and their health status.

Researchers who conduct stand-alone qualitative studies using just one or two
methods and who are not skilled could produce results that are less convincing. Of
the studies listed in Table 12.2, some researchers used only focus group discussions
(Palabrica-Costello et al., 1997; Zimmerman, Radeny and Abwao, 1996). Focus
group discussions yield plenty of group-level data but the researcher is limited in
his or her ability to provide substantial evidence for a particular research topic with
these data alone. Such data are usually normative (i.e. what people are expected to
do and say in their particular community vs. what people really do and say when
they are observed or individually interviewed). The inexperienced researcher will
often select focus group discussions as a quick and easy qualitative method, and will
invariably be overwhelmed during the analysis of these data.

Some researchers may try and complement data from a method with one subgroup with data from another method with another subgroup in their stand-alone
qualitative studies (Greene, 1996; Olukoya and Elias, 1996). Olukoya and Elias used
focus group discussions to interview men and women about their perceptions of
reproductive tract infections and the quality of family planning services in Lagos
and in-depth interviews with herb sellers. Individual-level data for herb sellers
combined with group-level data for men and women are not considered complete
or thorough data sets. The use of focus group discussions (to elicit men and
women's perceptions) and in-depth interviews (to interview herb sellers) is only a
starting point in qualitative data collection. Additional qualitative methods could
have been used with each subgroup to build on data from focus group discussions
and in-depth interviews to strengthen the quality of results.

Qualitative and quantitative research

Interlinked qualitative and quantitative research combines the use of qualitative
and quantitative methods. Researchers may use qualitative results to explain quantitative findings and vice versa, assist in the design of quantitative instruments, and
help address gaps that arise in quantitative research (see Chapter 13).

Guidelines

Use qualitative findings to explain quantitative findings

Researchers can include a qualitative component in a study of gynaecological morbidity to complement the results from a quantitative component. Examples from
the studies reviewed demonstrate how these methods may be combined effectively

and not so effectively. Khattab (1995) specifically used in-depth interviews and participant observation to develop a series of case studies in Egypt. The women selected for these case studies were 8 per cent of the total sample of women who participated in the clinical study and were found to have special health problems. By using in-depth interviews and participant observation, the researchers were able to follow up with these women and document the conditions under which they lived with their health problems and their interactions with the formal health system. By selecting two specific methods, it was possible to obtain women's perspectives on their health and cross-check the data with participant observations. The data revealed more in-depth information about the women, appropriately complementing the clinical findings.

The inappropriate choice of complementing quantitative findings with qualitative findings limited to focus group discussions appears to be common practice. Sanchez and Juarez (1995) used focus group discussions to interview adolescent girls, women of reproductive age and older women to complement a survey, and physical and laboratory examinations for a study of women's health in the Philippines. They found that women of reproductive age spoke a lot on practices and beliefs regarding abortion while adolescent girls spoke more on menstruation and family planning. Our interpretation of these results is that since adolescent girls believe that abortion is a taboo topic, they are unlikely to report their abortion experiences in a focus group discussion. Instead, they are likely to report only what they are expected to say and do by the society in which they live. Perhaps additional qualitative methods could have been used, such as in-depth interviews with women and adolescent girls. Data from these individual-level interviews could have revealed more personal accounts of women's illness and health-seeking episodes, including abortion, to better complement the results from the survey and physical and laboratory examinations.

In our view, it is inadequate to conduct a series of focus group discussions and present these data as the complementary qualitative component to a quantitative study. Instead, we recommend that researchers review the menu of qualitative methods available and select two or three methods that will provide meaningful data to enhance quantitative findings with multiple perspectives. While such a study may not require a full-time experienced anthropologist on the study team, we strongly recommend that researchers involve a team member who is trained in the use of qualitative methods rather than expect survey interviewers to complete the qualitative component.

Use qualitative data to assist in the formulation of quantitative instruments
Researchers may also use qualitative research to help design quantitative instruments. Oomman (1996) used a symptom survey form to elicit specific 'women's health' symptoms from women when they arrived for their clinical examination.

The symptom terms were derived from qualitative data from several methods (as noted earlier) rather than from translations of English terms for discharge, menstrual problems, prolapses and so on. For example, *dhola pani* (white water) was used instead of the word discharge when interviewing women about vaginal discharge. Qualitative data were also used to gather information that would assist in the phrasing of questions about sensitive issues such as abortion and miscarriage. Women referred to 'lost' pregnancies as *adhura* or incomplete, and not as abortion, whether they were induced or spontaneous; the translation of abortion into the local language was not an appropriate term to use in the survey form. Bulut et al. (1995) specifically used focus group discussions for input to design the questionnaire on self-reported symptoms that might signal reproductive morbidity. They also prepared a checklist of symptoms from the qualitative data to probe women further about their reproductive morbidity.

We recommend that, where possible, researchers use data from the qualitative phase to design quantitative instruments. Using local terminology can enhance the validity of the responses because the questions are more meaningful to the respondents. Qualitative methods that are particularly useful in eliciting local terminology are focus group discussions, key informant interviews and free listing. It should be pointed out, however, that just one focus group discussion is insufficient; several group discussions should be conducted to understand the range of terms and issues that could be used in quantitative instruments.

Use qualitative methods to help address gaps that arise in quantitative research
Sometimes researchers may wish to investigate the results and questions from a quantitative study with a qualitative study. This usually occurs in the form of focused qualitative research (see, for example, Bang and Bang, 1994). After conducting a clinical study, the researchers reported very high prevalence figures for gynaecological morbidity in their study area. To investigate this further, a structured survey to record women's perceptions of white discharge and a series of focus group discussions, in-depth interviews and open-ended structured interviews were conducted.

Guidelines for the use of qualitative methods for specific dimensions of gynaecological morbidity

In this section we discuss how qualitative methods may be selected and combined to collect data on different dimensions of gynaecological morbidity. In general, basic guidelines for the choice of methods are:

- Get narratives of actual behaviours as well as hypothesized behaviours and observed behaviours.

- Combine group with individual methods.
- Use less structured methods to explore topics.
- Use more structured methods to confirm findings.
- Use creative methods (like body mapping) and participatory methods (like role playing) to involve participants in the data collection process.

To illustrate how each of these dimensions may be investigated with specific methods, we use Oomman's study (1996) for a first-hand account of how qualitative methods can be used extensively as part of a larger study on gynaecological morbidity. This study will be referred to as the Rajasthan study. Ideally, one should investigate the dimensions of gynaecological morbidity sequentially as described below, but this decision will depend on the study objectives, time period and budget.

Building rapport and social context

- *Purpose*: To establish rapport with the community, to explain the objectives of the study and to understand the larger context of gynaecological morbidity in the study area.
- *Methods*: Community mapping techniques, discussions with key community leaders and participant observation of village and other subgroup gatherings.

Health researchers interested in gynaecological morbidity often jump straight to the issue of reproductive health problems. They begin interviewing members of the study community without first building rapport or inquiring about the larger context of gynaecological morbidity. This may not be the best strategy since women and men are naturally reluctant to discuss sensitive issues with strangers at the first meeting.

Researchers should attempt to build rapport and understand the social context. In the Rajasthan study, the research team began with village mapping methods to document the context in terms of geographic details as well as the social structure and location of health providers in the community. Researchers also met with village elders, teachers, health providers and traditional healers to explain the purpose of the study and discuss women's health problems in the village.

Understanding gynaecological morbidity from the study sample's perspective

- *Purpose*: To explore a domain or category of illness similar to the biomedical category of gynaecological morbidity.
- *Methods*: Focus group discussions, key informant and in-depth interviews, body mapping.

Since women (or men) may not perceive gynaecological morbidity as a specific category of illness, it is important to explore their perceptions of ill health that relate to the biomedical construct of gynaecological morbidity. In the Rajasthan study, researchers used group and individual interview methods to explore this domain. Key informant interviews were conducted with traditional birth attendants, local traditional healers, older, knowledgeable women and health centre staff. Topics that emerged from these interviews include a range of 'women's, men's and children's illnesses', their causes and treatments, women's work patterns, traditional birth attendants' delivery practices, menstruation and menstrual practices, sexual behaviour patterns, and the relationship between food, weakness and illness.

Focus group discussions were used to explore normative ideas about women's health problems. These discussions were conducted with village women's councils and traditional birth attendants' groups. Discussion in these groups centred on illnesses: treatments that women used, illnesses that were more problematic for women and the reasons for these illnesses. Body mapping sessions were also conducted with some focus group sessions to obtain visual representations of women's perceptions about their bodies and illness. This method is particularly useful to document the ethnoanatomy and ethnophysiology of women's bodies. A body map served as a template for further discussion on topics like menstruation, pregnancy and childbirth and 'women's illnesses'. This research phase enabled researchers to establish that women used the term 'women's illnesses' rather than translations of the terms gynaecological or reproductive illnesses.

Describing women's perceptions of illness

- *Purpose*: To describe women's perceptions of illness, explore relationships between illnesses and the severity of illnesses, and probe women about sensitive topics.
- *Methods*: Repeated in-depth and key informant interviews, focus group discussions, free listing, pile sorting, triads and severity ratings.

Once researchers have identified certain categories of illness in the community, they can describe these further by using other qualitative methods. In the Rajasthan study, researchers turned to methods such as free listing and in-depth interviews with traditional birth attendants and other women to describe fully the symptoms in the domain of 'women's illnesses'. The free listing method was relatively unsuccessful as women were unable to list illnesses. Instead, they mentioned one or two illnesses, and went into lengthy explanations about issues related to those illnesses. As the free listing method was not fruitful, researchers decided to be flexible and modify the method. A list of women's illnesses was compiled from data from earlier interviews and body mapping sessions, and was used as a checklist of illnesses and symptoms. Women were randomly chosen from the village and asked specific questions about items on the checklist: for example, 'can you describe what happens when a woman has this illness?'; 'can you tell me the cause of this illness – why do women get this illness? What do women do to make themselves better when they have this illness?'

This process was found to be very useful as it prompted women to describe illnesses that they would otherwise have been reluctant to discuss in detail. Further key informant interviews, in-depth interviews and focus group discussions were conducted with women to establish the criteria for the severity of symptoms. Women were asked if they thought a particular illness occurred frequently and whether a few or several women experienced it.

Describing women's illness experiences and health-seeking behaviours

- *Purpose*: To understand women's illness experiences and health-seeking behaviours as reported by women and as observed by the researcher.
- *Methods*: In-depth interviews, semi-structured interviews such as illness narratives, and observation methods.

Women may describe symptoms of illness as they have occurred in the past or as experienced by other women. However, to obtain more valid data it is useful to document actual illness experiences as they occur. These may be documented as they are reported by women who are currently experiencing an illness episode and/or by researchers' observations of women who are currently ill. In the Rajasthan study, semi-structured interviews in the form of past illness narrative interviews were found to be an excellent method to interview women who were currently (or had recently been) experiencing an illness episode. These interviews enabled the researchers to examine the perceived causes of illness, the progression of illness, the treatments sought for illness, and whom the women spoke to about these sensitive health problems. Participant observation was used to document local treatments for women's illnesses and childbirth practices to cross-check the information women had reported in earlier interviews. Similar semi-structured interviews were also conducted with providers to describe the patterns of illness causes and treatment-seeking behaviour.

Documenting determinants and consequences of gynaecological morbidity

- *Purpose*: To document and examine the determinants and consequences of gynaecological morbidity.
- *Methods*: Key informant and in-depth interviews, semi-structured interviews, focus group discussions, observations, case studies.

During individual interviews and group discussions, researchers typically explore the perceived and reported causes and consequences of gynaecological morbidity. These need to be probed further to understand how such illnesses and their consequences may be effectively prevented in this community. In this regard, various interview methods to obtain women's and providers' perspectives on these issues are particularly useful. Observation methods help document information on women's lives that might make them susceptible to gynaecological problems. In the Rajasthan study, women and providers were specifically asked, using different interview methods, about the causes and consequences of 'women's illnesses'. Observation methods were also used to gather information on topics related to women's illnesses; direct observation was used to document women's household and field activities during the day, to document visits to local health providers, and to observe households of different economic strata. In addition, participant observation methods were also used to document sterilization camps conducted by government health services (since several women mentioned sterilization operations as a cause of vaginal discharge and menstrual irregularities).

Having discussed the models and methods that are appropriate for qualitative research in gynaecological morbidity, some general guidelines for the implementation of a qualitative study are proposed.

Guidelines to implement a qualitative study

The following steps can guide researchers in the implementation of a qualitative study.

1 Hire skilled interviewers, data collectors and data analysts

While this may seem an obvious and unimportant step, it is crucial to have skilled team members who are intensively trained in qualitative data collection and analysis. A senior, skilled qualitative researcher should train and supervise the data collectors. The researcher would work with data collectors throughout the study to develop field research guides, conduct the actual interviews and observations, and analyse data (read and code data and begin to develop coding schemes for final analysis). It is important for qualitative research that data collectors be more than data gatherers; they need to be good listeners, have adequate writing skills, and have the ability to probe issues and follow up. Data collectors should concentrate on recording (and not interpreting) the findings as the informant is speaking. In fact, even before interviewers are trained in specific qualitative methods, they should understand the critical aspects of the qualitative approach, namely triangulation, iteration, flexibility and contextualization.

2 Incorporate an exploratory or preparatory phase

The following four steps will facilitate future activity in the community/facility and assist in setting up a detailed qualitative component.

(i) Identify informants and the best time to approach them. Brief guidelines for sampling are:

  (a) Select a purposive sample of key informants during an initial exploratory stage of research. Use less structured methods, such as key informant interviews and in-depth interviews, to gather in-depth information on a range of topics. Each key informant should be interviewed at least three to five times for detailed information on particular topics over a period of time (Gittelsohn et al., 1998). While purposive sampling does not allow generalization of findings, every attempt should be made to ensure that informants are selected from the entire range of subgroups of the relevant population. This step allows more complete coverage of the topic. For example, if women are being interviewed in an Indian village about birthing experiences, key informants should be selected from different economic and social backgrounds.

  (b) Select a random or purposive sample for more structured methods (such as pile sorting and free listing). The random selection of respondents will strengthen the representativeness of findings and ensure adequate coverage. Informants should be interviewed only once or twice (Gittelsohn et al., 1988). Random sampling may be easily executed if a list of people/households is available for a particular community. Where such lists are not available, a community mapping exercise can be used and the resulting map can be used as a framework from which a systematic sample may be drawn.

(ii) Explain the purpose of the study to the community/facility.

(iii) Gain consent of key leaders/personnel and build rapport with the community/providers.

(iv) Identify the issues to assist in the setting up of qualitative field guides for data collection and determine whether certain questions may be too sensitive to ask in a particular setting.

3 Implement a data collection phase

This will allow continual (iterative) and flexible use of qualitative data to inform the next steps.

(i) Identify and describe domains related to gynaecological morbidity using methodological triangulation for key topics.

(ii) Use qualitative methods to describe the context of gynaecological morbidity in the community.

(iii) Design the quantitative study (surveys) to ensure maximum participation.

(iv) Continually use qualitative data to formulate questions for further qualitative data collection, and design more valid quantitative survey instruments using specific local terminology and phrasing.

4 Conduct data analysis on an ongoing basis

(i)   Analyse qualitative data as they are being collected.

(ii) Code data and discuss this with the entire team at the end of each week of data collection.

(iii) Follow up on themes, questions and issues that have emerged from the data using additional qualitative methods, interviewing more informants and probing specific topics.

(iv) Assess the quality and quantity of data collected on an ongoing basis to assist researchers in recognizing information categories and thematic patterns that recur. In the process, they will recognize that there are multiple perspectives on a topic that may or may not need to be explored further.

(v)   Do not leave data analysis to the end. Not only do the volumes of textual data become overwhelming, but the advantage of iteration that is critical for good qualitative research is lost.

(vi) Integrate qualitative and quantitative data by comparison, where applicable; explain quantitative results with qualitative results and vice versa. Researchers should note and explain convergence, divergence and inconsistencies between data from different sources, rather than only report convergent points of interest. At this stage, if necessary and if possible, further qualitative data may be obtained to explain/confirm quantitative results (see Chapter 13 for discussion on integrating qualitative and quantitative data).

Conclusion

Based on our review of available qualitative studies of gynaecological morbidity and our research experience, we find that the qualitative approach could be better used and understood. The use of qualitative instruments tends to be limited to a few methods such as focus group discussions and in-depth interviews. Furthermore, we find that most qualitative research in this field has focused more on describing women's perceptions of their gynaecological problems, and less on health-seeking behaviours and the determinants and consequences of gynaecological morbidity. Hence we have recommended a more methodologically rigorous and systematic use of qualitative methods through two models, and appropriate qualitative methods to investigate specific dimensions of gynaecological morbidity. We also suggest some practical steps that may guide researchers in the implementation of a qualitative study.

REFERENCES

Bang R, Bang A (1994) Women's perceptions of white vaginal discharge: ethnographic data from rural Maharashtra. In: Gittelsohn J et al., eds. *Listening to women talk about their health*, pp. 79–94. New Delhi, Har Anand Publications.

Bang R, Bang AT, Baitule M et al. (1989) High prevalence of gynaecological diseases in rural Indian women. *Lancet*, 1(8629): 85–88.

Bentley ME, Gittelsohn J, Nag M et al. (1992) Use of qualitative research methodologies for women's reproductive health data in India. In: Scrimshaw NS, Gleason GR, eds. *RAP: Rapid Assessment Procedures: qualitative methodologies for planning and evaluation of health related programmes*, pp. 241–249. Boston, International Nutrition Foundation for Developing Countries.

Bernard HR (1988) *Research methods in cultural anthropology*. Newbury Park, CA, Sage Publications.

Bulut A, Yolsal N, Filippi V et al. (1995) In search of truth: comparing alternative sources of information on reproductive tract infection. *Reproductive health matters*, 3(6): 31–39.

Chapple A (1998) Iron deficiency anaemia in women of South Asian descent: a qualitative study. *Ethnicity and health*, 3(3): 199–212.

Erwin JO (1993) Reproductive tract infections among women in Ado-Ekiti, Nigeria: symptoms recognition, perceived causes and treatment choices. *Health transition review*, 3(Suppl.): 135–149.

Ford NJ, Manlagnit AB (1994) Social factors associated with abortion related morbidity in the Philippines. *British journal of family planning*, 20: 92–95.

Gittelsohn J, Pelto P, Bentley ME et al. (1998) *Rapid Assessment Procedures (RAP): ethnographic methods to investigate women's health*. Boston, International Nutrition Foundation.

Gittelsohn J, Bentley ME, Pelto P et al. (Eds) (1994) *Listening to women talk about their health: issues and evidence from India*. New Delhi, Har Anand Publications.

Gorbach PM, Hoa TK, Eng E et al. (1997) The meaning of RTI in Vietnam: a qualitative study of illness representation: collaboration or self-regulation? *Journal of health education and behavior*, 24(6): 773–785.

Greene PAS (1996) Synopsis of a report on a qualitative research study on knowledge, attitude and practice related to female genital mutilation in the northern province of Sierra Leone. The Wesleyan Church of Sierra Leone. (Unpublished.)

Jaswal SKP, Harpham T (1997). Getting sensitive information on sensitive issues: gynaecological morbidity. *Health policy and planning*, 12(2): 173–178.

Kanani SJ (1992) Application of rapid assessment procedures in the context of women's morbidity: experiences of a non-government organization in India. In: Scrimshaw NS, Gleason GR, eds. *RAP: Rapid Assessment Procedures: qualitative methodologies for planning and evaluation of health related programmes*, pp. 123–136. Boston, International Nutrition Foundation for Developing Countries.

Kanani S, Latha K, Shah M (1994) Application of qualitative methodologies to investigate perceptions of women and health practitioners regarding women's health disorders in Baroda slums. In: Gittelsohn J et al., eds. *Listening to women talk about their health*, pp. 116–130. New Delhi, Har Anand Publications.

Khattab HAS (1995) *The silent endurance: social conditions of women's reproductive health in rural Egypt*. 2nd edn. UNICEF/The Population Council, Middle East and North Africa.

Koenig M, Jejeebhoy S, Singh S et al. (1998) Investigating women's gynaecological morbidity in India: not just another KAP survey. *Reproductive health matters*, 6(11): 84–97.

Lane S, Meleis AI (1991) Roles, work, health perceptions and health resources of women: a study in an Egyptian delta hamlet. *Social science and medicine*, 33(10): 1197–1208.

Mathison S (1988) Why triangulate? *Educational Researcher*, 17(2): 13–17.

Narayan KA, Srinivasa DK (1994) Some experiences in the rapid assessment of women's perceptions of illness in rural and urban areas of Tamil Nadu. In: Gittelsohn J et al., eds. *Listening to women talk about their health*, pp. 67–78. New Delhi, Har Anand Publications.

Olukoya AA, Elias C (1996) Perceptions of reproductive tract morbidity among Nigerian women and men. *Reproductive health matters*, 4(7): 56–65.

Oomman NM (1996) *Poverty and pathology: comparing rural Rajasthani women's ethnomedical models with biomedical models of reproductive morbidity: implications for women's health in India*. PhD dissertation, The Johns Hopkins School of Hygiene and Public Health, Baltimore.

Palabrica-Costello M, Chaves CM, Conaco C et al. (1997) *Beliefs and practices about reproductive tract infections: findings from a series of Philippine FGDs*. RTI Integration Project Report No. 1 Population Council, Manila, in collaboration with the Department of Health, The Philippines.

Patel P (1994) Illness beliefs and health-seeking behaviour of the Bhil women of Panchmahal district, Gujarat state. In: Gittelsohn J et al., eds. *Listening to women talk about their health*, pp. 55–66. New Delhi, Har Anand Publications.

Patel BC, Barge S, Kolhe R et al. (1994) Listening to women talk about their reproductive health problems in the urban slums and rural areas of Baroda. In: Gittelsohn J et al., eds. *Listening to women talk about their health*, pp. 131–144. New Delhi, Har Anand Publications.

Population Council (1996) *Research related to the assessment and management of reproductive tract infections and sexually transmitted diseases in the Indian context. A report*. New Delhi, The Population Council Regional Office South and East Asia.

Ross JR, Laston SL, Nahar K et al. (1998) Women's health priorities: cultural perspectives on illness in rural Bangladesh. *Health*, 2(1): 91–110.

Sanchez RD, Juarez MP (1995) Community-based research and advocacy on health among poor women in Davao City, Philippines. *Reproductive health matters*, 5: 89–94.

Vuylsteke B, Laga M, Alary M et al. (1993) Clinical algorithms for the screening of women for gonococcal and chlamydial infection: evaluation of pregnant women and prostitutes in Zaire. *Clinical infectious diseases*, 17: 82–88.

Younis N, Khattab H, Zurayk H (1993) A community study of gynaecological and related morbidities in rural Egypt. *Studies in family planning*, 24(3): 175–186.

Zimmerman M, Radeny S, Abwao S (1996) Female circumcision: a report on the focus group discussions from Embu, Nyeri, and Machakos districts of Kenya. (Report prepared for PATH, Kenya.)

Zurayk H, Khattab HAS (1995) Comparing women's reports with medical diagnoses of reproductive morbidity conditions in rural Egypt. *Studies in family planning*, 26(1): 14–21.

Appendix 12.1

Recommended manuals for the use of qualitative methods in gynaecological morbidity research

Rapid Assessment Procedures (RAP): Ethnographic Methods to Investigate Women's Health

Joel Gittelsohn, Pertti Pelto, Margaret Bentley, Karabi Bhattacharyya, Joan Jensen
1998, 196 pages

Purpose

This book is adapted from a protocol for the Ford Foundation India Project entitled 'Building Social Science Research for Women's Reproductive Health in India'. A companion book, *Listening to Women Talk About Their Health: Issues and Evidence from India*, discusses the experience of using the protocol and strategies to incorporate the findings into programme goals.

The manual's strengths include supporting the use of qualitative as well as quantitative methods of data collection, providing both manual and computerized options for data managing and analysing, and emphasizing the development of a qualitative database that can become an expanding resource for an organization. An additional aspect of this RAP, and where it differs from other manuals, is that it addresses a wide range of women's health problems rather that focusing on a specific disease or cluster of highly related illnesses.

Organization of the manual

The manual is organized in four sections:
Section 1: Overview of the protocol
Section 2: Protocol procedures
    Part 1 – Training exercises
    Part 2 – Data collection
    Part 3 – Applying data to programmes
Section 3: Appendices
Section 4: Blank data collection and data analysis forms

Experiences with using this manual

The manual was developed and refined from experiences the authors had working with NGOs and academic organizations in India. NGOs, inexperienced in formative, qualitative research methods, wanted to learn how to collect, manage and analyse information about women's reproductive health that could be used in planning and implementing intervention programmes, and shared with other NGOs.

Experience with this manual in India indicates that within one year, research teams with no previous qualitative research experience have generated substantial information on women's health. In addition, after reviewing how several NGOs in India used the manual, the authors state, 'Unlike many other manuals, the emphasis is as much on transfer of methodology as it is on collecting a particular set of data'.

Available from:

International Nutrition Foundation
P.O. Box 500
Charles Street Station
Boston, MA 02114–0500
USA

Telephone: 1–617–227–8747
Fax: 1–617–227–9504

Assessing Safe Motherhood in the Community: A Guide to Formative Research

Nancy Nachbar, Carol Baume, Anjou Parekh, MotherCare/John Snow, Inc. 1998, 140 pages.

Purpose

This guide is intended for investigators designing community research on safe motherhood and programme managers who will ensure that the research is directed toward programme needs. The guide assumes that users have a knowledge of qualitative research methods and an understanding of health behaviour change programmes as well as community interventions. Therefore, training in formative research is not a component of this manual. Instead, the guide is a tool for researchers working with programme managers, who are interested in designing formative research on community aspects of safe motherhood.

Available from:

> John Snow, Inc.
> 1616 N. Fort Myer Drive
> 11th Floor
> Arlington, VA 22209
> USA
>
> Telephone: 1–703– 528–7474
> Fax: 1–703– 528–7480
> E-mail: mothercare_project@jsi.com
> Web site: http://www.jsi.com/intl/mothercare

Qualitative Research for Family Planning Programs in Africa

> Compiled and edited by Adrienne Kols
> 1993, 63 pages.
> Center for Communication Programs, Johns Hopkins University.

Purpose

This report was published as part of an Occasional Paper Series of the Center for Communication Programs of Johns Hopkins School of Public Health (JHU/CCP). It disseminates results of fieldwork and research conducted in Africa by the staff of JHU/CCP.

The objective of this report is to demonstrate the importance of qualitative research when conducting campaigns to promote family planning. It discusses how seven African projects used focus groups and in-depth interviews to design new family planning communication campaigns, evaluate ongoing programmes and explore suspected problem areas. The report presents case studies and findings from Burkina Faso, Cameroon, Côte d'Ivoire, The Gambia, Ghana, Kenya and Nigeria.

Ordering information

The report is available free to organizations and individuals working in developing countries. The cost for readers in developed countries is US $5 a copy.

Available from:

Center Publications
Johns Hopkins Center for Communication Programs
111 Market Place, Suite 310
Baltimore
MD 21202–4024
USA

Telephone: 1-410-659-6300
Fax: 1-410-659-6266
E-mail: webadmin@jhuccp.org
Web site: http://www.jhuccp.org/occastwo.stm
Internet order form: http://www.jhuccp.org/puborder.stm

Qualitative Research for Improved Program Design: A Guide to Manuals for Qualitative Research on Child Health and Nutrition and Reproductive Health

Peter J. Winch, Jennifer A. Wagman, Rebecca A. Malouin, Garrett L. Mehl
January 2000, 182 pages

Support for Analysis and Research in Africa (SARA) Project Health and Human Resources Analysis for Africa (HHRAA) Project U.S. Agency for International Development, Africa Bureau, Office of Sustainable Development in collaboration with Department of International Health, Johns Hopkins University, School of Hygiene and Public Health.

Purpose

This guide is designed for programme managers, researchers, health programme funders and others who are considering using qualitative research methods to help them design more effective health programmes, or evaluate the strengths and weaknesses of existing programmes. It is assumed that the reader already has some familiarity with the basic methods in the 'qualitative research toolbox', such as in-depth interviews, focus groups and participant observation.

This guide describes some of the existing manuals for conducting qualitative research on health, and provides information to help would-be users select the manual that is most appropriate to their needs. This guide does not review the available qualitative research tools related to prevention and treatment of chronic and non-infectious diseases, including tobacco control, obesity prevention and management of diseases like diabetes or epilepsy.

Organization of the manual

This guide is divided into three sections. The first section reviews manuals on qualitative research in health and discusses computer software available for qualitative data analysis. The next section reviews manuals of methods and training for participatory research. Finally, available manuals on specific health topics in child health and nutrition, and reproductive health are reviewed. Ordering information for the manuals and tools discussed in each chapter are found at the end of that chapter.

Ordering information

The manual is available free of charge from:

Support for Analysis and Research in Africa (SARA) Project Academy for Educational Development

1825 Connecticut Avenue NW

Washington DC 20009

USA

Telephone: 1–202–884–8700

Fax: 1–202–884–8701

E-mail: sara@aed.org

Web site: http://www.aed.org

13

Integrating qualitative and quantitative methods in research on reproductive health

Pertti Pelto[1] and John Cleland[2]

[1] Pune, India; [2] Centre for Population Studies, London School of Hygiene and Tropical Medicine, London, UK

The purpose of this chapter is to examine the ways in which qualitative and quantitative methods have been used together in reproductive health research. Before discussing the ways in which the two research approaches have been combined, a brief summary of the relative strengths and weaknesses of the two methods is presented. After reviewing the various approaches to integrating qualitative and quantitative data, we will present some of the ways in which the triangulation of different types of data can be effectively presented and interpreted.

In earlier decades, social scientists and other health care researchers tended to divide into competing methodological-cum-theoretical camps, creating an antithesis between quantitative versus qualitative paradigms for research. Some qualitative researchers took a basically anti-science position, and argued that the use of statistics and measurement in human behaviour was misconceived and misleading. Philosophical ideas associated with phenomenology, hermeneutics and 'postmodernism' argued for 'other ways of knowing' that needed no numerical treatment or other standardized presentation of empirical data. On the other side of the argument, a few quantitatively oriented researchers have appeared to equate the concept of 'science' with numerical analysis of data, particularly when associated with the 'experimental method'. For example, in describing evaluation research, Rossi and Wright (1977:13) have claimed that 'there is almost universal agreement among evaluation researchers that the randomized controlled experiment is the ideal model for evaluating the effectiveness of public policy'.

Reichardt and Cook (1979: 9–10) have discussed the 'confrontation' of the two research philosophies, noting that 'the quantitative paradigm is said to have a positivistic, hypothetico-deductive, particularistic, objective, outcome-oriented and natural science worldview. In contrast, the qualitative paradigm is said to subscribe to a phenomenological, inductive, holistic, subjective, process-oriented . . . worldview'.

However, the authors go on to say that 'the conceptualization of the method-types as antagonistic may well be leading astray current methodological debate and practice. It is our view that the paradigmatic perspective which promotes this incompatibility between the method-types is in error' (Reichardt and Cook, 1979:11). In a similar vein, sociologists Glaser and Strauss, whose 'grounded theory' has been a veritable Bible for qualitative studies in sociology, wrote that 'there is no fundamental clash between the purposes and capacities of qualitative and quantitative methods or data . . . We believe that *each form of data is useful for both verification and generation of theory*' (Glaser and Strauss, 1967: 23, emphasis in original). Reichardt and Cook partly agree with Glaser and Strauss, but go on to suggest that there are differences in the main aims and strategies of the two research styles. 'It appears that quantitative methods have been developed most directly for the task of verifying or confirming theories and that to a large extent qualitative methods were purposely developed for the task of discovering or generating theories' (Reichardt and Cook, 1979:17).

While these arguments on qualitative versus quantitative approaches were current in anthropology, psychology and sociology in the 1960s and 1970s, the adoption of qualitative methods (and arguments about the two research approaches) have been somewhat more recent in epidemiological and demographic research and other studies related to reproductive health issues. It appears that definitions of appropriate ways of using qualitative techniques in relation to quantitative methods are still being worked out in various sectors of health care research.

It is worthwhile to introduce another historical note here. Historians of science are well aware that most branches of science have included very large sectors of qualitative, descriptive study, particularly in early phases of theory-building. There are a wide range of scientific works that contain little or no quantitative materials. Charles Darwin's famous book, *The Origins of Species,* is only one of a long list of basically qualitative works in the history of biology, medical science, geology and other bodies of knowledge, that illustrate this fundamental aspect of the scientific enterprise. It can be suggested that, just as the histories of many branches of science have moved from early qualitative explorations to later phases involving quantitative modelling and hypothesis testing, so the developmental sequences of individual research projects can often follow that same sequence.

Some methodologists have pointed to the many ways in which quantitative scientific work relies on qualitative presentation. Campbell (1979: 51) has argued that,

[S]cience depends upon qualitative, common-sense knowing even though at best it goes beyond it . . . Let us take . . . a scientific paper containing theory and experimental results demonstrating the particulate nature of light, in dramatic contrast to common-sense understanding . . . Were such a paper to limit itself to mathematical symbols and purely scientific terms, omitting ordinary language, it would fail to communicate to another scientist in such a way as to enable him to replicate the experiment and verify the observations. Instead, the few scientific terms have been imbedded in a discourse of elliptical prescientific ordinary language.

What applies to physics applies with even greater force to quantitative studies of human behaviour. The numbers by themselves often convey rather little. To imbue them with meaning, in other words to interpret them, typically requires an intimate knowledge of the subject and the study population that goes far deeper than the statistical results themselves. In the discussion sections of most complex statistical analyses may be found an unacknowledged qualitative component, in which the analyst attempts to place the results in their human context.

The field of sociocultural anthropology is perhaps the best example of a research discipline that was, until recently, almost wholly dominated by qualitative research paradigms. Quantitative data played almost no role in most ethnographic projects, even in research directed to illness and health care. However, the earlier qualitative emphasis in anthropology was not intended as an attack on quantitative methods. Cultural anthropologists did not consider themselves to be 'anti-science'.

The philosophical and methodological arguments for qualitative data-gathering in anthropological research have generally involved three inter-related assumptions. Data concerning 'cultural meanings', values and culturally prescribed behavioural patterns cannot be understood simply from numerical analysis, but require 'in-depth cultural explanations' from persons who are native speakers and practitioners of the cultures under study. Cultural patterns of behaviours and knowledge systems must be studied 'holistically', because each 'cultural element' or behaviour pattern is connected to a wide range of other parts of the 'overall cultural and social system'. The third assumption was often left unstated: that in given social groups and communities, there is a uniformity or homogeneity of cultural patterns, so that cultural information given by one or a few informants, regardless of their specific life circumstances, could 'speak for' and give accurate information generalizable to major portions of the entire community or reference group to which they belong.

The third assumption seemed to fit with cultural data in traditional, relatively slow-changing societies. The homogeneity assumption also fits relatively well with the study of language patterns (grammar, syntax, etc.) and highly ritualized activities such as weddings, funerals and other ceremonial behaviour. However, anthropologists, like other types of researchers, encounter traditional, slow-changing populations very rarely in these times of revolutionary change in transportation and communication.

During the past three decades, anthropologists, particularly those involved in applied research in health fields, have largely adopted a paradigm combining quantitative and qualitative data-gathering methods. The concept of a 'qualitative–

quantitative mix' of methods was set forth extensively in one of the first comprehensive books on anthropological research (Pelto, 1970).

Most of the qualitative data-gathering tools that have become increasingly familiar in studies of reproductive health issues were first developed and refined by
cultural anthropologists and qualitative-oriented sociologists. However, careful
assessment of qualitative methods and comparisons among different data-
gathering techniques is a recent phenomenon.

Just as social anthropology has become more receptive to quantitative data gathering in recent decades, so the more numerical branches of social science have
become more open to qualitative methods. Consider demography, for instance, a
quintessentially quantitative discipline. Twenty-five years ago, demography was
entirely dominated by analysis of large data sets, such as censuses and surveys. This
situation has been transformed thanks partly to the pioneering efforts of John
Knodel, John Caldwell and others. Qualitative techniques have been borrowed from
market research and applied to population issues (Knodel, Chramratrithirong and
Debavalya, 1987). Similarly, anthropological methods of observation and unstructured interviewing have been successfully deployed in preference to classical demographic surveys (Caldwell, Reddy and Caldwell, 1982). In the last 10 years
there has been a spate of volumes specifically dedicated to the contribution of non-
quantitative methods to population research (Basu and Aaby, 1998: Caldwell, Hill
and Hull, 1988; Greenhalgh, 1995; Yoddumnern-Attig et al., 1993).

The relatively new field of reproductive health research has benefited from this
movement towards greater eclecticism of methods in its contributory disciplines.
There is no need to re-enact the old confrontations. Rather, there is a wide, if not
universal, consensus among researchers active in the arena of reproductive health
that both qualitative and quantitative methods have distinct and equally valuable
contributions to make.

Quantitative and qualitative methods: strengths and weaknesses

Quantitative methods subsume a range of possibilities: structured interview
surveys, self-administered questionnaires, structured observation, diaries and
analysis of health facilities or other types of records. Similarly, the tool box of qualitative methods contains many types of instruments: unstructured or semi-
structured individual interviews, group discussions, various types of observation
and the more structured techniques of free listing, pile sorting, paired comparisons, rating and ranking. In reproductive health research, the dominant quantitative method is the single-round structured interview survey and the dominant
qualitative method involves relatively unstructured individual interviewing or
focus group discussions. To simplify the ensuing discussion, quantitative and

qualitative methods will be represented by their respective dominant paradigms and other variants will be ignored.

To a very large extent, of course, the choice or blend of methods depends on the nature of the research question. Many research questions can only be properly answered by results in numerical form (though this does not imply that surveys are always feasible). For instance, when the magnitude of a problem (e.g. the prevalence of reproductive tract infection) needs to be ascertained, when the impact of an intervention has to be assessed (e.g. the effect of in-school sex education on the incidence of unprotected intercourse) or when the strength of a specified link (e.g. between a woman's schooling and her ability to avoid unwanted pregnancy) needs to be measured, numerical data are required. Conversely, other research questions, particularly those involving a deeper or more holistic explanation of why people act as they do, will often be better answered by qualitative methods. Examples include: Why do couples who want no more children not use contraception? Why do some women suffering from reproductive tract infections not seek help from health services?

However, skilful choice of research methodology depends not only on the nature of the research question. It should also be informed by an awareness of the inherent relative strengths and limitations of the methods themselves. Consider first the assumptions underlying, and constraints of, a structured interview survey. The number of subjects or respondents is usually large (hundreds or thousands) and they are selected to be representative of a specified population. The instrument consists of a pre-prepared list of questions, typically with pre-coded answers. It is usually administered during a single session lasting 20 to 60 minutes, by an interviewer who has been trained to ask questions in the same way and in the same order to all respondents. The nature and sequence of questions has to be relatively simple and straightforward. The overall number of questions has to be restricted. While probing and clarification are part of the interviewer's mandate, there is no opportunity to deviate from the pre-set blueprint by pursuing interesting leads or unusual replies. Once data collection is over, answers may be combined or transformed in various ways to form variables, which then form the building blocks of statistical analysis, in which the strength of association between variables is assessed in a variety of ways.

From this characterization, it is relatively straightforward to identify the conditions under which a survey is likely to yield valuable information. First, the ability of surveys to deliver representative results is most easily fulfilled when probability sampling is possible and the willingness of individuals to participate is high. For many types of population of interest in reproductive and sexual health research (e.g. sex workers, patients with sexually transmitted infections – STIs), these conditions do not apply and thus this advantage is lost. Second, the subject matter of the inquiry must be familiar and relatively well explored. Unless this holds true, the selection of variables to be included is likely to be both arbitrary and incomplete. Sound judgements have to be made on the extent to which complex or subtle concepts, such as inter-spousal communication or health seeking responses to illness, can be adequately represented in a succinct manner without distortion.

A second and related condition concerns means of measurement. For a survey to be successful, the variables of interest have to be measured with reasonable reliability (or repeatability) and validity by a simple process of question and answer. This implies for instance that the design, phraseology and vocabulary of questions is appropriate; that ways of overcoming or minimizing the reluctance of individuals to report sensitive or socially disapproved behaviour have been devised; and that the ability of respondents to recall past events with sufficient precision has been ascertained. Ideally, formal tests of reliability and validity should be performed before the fielding of a major survey, but in practice these are rarely done by social scientists (though they are commonplace in epidemiology). More frequently, the accumulated experience of past research acts as a guide to expected levels of data quality. For instance, it is now accepted with good reason that well conducted surveys generally yield reasonably valid information on contraceptive use but rarely give accurate data on induced abortion. Survey data quality can also be assessed in other post-facto ways: by critical examination of the coherence and plausibility of results; by comparison of results with independent sources of information; by intensive re-interviewing of sub-samples; and by seeking the same information in different parts of the same interview (for application to sexual behaviour see Dare and Cleland, 1994; Schopper, Doussantousse and Orav, 1993).

Consider the situation of an unstructured interview or group discussion. Partly because each interview or discussion generates so much information but also because of the need for highly skilled investigators, the number of units is small, ranging typically from a handful to 50. The investigator has a list of topics or themes to be addressed that define the rough boundaries of the domain of study, but there is no predetermined menu of variables. Interrogation is open-ended and flexible and less time-bound than in a survey. Leads can be pursued in detail. Respondents are encouraged to relate experiences or feelings in their own words and at their own pace. Complex sequences of events (as in the formation of a sexual relationship or an illness episode) can be expressed and social interactions described. The investigator has the opportunity to cross-check different parts of the narrative and to resolve apparent contradictions. Repeated interviews with the same individual, a common strategy with qualitative research, may allow trust and rapport between respondent and investigator to grow, and this in turn may encourage greater openness in the reporting of sensitive issues. Information given in unstructured individual interviews or group discussions may be tape-recorded or summarized in note form and expanded later. The raw material for analysis comprises text and the analysis proceeds in an inductive manner by repeated examination of the text to detect important themes, dimensions and interrelationships. Validity is enhanced by careful checking that the interpretation and conclusions are consistently supported by different strands of the evidence. Results of qualitative work are usually presented not in the form of numerical results but as a set of interpretations, supported by direct quotations.

It is clear from this brief description of the salient features of qualitative work that its strengths and weaknesses are, to a large extent, the opposite of those of a structured survey. Thus qualitative research is vastly superior to surveys in exploring new frontiers of knowledge about human behaviour, documenting detailed and complex processes and elaborating subjective rationales for behaviour. Conversely, it is much more difficult to ensure representativeness of results or to measure variations in belief or behaviour between different population strata because of the small number of observations. It is this complementarity that makes methodological mixes such an appealing option in reproductive and sexual health research, as indeed in other branches of the social sciences. In the following sections, various ways in which both approaches can be combined are outlined.

Combining quantitative and qualitative approaches

Model A: qualitative and quantitative approaches are integrated in a single instrument

In structured survey research, it is common to encounter instruments with qualitative elements. The latter typically take the form of open-ended questions to which answers are supposed to be recorded in verbatim form by the interviewer. Such questions often concern motives. For instance, why did you do . . .? Why are you not doing . . .?

The intention of these additions is clear. It is to obtain richer insights than those usually obtained from a totally structured approach by borrowing some of the inherent advantages of the qualitative method. For several reasons, the net result is nearly always disappointing. The assumption that complex motivations can be adequately captured by a single question is mistaken. Indeed their thrust is sometimes implicitly aggressive, as in questions about reasons for non-use of services, and thereby disposes respondents to supply defensive reasons that bear little relation to reality. Interviewers are usually poorly equipped to probe in sufficient depth or to record verbatim answers with speed and accuracy. The amount of space allocated for recording of answers may be so small that it invites meagre recording. And even if interesting data are captured, they are usually converted to numerical codes for processing and thus lose the very richness of detail and expression that were part of the original purpose.

In the hands of experienced researchers and skilled interviewers, however, it is possible to fuse the techniques of structured and less structured interviewing in a single instrument, so that both numerical and textual results of value are obtained. For instance, in a study of sexual networking in Thailand, Havanon, Bennett and Knodel (1993) studied a purposive sample of 201 men and 50 women. Detailed and systematic interview guidelines were developed but most questions were open-ended. Questions were asked in a conversational style and interviewers were free to engage in conversation about other topics when appropriate to enhance rapport. Data capture took the form of notes, which were expanded into detailed accounts shortly after the completion of each interview. Interviewers were also encouraged to write down verbatim comments that they considered to be of special interest or value.

This approach yielded numerical results, for instance on the number of commercial sex encounters in the preceding 12 months, number of non-commercial sex partners and regularity of condom use. At the same time, extensive qualitative results are presented that provide insights into the role of commercial sex in Thai culture.

Research concerning the situations and behaviours of health providers (doctors, nurses and community health workers) is often structured as mixed qualitative–quantitative studies, probably because the available samples are relatively small and no attempt is made to get random samples. A study by Iyer and Jesani (1999) in four districts of Maharashtra, India, consisted of in-depth interviews with 183 auxiliary nurse midwives (ANMs). The qualitative materials included reports of sexual harassment, the poor quality of supervision, and the many problems caused by the 'target system' of generating family planning acceptors. Quantitative tables, developed from the same interviews, included time utilization estimates in hours and 'per cent of workday', summaries of accommodations and facilities, tabulation of strategies used by ANMs to motivate women to accept family planning services, and the ANM's 'votes' concerning the expected effects of removal of family planning targets.

A similar study by Khan, Patel and Gupta (1999) in two districts of Uttar Pradesh consisted of in-depth interviews and focus group discussions with a total of 54 ANMs. Quantitative data were presented concerning the equipment available to the ANMs; supplies of medicines; and the percentages of intrauterine contraceptive devices and sterilization targets reportedly met by the ANMs. The study gives numerous quotes from ANMs concerning their weekly rounds of work, their physical surroundings and supplies, their perceptions of the quality of care provided to clients, and problems in meeting their 'targets' in family planning. In this study it is clear that the basic data-gathering was conceptualized as qualitative in nature, with the expectation that many features could be presented in numerical form.

It is relatively easy to devise other ways in which structured and less structured approaches might be integrated. For instance, the administration of a short structured interview might be followed by more discursive open-ended interviews, or vice versa. An example of the latter may be found in MacCormack (1985). Largely qualitative interviews with Jamaican women on lay concepts of reproductive physiology which used anatomical drawings ended with structured questions on age, education, socio-economic status and so on. The relative dearth of such approaches no doubt reflects practical constraints. Many researchers are not equally conversant with both quantitative and qualitative methods and it is not easy to recruit and train interviewers of sufficient calibre for the task.

Model B: studies in which qualitative and quantitative approaches are separate but complementary

Studies in which qualitative and quantitative methods are used separately but in a complementary fashion, encompass a range of possibilities. In many instances, one approach is clearly subservient to the other. For instance, ethnographic research often includes a census or survey of the study population to provide a statistical background that will strengthen interpretations of the qualitative data. This is the method favoured by Caldwell and associates.

In India, the research began with an initial census of the study population, which serves as the baseline data for all future work. Many original results are mapped. Vital events are recorded. As new information becomes available, smaller surveys are conducted to examine particular sets of relationships. Yet the core of the work is essentially anthropological (Caldwell and Hill, 1988: 7).

It has also been used effectively by Patricia and Roger Jeffery in their extensive series of studies of reproduction and related issues in north India (Jeffery and Jeffery, 1996; Jeffery, Jeffery and Lyon, 1989). Their work was also essentially ethnographic but they did collect and present statistical data, for instance on fertility and infant mortality, cross-classified by caste and religion. Similarly, the reverse situation is common. Quantitative research teams may collect and present qualitative data to provide a cultural context for the interpretation of numerical results.

Studies in which both the qualitative and numerical component carry equal weight are relatively uncommon. The work by Sarah Salway and Sufia Nurani in Bangladesh provides a good example (Salway and Nurani, 1998a,b). They conducted in-depth interviews among rural and urban Bangladeshi women in order to examine the cultural ideas and motives concerning the adoption or non-adoption of contraception during postpartum amenorrhoea. They noted that both urban and rural women usually waited until the onset of menses before adopting contraception, despite the efforts of family planning workers who promote immediate postpartum contraception. These data served to throw light on quantitative data from surveillance of childbirth cases, in which there was a strong tendency for women to delay the adoption of contraception until the onset of menstruation.

The qualitative interviews were not directly linked to quantitative data collection. Interviews were carried out with 39 rural women in the Matlab area, and 34 urban women (Dhaka). Their samples were selected from among women who adopted contraception after childbirth, with approximately half adopting contraception before onset of menstruation and the rest after menstruation had resumed. The qualitative data were gathered during the period from November 1993 to May 1994. Quantitative data were taken from available childbirth and health care utilization records in the two areas – the record keeping system in the rural Matlab area and the urban surveillance system in Dhaka. A special add-on questionnaire was administered for the urban sample, linked to the urban surveillance system. The quantitative data consisted of 5483 women (childbirths) in the rural area (1990–91) and 1151 cases in the urban area (1992–93).

From the qualitative interviews Salway and Nurani found that both urban and rural women have strong and coherent beliefs concerning the negative effects of contraceptives, which are particularly serious in relation to their perceptions of the extreme vulnerability of women in the postpartum period. Thus avoidance of early adoption of contraception was mainly due to the women's concerns about their own weakened health conditions. The researchers found that the Bangladeshi women recognize conception to be considerably less likely (though not impossible) during postpartum amenorrhoea; however, they showed rather scant knowledge of the significance of breastfeeding in the postpartum process. They also found that women believe that the gap between births should be at least three years. The quantitative data demonstrated a very strong relationship between onset of menses and adoption of contraception, which was more pronounced in the urban population. In this study, the qualitative data give clear and useful cultural explanations for the sharp peak of contraception adoption around the time of renewed menstruation (a major pattern in the quantitative data). They also strengthen the credibility of the researchers' policy recommendations. Salway and associates feel that the policy of promoting contraception in the immediate postpartum period is ill-advised.

The model of qualitative–quantitative integration in this study does not require a specific time sequence, as the researchers were already aware of the relationship between onset of menstruation and adoption of contraception before beginning their research. However, it appears that the qualitative data were collected during the collection of the special add-on questionnaire in the urban sample. This model of concurrent collection of the qualitative and quantitative materials is conceptually similar to those studies in which qualitative and quantitative materials are incorporated into a single data gathering instrument.

Model C: studies in which qualitative data-gathering is used to sharpen the quantitative instrument, and to provide appropriate local language and content for the questions

Many studies, particularly those exploring relatively new territory, begin with key informant interviews, group discussions and other qualitative data gathering, and then go on to develop appropriate questions and effective vernacular language for the structured survey phase of the project. This is probably the most common way in which the two types of data collection are combined. In most instances, the exploratory, qualitative phase is totally subservient to the quantitative phase, is often perfunctory and serves mainly to imbue the research proposal with superficial appeal. In these circumstances, qualitative results are rarely reported.

However, there are increasing numbers of studies on reproductive and sexual health in which the initial qualitative phase is taken seriously and executed with sufficient skill to generate important results, while still serving the primary purpose of sharpening instruments for a structured survey. A large-scale project in Orissa (India) concerning male sexual behaviours, health problems and promotion of safer sexual practices, began with the mapping of locations where men go for sexual contact, a free listing of men's sex-related health problems and an in-depth collection of young men's sexual histories (Collumbien et al., 1999)

The qualitative phase of the research provided considerable vocabulary related to sexual behaviours, as well as insights into specific forms of questions to be quantified. At the same time, the qualitative phase of research was seen as giving a descriptive, contextual framework for understanding the kinds of answers that would be forthcoming in the survey. For example, for all those men (whatever the frequencies) who reported contacts with sex workers, the descriptive data provided information on the varieties of situations in which such sexual contacts take place. Those data also gave clues, for example, to the variations in situations that influenced degree of use of condoms.

To the extent that the contents of the quantitative survey, and the language used in questions, were made to be more culturally appropriate, it was of course essential that the qualitative research took place before the formulation of the survey instrument. On the other hand, the explanatory and illustrative aspect of the qualitative fieldwork could as easily have been delayed until after the survey was completed. Thus, the two separate functions of this kind of qualitative research can be conceptually distinguished, and portions of qualitative work could be delayed until after some survey results are available.

A study of inter-spousal negotiation about reproduction is another good example of an investigation where equal weight is given to the prior qualitative and the following quantitative phases (Blanc et al., 1996). The first part of the study comprised 34 focus group discussions among different population strata. This was followed by a survey of a sample of over 3000 individuals. The main report combines tabular material with analysis of text from the discussions. Moreover, the qualitative phase provided fresh insights into customs and vocabulary that could be further pursued in the survey. Sporadic abstinence, rather than rigid adherence to some variant of the rhythm method, emerged in group discussions as an important method of birth control. One commonly understood phrase to describe this behaviour referred to women 'facing the wall'. Husbands would also take short trips away from home at times when they were particularly keen to avoid pregnancy. The structured survey was able to exploit this new information and thus obtain better measures of pregnancy avoidance in this population.

A study by Watts et al. (1998) of domestic violence against women in Zimbabwe gives another interesting example of how the initial qualitative phase of research led to significant modifications of the quantitative survey. The study was carried out in the Musasa Project in Harare in 1995–97. During the qualitative phase of research, an unforeseen issue emerged concerning the extent to which women's husbands/regular partners not only forced them to have sex (25 per cent), but also sometimes *stopped* having sex with them (17 per cent). Both forms of coercion were apparently used by men as a means of punishing or controlling their partners (Watts et al., 1998). The researchers found that among the cases in which sexual violence occurred, there was a significant overlap of coercive sex and withholding of sex.

A final example comes from a Nigerian study by Elisha Renne (1993). The research began with a household census of an entire village. This was followed by open-ended interviews of 70 women and 66 men. These were tape-recorded and transcribed and those qualitative materials were used to design a survey instrument that was subsequently administered to a sample of about 600 men and women. The results reported from this inquiry draw upon both the preliminary and the survey phase.

Model D: research model in which the quantitative survey is developed to test specific hypotheses arising in the course of prior qualitative research

A study by Stephen and Jay Schensul and associates (1994) in Mauritius provides a particularly good example of this type of integrated qualitative to quantitative research. Their research was carried out in the export processing zone (EPZ), where large numbers of young single women come to work to augment meagre family incomes and accumulate funds for their personal use and future marriage. The researchers began with key informant interviews in order to explore information on working conditions, workers' living situations and other contextual data. Informal observations in the workplace and off-hour socializing locations were also carried out.

Their second phase of qualitative data-gathering consisted of in-depth open-ended interviews with a purposive sample of 90 women and 30 men. Here the aim

Table 13.1. Progression of sexual intimacy in Mauritius

Sexual activity	Frequency in survey (%)
Holding hands	68
Hugging	61
Kissing	64
Caressing the woman's breasts	48
Man strokes her genital area	31
Man puts finger in her vagina	26
She strokes his penis	24
She masturbates the man	17
Rubs his penis on her genital area	16
Penis slightly inserted in vagina	14
Full penetration	7
Oral sex	4

Source: Schensul et al. (1994).

was to elicit extensive descriptive information on sexual behaviours and reproductive health. The informants were selected from six of the larger factories in the EPZ. In the qualitative interviews, the young women were open when discussing 'stories, concerns, questions and myths about sex, reproductive functions and reproductive health' (Schensul et al., 1994: 87). The researchers 'drew sketches of male and female anatomy, shared problems, discussed virginity, and commiserated over lost love affairs'. From these informal, open-ended discussions the research team gained two important products:

- The vocabulary used by the young women in discussing sexual behaviours, ranging from *attrape la main* (holding hands) and *embrasse* (kissing) to more sexually intimate actions such as *mette dans bord dans bord* (penis slightly inserted into vagina) and *gagne relations sexuelles* (full penetrative sex).
- A hypothesized sequence of the sexual behaviours, which constituted a script for gradual (sometimes not so gradual) development from the less intimate behaviours leading up to more physically intimate sexual relations. The Schensuls and their colleagues hypothesized that this script for sexual behaviour is sufficiently rigid so that the pattern of frequencies of the behavioural items, and the reported experiences of the women, will take the form of a Guttman Scale.

This hypothesis concerning the script was tested as one part of their quantitative survey of 498 young women – a random sample stratified by ethnicity (Hindus, Creoles and Muslims). The results of the survey (Table 13.1) gave numerical support to the hypothesized sexual script.

Using the Guttman Scale statistical procedure, these items were aggregated into a complex variable (degree of involvement in potentially risky sex) to test hypotheses about relationships among exposure factors, family variables and other predictor variables. This composite dependent variable has strong construct validity as well as ethnographic face validity because of the qualitative procedures that identified the individual behavioural items.

The quantitative survey contained a large amount of other information on demographic and family background factors, having boyfriends, education and condom use, and knowledge of STIs, HIV and other risk factors. A major point that emerged from this research design was the importance of the vocabulary materials for ensuring good understanding and validity in the structured interview process. The Schensuls used the same basic qualitative-to-quantitative research design in Sri Lanka, where they were able to get very important data on male-to-male sexual behaviours, in addition to the sexual behaviour scripts in heterosexual relations (Silva et al., 1997).

A study by Helitzer-Allen and Makhambera (1993) on sexual behaviour and initiation among Malawi girls illustrates a truly in-depth combination of qualitative and quantitative research:

'From 1991 to 1992, we conducted research involving almost 600 young females, ages 10 to 18. First we lived in two villages and worked with 258 girls. We held in-depth interviews with the girls, their mothers and grandmothers; observed the girls in their daily activities; attended initiation ceremonies; talked with village leaders, male and female; and held focus group discussions on questions of reproductive health, sex and STD/HIV/AIDS prevention. From that work, we then developed several hypotheses, which we tested through a survey of 300 adolescents in 10 other villages' (Helitzer-Allen and Makhambera, 1993: 7).

Model E: qualitative studies after quantitative data collection, to seek explanations and understanding of the results found in the quantitative phase of research

There are several ways in which qualitative work may follow a quantitative investigation and seek to provide explanations and further understanding of numerical patterns. The survey may bring to light unexpected or surprising results that evoke the need for a further unplanned phase of in-depth fieldwork. A particularly fine example comes from studies of the Tamasheq of Mali, where survey evidence suggested the children of the dominant noble caste suffered higher mortality than the offspring of Bellas, the descendants of slaves (Hilderbrand et al., 1985). Subsequent ethnographic study provided an obvious explanation: the children of the noble class by tradition were fostered out to Bella women, a situation with striking parallels in nineteenth century France where children of the aristocracy were often sent out to wet nurses, with devastating consequences for survival (Hilderbrand et al., 1985).

A recent study of abortion services in two public sector hospitals in Istanbul, Turkey consisted of a quantitative phase during which '550 women were interviewed immediately before and after their abortion [six months later]' (Bulut and Toubia, 1999: 263). After the quantitative materials had been examined, small samples of women were selected for focus group discussions. 'Based on their initial questionnaires, women with different types of post-abortion experiences were chosen' (Bulut and Toubia, 1999: 264). The quantitative data in this study showed that there were serious complaints about the quality of care. They also showed dramatic differences between the two hospitals in the perceptions of the interpersonal relations with the health providers: only 6 per cent reported the relations with the doctor to be very good in Bakirkoy Hospital, compared with 37 per cent in Sisli Hospital. The focus group interviews that followed were rather few in number (two in each hospital), but were useful in highlighting some important features. All the women in the focus groups complained about lack of individual attention from the providers, including lack of follow-up services. Another interesting finding from the focus groups was that all the women 'affirmed that they did not look upon induced abortion as a method of contraception' (Bulut and Toubia, 1999:266).

Good examples of this reactive sequence are relatively rare, presumably because an additional phase of qualitative data collection after the quantitative survey often requires successful application for fresh research funds and perhaps the assembly of new research skills. These practical barriers are largely overcome when a final qualitative phase is part of an overall pre-planned research strategy. For example, a sub-sample may be selected at random from a large survey for in-depth or intensive interviewing to provide additional depth of understanding. Alternatively, the survey can be used to identify particular categories of individuals, which are then sub-sampled for in-depth work. An ongoing multi-site study funded by the World Health Organization's Department of Reproductive Health and Research, on the interface between birth prevention and HIV prevention, provides an example. A survey will be used to identify four main types of respondents, according to their degree of apparent risk of HIV or STIs and their risk of having an unwanted pregnancy. While the survey data will be used to perform a statistical analysis of factors associated with specified behaviours, unstructured interviews will be conducted with a sub-sample of each of the risk categories to provide additional explanatory depth.

This principle can easily be extended to nest matched case-control designs into the framework of a prior survey. Under this design, cases might be individuals with a specified reproductive health problem or a specified type of behaviour, and controls would be similar persons (e.g. matched on sex, age and marital status) who lacked the specified illness or behaviour. Unstructured interviewing would then seek to provide explanations for this divergence.

Model F: qualitative work is used to develop a sample for structured investigation

As mentioned earlier, some populations of particular interest in reproductive and sexual health research are extremely difficult to approach because some of their behaviours are illegal or invoke strong social disapproval. Examples include intravenous drug users, prostitutes and clients, abortionists and their clients and men who have sex with men. For research among these types of people, the qualitative approach may prove an invaluable precursor to more quantitative investigation. Qualitative work, be it in the form of interviewing, observation or participatory methods, typically involves prolonged engagement of the research team with the study community. Over time, mutual trust and respect should increase. Close relationships with key informants may develop. In these and other ways, opportunities may arise to generate a sample, perhaps by the snowballing technique, among whom a structured quantitative interview can then be developed.

A study of sexual behaviour and HIV transmission in Uganda provides an unusual example of the use of ethnographic work to generate samples for further investigation. Prolonged observation and informal interviewing by Pickering, the anthropologist on the research team, identified different sexual networks. For instance, different types of sex workers were identified on the basis of the characteristics of clients and prices charged. Similarly, rural men who visited a town frequently for casual labour or trade were followed up for six months and those exhibiting high rates of partner change were also identified (Pickering et al., 1996, 1997). Subsequently, blood samples were obtained from 54 such individuals belonging to three distinct sexual networks in order to test the suitability of HIV sequence analysis to characterize the different networks (Yirrel et al., 1998).

Model G: structured content analysis of qualitative (in-depth) case studies is used to provide some numerical perspectives on the categories of cases and types of situations

The qualitative study of treatment-seeking sexual behaviours and other reproductive health issues in various communities has often taken the form of case studies in which in-depth interviews are carried out in multiple visits to each person (case). Repeated visits to the same individuals allow for collection of large amounts of detail concerning each behaviour, thus contributing to strong validity of the data. For example, Joshi and colleagues collected data from a sample of 69 women who reported reproductive health problems (Joshi and Dhampola, 1999). The study was carried out in eight villages in a rural area of Baroda district, Gujarat (India). Each woman was visited approximately five times to collect information on the woman's experience of symptoms, treatment-seeking experiences and other information related to reproductive health. These data were supplemented by group interviews in the villages, as well as interviews with selected health providers.

The rich store of qualitative case materials was analysed using structured content analysis in order to identify key variables and provide frequencies for the main variations. For example, out of 119 treatment events, the women reported going to private practitioners on 51 occasions, and only 16 visits to government primary health facilities. Thirty-six instances of home remedies were also reported by the women, with some reporting multiple resort to home treatment. (Only five women relied exclusively on home remedies.) Although the relative percentages must be regarded as only rough estimates, these quantitative data, taken together with the information from group discussions, give strong evidence of the women's preferences for private practitioners (most of whom are unqualified or less qualified in terms of their training credentials). The preferences for private practitioners are, of course, illustrated by numerous statements from the women. For example, though private doctors charge money, 'they give strong medicines [powerful *goli*], which cures in 2–3 days. They are bound to give good treatment as they take money. I prefer private to government doctors'.

Careful content analysis of qualitative case studies is extremely useful, provided the content analysis (counting of instances) is carefully done. For example, in the study from Baroda, Gujarat, the fact that visits to private practitioners are reported three times as often as visits to government facilities gives the reader much more information (and confidence) than vague statements such as 'most of the women prefer private doctors'.

Model H: qualitative – quantitative – and back to intensive qualitative data-gathering

In a clinical study of reproductive pathologies in a slum population in New Delhi, Garg and associates (2000) found surprisingly high rates of reproductive tract infections and STIs. The researchers had already carried out in-depth interviews and other qualitative data gathering early in the study before the quantitative (clinical) morbidity survey. Based on the findings from the clinical survey, they felt it useful to select a small sample of STI cases from the quantitative study in order to explore in greater depth some of the risk factors for STIs as well as the treatment seeking behaviours of the affected women. In this research model, the quantitative study raised a number of questions about the unusually high frequency of STIs in the slum population. The quantitative data also suggested that certain parts of the community were particularly high-risk microenvironments. In-depth interviewing in these clusters of households revealed additional information on their multi-partner sexual activities.

Qualitative data and sample sizes

A half century ago the famous anthropologist, Margaret Mead ridiculed the idea of sampling, and said that a single individual (informant) was sometimes sufficient, provided his or her demographic/ethnic and cultural origins were fully presented. Nowadays no serious researcher would accept that extreme view. On the other hand, practically all qualitative research involves small samples, compared with the hundreds and thousands of individual units in demographic, epidemiological and other research in human behaviours. Most qualitative researchers are keenly aware of sources of variation in populations, such that issues of representativeness must be addressed no matter how small scale the individual study. If the sample sizes are small, how can the data be taken seriously? How many cases (informants, group discussions, etc.) are sufficient to present the qualitative, descriptive materials in a convincing manner? Are there types of data for which small numbers of cases or informants can provide sufficient credible and useful information?

Our common sense tells us that there are indeed types of information for which large samples are not required. Some obvious examples of questions for which small numbers of informants would suffice to give us fairly accurate, credible data are:

- What substances do worshippers ingest in the Catholic Communion service?
- On what day will Ramadan begin in the year 2002?
- Is there a tram service in the city of Melbourne, Australia?
- Does this village have a school?
- (In a rural region in India) Does the primary health centre charge money for the doctor's consultation?
- (In the English language) What is the plural form of cow? Sheep? House? Woman?
- (In a small city, anywhere) What are the main ethnic and religious groups in this city?
- What brands of condoms are available in this community (or region)?
- (In a village) What are the main illnesses and health problems suffered by women in this community?
- (In a village) What are the persons/places to which people go for treatment of health problems around here?

Most of the fore-mentioned examples refer to points of information that could be supplied by one or two individuals who are experts in one sense or another. Regarding the Catholic Communion or Ramadan for the year 2002, we would look for key informants who are associated with a specific religion, though they need not be highly specialized. For the item regarding a tram service in Melbourne, our expert informant needs only to be a resident of, or have visited, Melbourne. The last four examples concern information for which we would like to have more than one or two informants, though a fairly adequate answer to the questions could be had from a sample of less than 10 persons, provided they are at least moderately well-informed local residents. The item on condoms would best be answered by young male informants, preferably those experienced in these matters. For the item on women's health we would of course prefer female informants.

More ambiguity arises when we gather data about attitudes and local knowledge that are strongly shaped by cultural and social norms. So-called KAP (knowledge, attitudes and practices) surveys often include questions about local cultural items for which the K(nowledge) and A(ttitudes) display rather little variation because they are part of local cultural knowledge.

Handwerker and others have argued that such cultural data do not require conventional random sampling, and in fact the model of random sampling and statistical analysis is wrongly applied to such data. Handwerker and Wozniak note that peoples' cultural knowledge and attitudes are socially constructed and widely shared within and across communities and populations. The processes of interpersonal communication in the social construction of knowledge mean that individual instances of cultural knowledge are not independent events, as required in classical statistical modelling. The socially constructed nature of cultural phenomena makes the classical sampling criterion of independent case selection not only impossible to attain, but also undesirable (Handwerker and Wozniak, 1997).

Handwerker and Wozniak thus distinguish between life experience data (such as age, number of children, marital status, health status) and culturally constructed data (which violate the criterion of independent events). In their study of foster mothers in Connecticut, Handwerker and Wozniak demonstrated that life experience data were correctly estimated only from random samples in the population, whereas culturally constructed data were effectively estimated using small convenience samples. The researchers pointed out that the convenience samples produced serious errors in estimating the average age of the mothers, as well as the percentage of white and black (ethnicity) in the population. The average agreement among informants for the culturally constructed data (criteria of familyness and motherhood) ranged from 0.54 to 0.82, whereas the agreement concerning life experience data was much lower.

The argument presented by these theoreticians concerning socially and culturally constructed information (cultural knowledge and attitudes, etc.) leads to the conclusion that effective cultural data can be gathered from relatively small, non-random samples of informants, although researchers should always be careful to include representation from major cultural sources of variation, including male–female differences, intra-community ethnic differences and caste differences. The argument concerning culturally constructed data does not eliminate the need for attending to general representativeness and sampling. The cultural argument also suggests that one searches out persons who are local experts concerning whatever topical areas are the focus of study.

The argument for the use of relatively small convenience samples of informants was greatly strengthened by the development of mathematical proofs for consensus modelling of cultural data by Romney and associates (1986). The concept of cultural consensus, or knowledge consensus, is best illustrated from a well-known information model: a test given by a teacher to students in a classroom. The teacher has distributed (and socially constructed) items of knowledge and information in her lectures, plus the required readings on the subject – geography, history or whatever. Suppose the teacher gives the students 100 questions and several students have studied and learned so well that they answer all 100 questions correctly. Suppose also that the teacher has lost the answer key, but she is well aware of which students are the best and brightest in the classroom. Logically (mathematically), the students who have answered all the questions correctly will show a 100 per cent correlation in their answer sheets. More generally, the students who have higher numbers of right answers are more highly correlated with each other, whereas the students with many wrong answers are less correlated with the good students, and less correlated with each other. Romney and associates demonstrated mathematically that the teacher who has lost her answer key can reconstruct the set of correct answers from the analysis of the pattern of intercorrelations among the students. The solution to the problem is an application of factor analysis of the respondents (rather than the interrelations among the items in the test).

Borgatti (1992) developed the computer software for consensus modelling, based on the work of Romney and associates, making it possible to identify the degree of cultural consensus in any body of culturally constructed data. In addition to the application of consensus analysis procedures to knowledge and attitudes, the procedures apply equally well to the behaviour isomorphic with a given body of knowledge (observations on how women give birth, how puberty rites are carried out, how people marry). Data appropriate for consensus analysis might come from text collected by various forms of informal or semi-structured interviews (so long as all informants responded to the same questions), from structured observations, or from structured interview formats like sentence frames, pile sorts, triads tests or rating scales (Handwerker and Wozniak, 1997; Weller and Romney, 1988).

The literature and various applications of consensus modelling have produced a set of guidelines for the number of informants needed to establish confidence intervals and similar statistical criteria, with different levels of inter-informant agreement. Logically (mathematically), the higher the inter-informant agreement, the smaller the required sample (Weller and Romney, 1988). In many cases, when inter-informant agreement is 0.60 and above, high degrees of statistical confidence are reached with 10 to 20 informants. In all cases, however, researchers must be quite clear that these methods and models do not apply to life experience data. Actual cases of illness, treatment-seeking events, individual sexual behaviours and many other types of data do not conform to the logical requirements of consensus modelling because they are subject to a wide range of different determinants and contextual variables affecting individual histories. In some behaviour settings, on the other hand, the sources of variation may be sharply constricted by a variety of factors. For example, the steps of procedure in laparoscopic sterilization camps in India are highly constrained by the surgical protocol and public health guidelines. A small number of observations (10 to 20 camps) is likely to demonstrate a high degree of consensus if tested with the Borgatti ANTHROPAC modelling software.

The concept of triangulation

Triangulation in research refers to the use of multiple sources and types of data, in order to 'validate' or give further support to the results from specific data sources. Thus, we often hear of researchers collecting qualitative data – from individual interviews and focus group discussions – in order to 'validate' the conclusions from quantitative surveys. The origin of this terminology, triangulation, is from navigation and surveying. The surveyor or navigator establishes a specific 'precise location' by sightings on several different reference points using mathematical calculations. In the social sciences, 'triangulation prevents the investigator from accepting too readily the validity of initial impressions; it enhances the scope, density, and clarity of constructs developed during the course of the investigation . . . It also assists in correcting biases' (Goetz and LeCompte, 1984:11).

Researchers often state that they have used triangulation in their analysis of several different kinds of data. For example, focus group discussions are used as triangulation with case studies and key informant interviews. Collections of qualitative data are sometimes used for triangulation with quantitative survey data. However, such procedures are often quite informal and ad hoc, without formal testing or careful analysis. Thus, the concept of triangulation in combined qualitative–quantitative research has remained vague and unsatisfactory, despite the impressive possibilities.

The example of the Schensuls' research in Mauritius, described in the foregoing, can be regarded as an excellent model of one particular type of triangulation. Their quantitative results were carefully designed to test the hypotheses generated in the qualitative phase of the study. For such triangulation to be meaningful it is of course necessary that two (or more) different data-gathering methods are used to collect the same behavioural or ideational information. That elementary principle is sometimes violated when researchers use two different data-gathering methods and ask different types of questions. Sometimes even small changes in the wording of questions result in large differences in the answers. Such results cannot be regarded as triangulation.

Quite often the use of two or three different research techniques produces conflicting data. If those data are indeed focused on the same behaviours and attitudes, researchers must then decide which research technique produced more credible data. Helitzer-Allen's research among Malawi adolescent girls is an example of this type of situation. In-depth interviewing produced results that contradicted some of the data from focus group discussions. In this case, the researchers considered the two data sets to be a methodological test rather than simply triangulation. They concluded that the data from the focus group discussions were misleading with regard to actual sexual behaviours of the Malawi girls, particularly in the sense that 'focus group discussions elicited more socially "correct" answers and produced good data on social norms, but not very good data on deviations from those norms. By contrast, in-depth, one-on-one interviews were necessary for eliciting good data on actual knowledge and experience' (Helitzer-Allen, Makhambera and Wangel, 1994:80). The researchers concluded that both methods should be used – but the in-depth interviews should be first. Also, 'had we used focus group discussions alone, we might have concluded that the idealized norms regulating . . . information . . . and behaviour are adhered to much more so than proved to be the case' (Helitzer-Allen, Makhambera and Wangel, 1994: 7).

Qualitative methods are sometimes used as a means of checking on the validity of results of a quantitative investigation. The best-known published examples of this type of work have given results that are highly damaging to the survey approach (Bleek, 1987; Campbell and Stone, 1984). In view of the earlier rivalry between the two genres of research, there is a strong element of schadenfreude among ethnographers at this exposure of the frailties of surveys. Survey practitioners are quick to riposte that much qualitative work is impossible to validate in the same manner and thus refutability, that key characteristic of scientific progress, is missing.

Less commonly, the same research team uses qualitative methods as a check on the validity of their own survey results. Konings et al. (1995) applied in-depth interviewing to a random sub-sample ($n=75$) of a larger structured survey ($n=460$). Large and statistically significant differences in results from the two approaches were obtained. For instance, 70 per cent of male in-depth interviewees reported at least one non-regular partner in the previous 12 months, compared with about 50 per cent in the structured interview approach: the corresponding figures for women were 32 per cent and about 12 per cent. Key informant interviewing and observation in the study site strongly suggested that the results of the in-depth approach were more valid.

An evaluation study by Trend (1979) is often cited as an example of 'contradictions' between qualitative and quantitative data. His study was an evaluation of a housing subsidy programme in the US. The data from qualitative in-depth observations in a project site pointed to serious problems of worker morale, laxity of 'quality control' procedures and other process indicators. On the other hand, quantitative data showed that the project was successful in meeting its performance targets, and was at least as cost-effective as other parallel project sites. Trend identified additional data that helped in explaining the disjunctions between the (negative) qualitative picture and the (positive) quantitative indicators. Although he used the concept of triangulation in his discussion of these issues, we would argue that the specific contents of the two data sources are sufficiently different that the triangulation concept fits rather poorly.

Ward and associates have reported three case studies in which the data from focus group discussions were compared systematically with the results of quantitative surveys (Ward, Bertrand and Brown, 1991). The studies were all focused on peoples' responses to questions about family planning methods (primarily tubal ligation and vasectomy), to be used in the social marketing of contraceptives. The researchers made systematic comparisons of the general conclusions reached on a series of specific questions using the two methods. Their findings were summarized as follows.

Overall, for 28 per cent of the variables the results were similar; for 42 per cent the results were similar but focus groups provided additional detail; for 17 per cent the results were similar, but the survey provided more detail. In only 12 per cent of the variables were the results dissimilar.

They reported that the discrepancies tended to appear in topics that were somewhat sensitive and/or relatively less familiar to the respondents. For example, some questions about vasectomy resulted in discrepant results because many of the men in the study areas were unfamiliar with vasectomy. It would appear, then, that in the topical area of family planning, focus group discussions and surveys can be used for real triangulation (if needed), and in many situations focus group discussions can provide a broader range of information than is obtained in the surveys.

Wight and West (1999) have recently examined the sexual activity of young Scotsmen, including number of partners, as reported in in-depth interviews compared with the same information from the same interviews a year earlier in a structured survey. They found that the overall aggregate data showed relatively good concordance. On the other hand, 'the apparent similarity . . . conceals considerable change in the responses of *individuals* between the two time periods' (Wight and West, 1999: 61). The researchers felt that the in-depth interviews were, on the whole, more accurate than the survey data. However, another factor affecting the comparison was the fact that the earlier, more structured interviewing was carried out by female interviewers. Several of the respondents recalled their embarrassment (and falsification of data) as they apparently gave fuller, more accurate information in the in-depth interviews (male interviewers). This recent study is another example illustrating the multiple factors that affect the validity and reliability of data.

On the basis of our examination of a number of recent qualitative-cum-quantitative studies in reproductive health, we suggest that in most cases triangulation, in the narrow sense of cross-checking, is not a primary or important feature of the studies. In many cases, the types of data gathered in the qualitative phase of study are somewhat different from those in the quantitative operations. Sometimes the qualitative materials simply provide raw materials (key questions and hypotheses) for quantitative research. In other cases it is highly useful to use qualitative procedures to provide descriptive materials about the complex contexts, processes and other systematic patterns within which specific, measurable behaviours are seen to operate. Thus, the combination of qualitative and quantitative data-gathering is usually for getting complementary (hence richer) information, rather than simply 'validating' the results of a survey through qualitative data, or vice versa.

Assessing contradictory findings from triangulation

A brief set of guidelines is presented for interpreting and checking on the meanings of contradictory results arising from different data-gathering operations:

1 Carefully check to see that the two sets of data are truly dealing with the same information. For example, a quantitative survey question might indicate a high level of satisfaction with a specific health service, while qualitative interviews report much lower levels of client satisfaction. In many cases the discrepancy may be due to different levels of specificity. In this example, the survey question was focused on a specific service while the qualitative interview elicited an evaluation of overall services.

2 Check to see to what extent the differences in results come from different segments of the population. Always assume that there are subgroup differences in your population. The contradictory results may be representative of higher vs. lower socioeconomic status, for example; or simply different geographical neighbourhoods in the community.

3 If group discussions and/ or survey interviews give different results from in-depth individual interviews, the most likely explanation is that the group discussions and survey data represent 'socially accepted ideals' of behaviours while the in-depth interviews are likely to be closer to actual behavioural realities (cf. Helitzer-Allen, Makhambera and Wangel, 1994; Konings et al., 1995, discussed earlier). However, such assumptions should be carefully checked against contextual data.

4 Whenever possible, it is useful to present apparently contradictory results to key informants and to the field research team to ask for their assessments of the contradictions.

5 Explore the possibility that the two sets of data were collected at different times,

so that perspectives of respondents or informants have changed due to intervening events or circumstances.

6 Find out if the persons who collected the data were different in age, sex, ethnicity and so on. In the example cited by Wight and West (1999, see earlier discussion), different answers were given to male interviewers as compared with female interviewers.

7 Many other situational factors at the time of interviews, observations or other data collection activities can influence the quality and direction of results.

8 In complex qualitative data, such as group discussions and in-depth interviews, one goal is to have enough contextual information so that various details can be cross-checked.

9 In quantitative data, too, there are often points within the data that permit cross-checking to see that there is internal consistency.

10 When contradictory results arise from two different kinds of informants or groups, then one should assess the possible motivations or differences of perspective affecting answers from the two types of people. One common example occurs when data from community health workers are compared with statements from medical officers and other administrators. In such situations, the two groups are likely to have different definitions of 'quality of care', different priorities with regard to essential services and other differences in perspective.

11 When trying to triangulate data from different kinds of personnel in a system, such as a health care system, NGO or other organization, it is always important to consider the power relations within the system that may be producing contradictory results in data that are based on peoples' verbal descriptions. Often the contradictions will be most glaring at the level of broad generalizations. 'Our organization is doing a very good job of providing services to the people' vs. 'there are many serious gaps and failures in our performance'. In most such cases it is useful to seek data at a more concrete level.

12 Many seeming contradictions in data can be resolved, or at least brought into clearer perspective, if the focus of information is brought down to lower levels of abstraction. Go for the specific details instead of generalities.

13 Triangulation, and the assessment of contradictions in data, whether qualitative or quantitative (or both) should, as far as possible, be resolved during data collection. Often the field team and local key informants can be very helpful in resolving incongruities in the data.

Presenting the findings from integrated qualitative and quantitative research

The writing up of research is always difficult, and even more so if a study is composed of several different types of data. For some people the presentation of quan-

Table 13.2. Usual organization of a quantitative research report

A	B	C	D	E
Introduction of the problem, background and review of the relevant literature	Statement of research questions and hypotheses; study population and data-gathering methodology	One or more tables giving basic characteristics of the study population	Tables for each block of important results, including testing of hypotheses (relationships)	Discussion of the results and their significance; conclusions

titative data may seem easy, as the main information is contained in sets of more or less 'standard' statistical tables. The usual organization of a purely quantitative research report (in very simplified form) is presented in Table 13.2.

The simplest strategy to add in qualitative data is to quote from one or two informants, cases or focus groups, to illustrate each of the main results in 'D' concerning the numerical results. Thus, if the numerical data show that most of the respondents prefer laparascopic sterilization as their main family planning method, then it is common to include verbatim quotes from one or two or three 'cases', looking for quotes that give an explanation, or reasons for the particular choice.

Some additional suggestions that may apply for different combinations of qualitative and quantitative materials follow:

1 In some studies, extensive qualitative data have been collected concerning general patterns of behaviour, which provide a framework or interactional system within which the quantitative data give certain selected frequencies. For example, the system of behaviour of community health workers (ANMs, etc.) is usually very structured by the bureaucracy within which they work. The description of community health workers' weekly and monthly activity patterns (from key informants and cases) could be presented between B and C above, as a descriptive section, taking care to include information about bureaucratic pressures (e.g. family planning targets and similar performance pressures), which help to understand behaviours presented in numbers in section 'D'. The numerical results can be supplemented (as above) with brief case materials (especially quoted statements), that refer to the contextual framework in explaining individual actions (e.g. reasons for inflating numbers of intrauterine contraceptive device cases).

2 Numerical data can often be partitioned into several 'main types' of persons or types of problems. For example, a series of pregnant and postpartum cases might include those who had frequent antenatal care from private practitioners, frequent antenatal care from a community health worker and government clinic, very little antenatal care and many problems but no antenatal care. In this situation, some of the numerical data can be broken down into the subcategories to give quantitative profiles of the different 'types'. In connection with the quantitative profiles, one or two individual case descriptions can be given to illustrate some of the main characteristics of each subgroup.

3 In general, six main types of qualitative data are particularly useful:
   • Descriptions of systematic patterns, processes or interactions (relationships). For example, a description of a laparascopic camp in terms of organization, sequences of action, personnel and other components.
   • Descriptions of specific events that illustrate dynamics affecting a situation. For example, an individual treatment-seeking narrative.
   • Cases – individuals with specific characteristics, including their specific patterns of use of health services, family planning, sexual behaviours or other actions.
   • Verbatim quotes from individuals that illustrate and help us understand attitudes and explanations for specific actions and choices.
   • Maps and inventories of facilities, services, events, and so on. For example, the map of all the local health practitioners and facilities.
   • Vocabulary, statements of cultural 'rules', ceremonial patterns and other very structured cultural materials (e.g. 'the first time she conceives, the woman is expected to go to her mother's house [her natal home] when she is seven months pregnant').

   The cases and individual quotes are the types of materials that are often used in small pieces, selected to illustrate the main, quantitative tables.

4 Some studies are predominantly qualitative, with the quantitative materials playing a secondary role. For example, a set of cases (in-depth interviews) of men's sexual behaviours or sexual histories is best treated as a descriptive 'essay' in which numerical materials are injected here and there to provide descriptive frequencies. In such studies, the numbers of statistical tables are kept to a minimum.

5 There are two main strategies for presenting qualitative essays: (i) to organize the materials in a chronological or developmental sequence. For example, individual sexual histories can be organized in terms of 'first sexual awakenings', 'first experience with a sexual partner', 'further development, including multi-partner sexual activities', 'current patterns'; and (ii) identify several main 'types of persons' and 'main themes', and try to fit them into some sort of logical flow.

6 In general, qualitative descriptive writing should avoid stereotyping through biased selection of cases, verbatim quotations or other illustrative materials. It is much better to err on the side of diversity and contradictions. That is, it is useful to present exceptions and deviations from the main patterns, along with the 'typical cases'. Presentation of exceptions and contradictions can add richness to descriptive narratives.

Of course there are many other elements and strategies in the art of writing research reports. Here we have included a few ideas that arise from our review of the different types of studies. Researchers should always scan the works of others in the same field to identify the strong points and weaknesses in published articles and research reports. Writing up the conclusions from qualitative-cum-quantitative studies is a developing area in which it is useful to emulate some features from predecessors, while developing one's own unique style.

Summary and conclusions

The combining of qualitative and quantitative data gathering in reproductive health research is not new. Nonetheless we feel that the decade of the 1990s has seen a growth of greater sophistication, both in the types of qualitative methodologies employed, and in the methodological rigour of the overall research designs, on both the quantitative and qualitative sides. The rapid spread of acceptance of qualitative methods, particularly in reproductive health research, appears to be driven by a number of different dynamics, but is particularly affected by the need for research in hitherto less explored, sensitive areas of human behaviour. New topics and fields of study have required innovations in research approaches, which also have opened new data-gathering possibilities in established areas.

Researchers are responding to challenges thrown up by research needs in sensitive topics such as abortion, sexual behaviours, sexual health problems and other relatively newer areas. Another source of methodological innovation comes from the continuing pressures for understanding the sociocultural, economic and practical realities of populations from their own vantage points. In some cases, research is improved simply through better understanding of peoples' non-academic, practical vocabularies, including the naming and categorizing of illnesses and symptoms. However, generating greater understanding of 'the peoples' perspectives' can be much more than simply vocabulary. Just as agricultural development agents have belatedly learned that many (not all) 'rustic' traditional agricultural practices have important positive functions, so too, recent research has begun to explore the complex logics of peoples' varied reproductive health behaviours. For example, it seems that only recently researchers have begun to realize the complexity of peoples' visions concerning health care alternatives. The array of potential providers, in many rural peoples' experiences, is often much wider than supposed in earlier research.

The political impulses from women's movements have also played a part in changing international agendas in reproductive health. The changed programmatic agendas from influential meetings, such as the Cairo Conference of 1994, have had an effect on research agendas and research strategies. Another major source of change has a much more negative garb: the worldwide spread of the HIV/AIDS pandemic has forced reproductive health programmes to rethink and redesign operational strategies, and new demands for information have brought innovations in styles of data-gathering.

The examples and 'models' presented in this chapter are not exhaustive of all the innovations in qualitative–quantitative research designs. The field of reproductive health research is in a dynamic phase, and we can expect continuing experimentation and improvements in the inter-relating of quantitative and qualitative approaches to the gathering and analysis of useful data.

REFERENCES

Basu AM, Aaby P, (eds) (1998) *The methods and uses of anthropological demography*. Oxford, Oxford University Press.

Blanc AK, Wolff B, Gage AJ et al. (1996) *Negotiating reproductive outcomes in Uganda*. Calverton, Maryland, Macro Int. Inc.

Bleek W (1987) Lying informants: a fieldwork experience from Ghana. *Population and development review*, 13(2): 314–322.

Borgatti SP (1992) ANTHROPAC 4:0. Natick, MA, Analytic Technologies.

Bulut A, Toubia N (1999) Abortion services in two public sector hospitals in Istanbul, Turkey. How well do they meet women's needs? In: Mundigo A and Indriso C, eds. *Abortion in the developing world*, pp. 259–280. New Delhi, Vistaar Publications.

Caldwell JC, Hill AG, Hull VJ (Eds) (1988) *Micro-approaches to demographic research*. London, Kegan Paul International.

Caldwell JC, Hill AG (1988) Recent developments using micro-approaches to demographic research. In: Caldwell JC et al., eds. *Micro-approaches to demographic research*, pp.1–9. London, Kegan Paul International.

Caldwell JC, Reddy PH, Caldwell P (1982) The cause of demographic change in rural South India: a micro approach. *Population and development review*, 8(4): 689–727.

Campbell DT (1979) 'Degrees of Freedom' and the case study. In: Cook TD, Reichardt CS, eds. *Qualitative and quantitative methods in evaluation research*, pp. 49–67. Beverly Hills, Sage Publications.

Campbell J, Stone L (1984) The use and misuse of surveys in international development: an experiment from Nepal. *Human organization*, 43(1): 27–37.

Collumbien M, Das B, Bohidar N et al. (1999) Male sexual health concerns in Orissa – an emic perspective. IUSSP seminar on Social Categories in Population Studies, Cairo, Egypt.

Dare OO, Cleland J (1994) Reliability and validity of survey data on sexual behaviour. *Health transition review*, 4(Suppl.): 93–110.

Garg S (2000) An epidemiological and sociological study of symptomatic and asymptomatic reproductive tract infections and sexually transmitted infections among women in an urban slum. New Delhi, Maulana Azad Medical College, Dept. of Community Medicine.

Glaser B, Strauss L (1967) *The discovery of grounded theory.* Chicago, Aldine.

Goetz JP, LeCompte MD (1984) Ethnography and Qualitative Design in Educational Research. New York, Academic Press Inc.

Greenhalgh S (Ed.) (1995) *Situating fertility.* Cambridge, Cambridge University Press.

Handwerker WP, Wozniak DF (1997) Sampling strategies for the collection of cultural data: an extension of Boas's answer to Galton's problem. *Current anthropology*, 38(5): 869–875.

Havanon N, Bennett A, Knodel J (1993) Sexual networking in provincial Thailand. *Studies in family planning*, 24(1): 1–17.

Helitzer-Allen D, Makhambera M (1993) How can we help adolescent girls avoid HIV infection? *Network*, 13(4): 7.

Helitzer-Allen D, Makhambera M, Wangel A-M (1994) Obtaining sensitive information: the need for more than focus groups. *Reproductive health matters*, 3: 75–81.

Hilderbrand K, Hill AG, Randall S et al. (1985) Child mortality and care in children in rural Mali. In: Hill AG, ed. *Population, health and nutrition in the Sahel*, pp. 184–207. London, Kegan Paul International.

Iyer A, Jesani A (1999) Barriers to the quality of care: the experience of auxiliary nurse midwives in rural Maharashtra. In: Koenig M, Khan ME, eds. *Improving quality of care in India's family welfare programme: the challenge ahead*, pp. 210–237. New York, The Population Council.

Jeffery P, Jeffery R (1996) What's the benefit of being educated? Girl's schooling, women's autonomy and fertility outcomes in Bijnor. In: Jeffery R, Basu A, eds. *Girls schooling, women's autonomy and fertility change in South Asia*, pp. 150–183. New Delhi, Sage Publications.

Jeffery P, Jeffery R, Lyon A (1989) *Labour pains and labour power.* London, Zed Books Ltd.

Joshi A, Dhampola M (1999) Treatment seeking behaviour of rural Gujarati women. Ford Foundation Working Paper Series, New Delhi.

Khan ME, Patel B, Gupta RB (1999) The quality of family planning services in Uttar Pradesh from the perspective of service providers. In: Koenig M, Khan ME, eds. *Improving quality of care in India's family welfare programme: the challenge ahead*, pp. 238–272. New York, The Population Council.

Knodel J, Chamratrithirong A, Debavalya N (1987) Thailand's reproductive revolution: rapid fertility decline in third-world setting. Madison, University of Wisconsin Press.

Konings E, Bantebya G, Caraël M et al. (1995) Validating population surveys for measurement of HIV/STD prevention indicators. *AIDS*, 9: 375–382.

MacCormack CP (1985) Lay concepts of reproductive physiology related to contraceptive use: a method of investigation. *Journal of tropical medicine and hygiene*, 88: 281–285.

Pelto PJ (1970) *Anthropological research: the structure of inquiry.* New York, Harper and Row.

Pickering H, Okongo M, Bwanika K et al. (1996) Sexual mixing patterns in Uganda: small-time urban/rural traders. *AIDS*, **10**: 533–536.

Pickering H, Okongo M, Nnalusiba B et al. (1997) Sexual networks in Uganda: casual and commercial sex in a trading town. *AIDS care*, **9**: 199–207.

Reichardt CS, Cook TD (1979) Beyond qualitative versus quantitative methods. In: Cook TD, Reichardt CS, eds. *Qualitative and quantitative methods in evaluation research*, pp. 7–32. Beverly Hills, Sage Publications.

Renne EP (1993) Gender ideology and fertility strategies in an Ekiti Yoruba village. *Studies in family planning*, **24**(6): 343–353.

Romney AK, Weller S, Batchelder WH (1986) Culture as consensus. *American anthropologist*, **88**: 313–338.

Rossi PH, Wright SR (1977) Evaluation research: an assessment of theory, practice and politics. *Evaluation quarterly*, **1**: 5–52.

Salway S, Nurani S (1998a) Postpartum contraceptive use in Bangladesh: understanding users' perspectives. *Studies in family planning*, **29**(1): 41–57.

Salway S, Nurani S (1998b) Uptake of contraception during postpartum amenorrhoea: understandings and preferences of poor, urban women in Bangladesh. *Social science and medicine*, **47**: 899–909.

Schensul SL, Schensul JJ, Oodit G et al. (1994) Sexual intimacy and changing lifestyles in an era of AIDS: young women workers in Mauritius. *Reproductive health matters*, **3**: 83–92.

Schopper D, Doussantousse S, Orav J (1993) Sexual behaviours relevant to HIV transmission in a rural African population. *Social science and medicine*, **37**(3): 401–412.

Silva K, Tudor SL, Schensul JJ et al. (1997) Youth and sexual risk in Sri Lanka. ICRW Research Report Series No. 3 (Women and AIDS Research Program). Washington D.C., International Centre for Research on Women.

Trend MG (1979) On the reconciliation of qualitative and quantitative analyses: a case study. In: Cook, TD, Reichardt CS, eds. *Qualitative and quantitative methods in evaluation research*, pp. 68–86. Beverly Hills, Sage Publications.

Ward VM, Bertrand JT, Brown LF (1991) The comparability of focus group and survey results. *Evaluation review*, **15**: 266–283.

Watts C, Keogh E, Ndlovu M et al. (1998) Withholding of sex and forced sex: dimensions of violence against Zimbabwean women. *Reproductive health matters*, **6**(12): 57–65.

Weller S, Romney AK (1988) Systematic data collection. *Qualitative research methods*, Series 10. Newbury Park, Sage Publications.

Wight D, West P (1999) Poor recall, misunderstandings and embarrassment: interpreting discrepancies in young men's reported heterosexual behaviour. *Culture, health and sexuality*, **1**(1): 55–78.

Yirrel DL, Pickering H, Palmarini G et al. (1998) Molecular epidemiological analysis of HIV in sexual networks in Uganda. *AIDS*, **12**: 285–290.

Yoddumnern-Attig B, Attig GA, Boonchalaksi W et al. eds. (1993) Qualitative methods for population and health research. Mahidol University, Institute for Population and Social Research.

14

Interpreting results from different sources of data

Tom Marshall,[1] Véronique Filippi,[1] André Meheus[2] and Aysen Bulut[3]

[1] London School of Hygiene and Tropical Medicine, London, UK; [2] University of Antwerp, Belgium; [3] Institute of Child Health, Istanbul, Turkey

Diseases and illnesses are matters of classification, and they change as social values about 'normal' aspects of age, fitness, and gender change. Yes we all are born and die, and in that sense, biology dominates, but how we use and experience our bodily potential in between those bookends is no more dictated by biology than is the style of our hats. Thinking about the consequences of assigning categories, I am reminded that language does not name reality, it organizes reality. Topics within areas of health, mental health, and sexuality have been subject to repeated renaming and redefinition as social values have changed. Tiefer (1995).

Introduction

This chapter is concerned with the interpretation of data from quantitative, community-based epidemiological studies. In many developing countries, where the coverage of health services is low and the quality of information from routine statistics variable, such studies are commonly the only way to establish population-valid results concerning reproductive health. These studies also have an important role where service coverage and information quality is higher, as there are many questions that cannot be addressed using only health service data.

Morbidity data are gathered using instruments ranging from laboratory assays and tests to clinical examinations and questionnaires. Interpretation depends on the relationship between what is measured and what is required to be known. This relationship can be particularly intricate when responses to questions are used as indicators of disease states and related states.

An important theme is how data from different sources can be drawn together, but not replaced by each other, to give an understanding of a person's morbidity and ill health. This process of understanding of what is being measured is an essential prerequisite for any associations with risk factors or consequences to be fully understood, and any planning or evaluation of an intervention to be undertaken. This chapter specifies different outcome entities and how they are best measured, and introduces the epidemiological concepts of reliability and validity and their statistical parameters, including sensitivity, specificity and the kappa (κ) statistic.

Before considering these issues in detail, two examples are presented.

Example 1

A number of studies have been carried out to investigate the link between medically diagnosed and self-reported gynaecological morbidity. One such study is a cross-sectional survey of married women in Cobançesme, an area of new settlement in Istanbul, Turkey (Bulut et al., 1995; Filippi et al., 1997). Data on self-reported reproductive morbidity and contraceptive use were gathered by questionnaire at home, followed by a clinical assessment of morbidity by medical examination with laboratory tests during a clinic visit. At the start of the clinical assessment, the physician asked the same questions relating to symptoms as in the home questionnaire. Approximately 700 women took part in both sections of the survey.

The proportion of women reporting symptoms indicative of various morbidities and the proportion medically diagnosed for the same morbidities are shown in Table 14.1 (Filippi et al., 1997). These results show that symptoms are more frequently reported to a physician in a clinical setting than to an interviewer at home, suggesting that the reliability of the questionnaire is limited when used in different circumstances. There is considerable disagreement between questionnaire-derived morbidity and clinical diagnosis, with the former tending to be more common, except with prolapse; this shows an aspect of the validity of the questionnaire as a tool for indicating clinical diagnosis. A more detailed analysis would explore these differences completely; however, the purpose of this example is to illustrate the problems of matching diagnosis with respondent-reported symptoms. The authors comment on cultural factors contributing to the differences for prolapse and menstrual disorders, as well as on laboratory and medical diagnoses being based on stricter criteria for the two types of infection and on possible weaknesses in the questionnaire.

A study that led to a similar type of data was earlier carried out in Giza, Egypt (Younis et al., 1994). Both these studies will be referred to later in this chapter.

Example 2

Irving et al. (1998) investigated the association between psychological factors (including anxiety, depression, life satisfaction, self-esteem and stress) and vaginal candidiasis (culture-positive and treated at least twice in the previous six months) in an exploratory cross-sectional study comparing 28 culture-positive women with 16 controls. Despite the small sample size, the infected group showed, with statistical significance, more clinical depression, less satisfaction with life, poorer self-

Table 14.1. Women reporting morbidity and the proportion medically diagnosed with the same morbidity (percentage)

Morbidity condition	Reporting associated symptoms		Diagnosis
	Home	Clinic	
Reproductive tract infection	43	48	20
Menstrual disorder[a]	13	25	16
Pelvic relaxation (prolapse)	19	19	27
Urinary tract infection	19	24	7

Note:
[a] The infections tested are listed in Filippi et al. (1997).

esteem and greater perception of life as stressful. This shows evidence of association with infection, but interpreting these is uncertain because the study (the authors describe it as preliminary) was not longitudinal.

This example shows how different types of information provide insight in that they show how this form of morbidity and ill health has further, measurable consequences.

The limited degree of agreement brought out in the first example appears in many studies of gynaecological morbidity. Sadana (2000) presents a list of studies where questionnaires, laboratory tests and clinical data collection were applied. Koenig et al. (1998) discuss seven studies of this type in India. In both these papers, the authors point to problems in reconciling data from different instruments in many of these studies. In this chapter, an attempt is made to present some of the concepts involved, and to use these as a base for exploring the relationships between data and results from these different sources.

The basis of sound interpretation

Certain features of a study feed into the process of understanding results. These include:

1 *The objectives.* The objectives specify what is to be measured, why these variables are chosen (the purpose) and the population of interest in which the measurements will be made.

2 *The items or variables to be measured.* How they are defined and how they relate to the objectives.

3 *The instruments used to measure these items.* By 'instrument' is meant a question

or group of questions in a questionnaire, a clinical examination or similar assessment, or an objective measurement such as a laboratory test for an infective agent or a test (such as the ureodynamic assessment of urinary incontinence).

4 *The design of the study.* This term covers the formal 'type of design' (such as cross-sectional survey, cohort study), the sampling scheme used to select the subjects in the study from the population of interest and the size of the sample.

5 *The way the data are analysed.* The methods used in data analysis have a strong influence on interpretation. In particular, which of the measured quantities are taken as 'outcomes' and which of the other measured quantities are assessed for association with the outcomes is important. The analysis should be based on the objectives, which should lead to these choices, and should also be based on sound statistical techniques. It must deal adequately with random error and confounding. Analysis issues are considered here in the context of reliability and validity, and briefly in more general terms at the end of the chapter.

6 *The sequence of interpretation.* Conclusions from data, particularly those that relate to associations and links between the variables being measured, must always be checked for simpler alternative explanations before substantive conclusions are made. These start from selection and measurement bias, through the possible effects of confounding to random error (can the association observed be explained as a chance finding?) (see Beaglehole, Bonita and Kjellström, 1993). In this chapter, we return to a review of this sequence, highlighting the effects of misclassification.

This chapter chiefly focuses on points 2, 3 and partly 5, listed above.

Issues relating to objectives and definitions

Objectives

Three types of objectives are relevant to the issues of this chapter.

The first objective is to validate an instrument or technique for identifying women with a particular disease or condition. This implies comparing the technique with an established method, and accepting the established method as adequate as a gold standard. Examples are validating a new laboratory test for an infection with established methods (Morré et al., 1999) or validating syndromic diagnoses and screening algorithms for sexually transmitted infections (STIs) (Diallo et al., 1998).

The second is to estimate the prevalence or incidence of chosen outcomes, most frequently outcomes relating to disease, illness and impairment. Estimates of prevalence are important to estimate health service need, assess the importance of different types of morbidity in different communities and, consequently, for advocacy on behalf of women suffering from these diseases, illnesses and impairments.

They form a background to the assessment of disability adjusted life years (DALYs).

The third is the epidemiological investigation of the risk factors or the consequences of particular diseases, illnesses or disabilities. There may be multiple consequences; Example 2 above illustrates depression as a putative outcome of infection, but there are many others.

The first area is one where techniques are well defined, and where definitive guidelines can be made. For the second and third, one is essentially trying to throw light on separate and distinct states or conditions of the people being investigated, and on the prevalence or incidence and interrelations between these states.

Definitions, outcome entities and groups of entities

We use the word 'entities' for the conditions one is trying to investigate, and present a list of types of these entities, from exactly defined biomedical conditions to more generalized ones, covering ill health and its impact, to health and well-being. Some are based on the definitions of impairment, disability and handicap in the International Classification of Impairments, Disabilities and Handicaps (ICIDH) (World Health Organization, 1980). The last but one is health-related quality of life, and covers a growing body of instruments aimed to provide overall assessments of the individual's health and functional status and level of welfare.

In analysing and interpreting data, these entities are commonly taken as outcomes. Many are of primary interest as descriptors of ill health. They can also be determinants, as already mentioned, and as shown in Example 2.

The first three types of entities cover aspects of the individual's condition that are based on, and in principle measurable through, predetermined criteria. The summary descriptions here incorporate concepts from Harwood et al. (1998), Murray and Chen (1992) and World Health Organization (1980).

- *Current infection*, taken as any microbial infection. This may be highly pathogenic, such as HIV, or relatively benign, such as human papilloma virus (excluding the more serious oncogenic types) or candida. Several tests to measure microbial infection (for example, serological tests) also measure past infection.
- *Medically-defined diseases*. In principle, these are diseases defined in the International Classification of Diseases (ICD-10; World Health Organization, 1992). They are normally ascertained medically, and their definition and diagnosis are generally made on the basis of pathological criteria (although this does not imply that a diagnosis is always dependent on pathology testing). An example is pelvic inflammatory disease (PID).
- *Impairment* (loss or abnormality of function of organ systems or anatomical parts). The function may be physical or mental. Examples are vesicovaginal fistula, tubal occlusion and depression.

There is an overlap between current infection and disease. Most current infections are part of a disease or a process of disease. There is considerable overlap between disease and impairment, and many conditions listed in the ICIDH are also in the ICD. An example is depression.

Knowledge of prevalence and severity is useful in a community context in order to build an understanding of the extent of preventable and curable infections and diseases, the burden of disease and the degree to which women may be at risk of later consequences on account of infection and disease. An example is the prevalence of HIV infection.

The next group brings in how a respondent sees and perceives her own condition. This is important for understanding motivations, for example, for seeking health care or for accepting restrictions in lifestyle.

• *Illness* (the perception by the respondent of an adverse state). Illness and disease are words that may be used interchangeably in lay parlance, but are distinct in our context, where illness is based on the perception of the respondent of various states, such as pain, emotional disturbance and unease. Examples are headache, pain during intercourse, vaginal itching and menstrual pain. Illness is essentially an awareness of symptoms.

Helman (1990) gives an overview of illness as a distinct area. It is the subjective response to, or awareness of, being unwell. This awareness is linked to the meaning a person gives to her condition; the importance she (or he) attaches to it and to particular symptoms can vary greatly between places, cultural backgrounds and different social groups (see Murray and Chen, 1992, who show how self-perceived indicators of specific conditions vary widely between states in India). An important aspect of reporting of illness is whether the person views the symptoms as abnormal and exceptional, or not. In Example 1 above, prolapse was reported less by women than diagnosed by physicians, and Filippi et al. (1997) suggest that the respondents did not always rate it highly enough to merit reporting, even in answer to a prompted question. Awareness, and thus reporting, of symptoms, whether spontaneously or in reply to prompting, can depend on the respondent's perception of their importance, of how her life is affected and to what extent she reckons something can and should be done to relieve them. Sadana (2000) discusses the factors that may underlie a tendency not to report illnesses, and quotes Mechanic and Newton that reporting an illness is more likely in the absence of social and psychological barriers.

Particular symptoms or groups of symptoms may correspond to an illness construct specific to a particular cultural setting, which may not correspond, or may only partially correspond, to a particular biomedical disease. These constructs are 'folk illnesses' (Helman, 1990), and if a symptom belongs to a folk illness, the respondent will see it as part of that illness. If there are folk illnesses in the area of gynaecological morbidity in the community under investigation, knowledge of them is important for interpreting self-reports of symptoms and illnesses, and can also guide questionnaire design. This knowledge can be gained by qualitative methods, and the importance of this aspect is stressed by Koenig et al. (1998).

The relevance of this is that questions about symptoms address the area of illness. If the reason to ask these questions is to ascertain the extent of disease, there are potential problems. If it is to assess the perceived impact of disease or illness, or health care seeking and other behaviour, these problems matter less. To interpret results, however, it is important to understand the locally-relevant constructs and the extent to which particular symptoms are normally considered worthy of report, or subject to barriers to their reporting.

An example is given in the commentary of Trollope-Kumar (1999) on a study of syndromic management of reproductive tract infections among low-income Bangladeshi women (Hawkes et al., 1999). Trollope-Kumar remarks that self-reports of vaginal discharge are very common in South Asia, which in her own clinical experience are frequently associated with other symptoms such as 'dizziness, burning hands and feet, backache and weakness'. She writes that many women 'seemed to be having a culturally shaped illness . . . not necessarily associated with reproductive tract disease', and discusses this in relation to the cultural context.

A related example comes from Patel and Oomman (1999), who discuss the 'intersection of reproductive and mental health'. They point to a high prevalence of self-reported gynaecological symptoms among women in South Asia along with evidence of a high prevalence of depression and a high degree of disagreement between diagnoses of reproductive disease and these self-reported symptoms. Many women report the symptoms but appear to be free of diagnosed disease, and the authors discuss the role of depression in this discordance.

The entities so far have focused on the individual's own condition and not on her activities, her environment, the society she lives in, her roles in everyday life and the impact that ill health or good health may have on these. The next two groups of entities are in these areas.

- *Disability* (an abnormality in the performance of a discrete task or activity). Examples are inability to engage in sexual intercourse, and urinary or faecal incontinence.
- *Handicap* (a disadvantage resulting from an impairment or disability that limits or prevents a fulfilment that is normal for that person). A handicap is to be seen in a functional and social context. The term may be taken in common parlance to denote a physical limitation on some form of capacity, but that is not the meaning here (WHO, 1980). An example is a handicap in social integration that

may follow curtailment of sexual activity on account of an impairment, which may in turn be on account of a disease. Another is social handicap following urinary incontinence.

Disability and handicap may be, and often are, linked with infection and disease. An example of linkages between entities in the different groups is given in Box 14.1.

Box 14.1. Example of progression from infection to handicap

Chlamydia *(infection)*
  → Cervical inflammation *(physical change)*
    → Cervicitis *(disease)*
      → Pelvic inflammatory disease *(disease)*
        → Infertility *(impairment)*
          → Inability to have child *(disability)*
            → Social exclusion *(handicap)*

This illustrates several stages, all of which can in principle be identified and measured. The sequence implicit in Box 14.1 is not inevitable. Chlamydial infection, even if untreated, does not always lead to these consequences; whether inability to have a child has social consequences, and what these are, is culturally determined; infertility is a problem for women who wish to have a child, but not for those who do not. Disabilities and handicaps can result from more than one disease and from other factors; there are plenty of potential reasons for infertility as well as chlamydial infection and potentially many other factors feeding into social exclusion.

All the groups of entities listed so far, with the exception of handicap, address health as the absence of specific conditions of ill health. Health-related quality of life measurement takes an alternative approach, bringing in the 'measurement of the positive' as well. Bowling (1997) provides a comprehensive list of many quality of life indicators. They cover the areas of functional ability, broad health and illness status, psychological well being and its converse, social networks and support, and life satisfaction and morale. Most testing and development has been done in Western countries. There is a conceptual overlap between the approach embodied in the progression from impairment to handicap, and that of health-related quality of life. However, among the instruments listed by Bowling, none is orientated towards reproductive health or the consequences of gynaecological morbidity. Quality of life indicators are not considered further in this chapter.

To summarize, the groups of entities range from the specifically biological one of infection to those in the over-arching concept of quality of life. Broadly, the further down the list, the more one is concerned with direct impact on the person, on her perception of her own health, her ability to function effectively for herself, in her home and in her community, and on the extent to which she is reduced by infection, disease, illness or some other reason. A survey may seek to ascertain the extent of any of these entities in a community or a population. The ultimate aim may be to illuminate the entities lower down the list, and seen from the viewpoint of the community and of the individuals who make up the community, one can argue that this aspect matters a great deal.

A final type of entity that reflects on the individual's health is 'being at risk'. For example, a woman with an untreated chlamydial infection is at increased risk of PID (pelvic inflammatory disease), ectopic pregnancy and infertility and its sequela (see Box 14.1), or a woman (or man) who engages in unprotected sexual intercourse with multiple partners is at risk of HIV, STIs and their consequences.

Measurement instruments

Quantitative data are obtained using the three different types of instruments mentioned earlier. The first is laboratory results from specimens taken from individuals in the survey sample or results from other tests carried out on individuals, such as laparoscopy. The second is results of clinical assessments carried out by medically trained personnel (not necessarily physicians, but with training appropriate to the diagnostic task). These may take place in a health service setting or elsewhere, such as in the respondents' homes. The third is responses to structured questionnaires, in which the respondents' own accounts of their symptoms, signs, disabilities, handicap and quality of life can be asked. These are often, though not always, administered in respondents' homes.

Of the three different data sources, each tends to be best for a different type of entity. However, there is overlap in the use of data sources. For instance, laboratory results often contribute to a clinical diagnosis. Moreover, an important component of clinical diagnosis is the patient's history. Survey questions relating to clinically relevant signs and symptoms are asked in interviews. This is different from the more variable way clinical histories are taken in ordinary practice, although the history taking aspect of clinical assessment in a survey framework may be standardized.

Different sources tend to be best for particular uses. Laboratory tests are generally best (and come closest to providing the gold standard) for detecting the presence of an infective agent, or providing immunological evidence for a past or present infection. Other test-based measurements also tend to be best for particular conditions, such as ureodynamic assessment for incontinence or laparoscopy for PID.

Clinical assessment has the potential to allow a complete view of the diseases covered by the survey. It must be remembered that there is considerable variation in

Table 14.2. Relevance of different types of instruments to different entities

Entity group	Type of instrument		
	Laboratory or other test	Clinical assessment[a]	Self-report in reply to survey questions
Current infection	Yes	Occasionally	Occasionally
Disease	Sometimes	Yes	Sometimes
Impairment	Contributes	Yes	Sometimes
Illness	No	Occasionally	Yes
Disability	No	Contributes	Yes
Handicap	No	Occasionally	Yes
Quality of life	No	Occasionally	Yes
Being at risk[b]	Contributes	Contributes	Contributes

Notes:
[a] Can include history taking and physical examination in a clinical context, but excludes laboratory and other tests used in clinical assessment.
[b] Risk can arise from physical, environmental or behavioural factors.

the interpretation of clinical observations and findings among physicians, and standardization of the procedures and interpretations is important in a survey or research context. Ideally, detecting a disease known to be caused by a specific infection should incorporate evidence from laboratory testing, but this is not always feasible.

Self-reporting through questionnaires provides evidence of illness (as we have defined illness). This is important because illness denotes the state of ill health as perceived by the respondent, which underlies much in terms of the behaviour and well being of the women concerned. It should be remembered that the account of ill health given by a respondent in the context of a clinical assessment and of answering survey questions outside a clinical setting will not in general be the same (see Example 1 and Filippi et al., 1997).

Table 14.2 lists the extent to which different data sources can provide useful information for each group of entities.

Table 14.3 explores the relation between types of instruments and specific infections, impairments and handicaps, such as severe prolapse and infertility. Many of the entities listed in Table 14.3, such as reproductive tract infection, can be of more than one type; in this example, this can depend on whether a specific infection with the infective agent is specified, or if the description is more general, encompassing several other infective agents and conditions, such as inflammation.

The objectives of a study lead to the entities to be investigated. These, in turn, lead to the choice of instruments. As one goes down the list of entities, the role of

Table 14.3. Examples of conditions and relation to type of instrument

Entity or condition	Type of entity	Type of instrument		
		Laboratory or other test	Clinical assessment	Self-report in reply to survey questions
Chlamydia	Infection	Yes	Suggestive	No
Pelvic inflammatory disease	Disease	Contributes[a]	Yes	No
Urinary tract infection	Infection/disease[b]	Yes	Yes	No
Reproductive tract infection	Infection/disease[c]	Yes	Yes	No
Third-degree prolapse	Disease/handicap	No	Yes	Yes
Vaginal discharge	Disease/illness/ impairment	No	Yes	Yes
Menstrual disorder	Disease/illness/ impairment	No	Yes	Yes
Infertility	Impairment	Contributes[d]	Yes	Yes
Depression	Disease/impairment	No	Yes	Yes

Notes:

[a] Can indicate a possible infective agent.

[b] The description can apply specifically to infection with the agent specified, or to a disease condition such as urethritis, or to a combined set of criteria.

[c] The description can apply specifically to infection with the agent specified, or to a disease condition such as vaginal inflammation, or to a combined set of criteria.

[d] Indicates changes underlying infertility.

the questionnaire increases. But although estimating the extent of a particular handicap, for example, requires information from questionnaires directed to individuals, understanding the handicap will be more complete when these data are accompanied by information on the diseases, impairments and disabilities in the same respondents.

Finally, it must be emphasized that no data source is free from errors. Laboratory tests detect infective agents with different degrees of success, different physicians may reach different diagnoses, and survey questionnaires are more or less successful in measuring what they aim to measure. The errors can be random or systematic, the latter leading to bias. Statistical tests address the former, but not the latter. A researcher must take all this into account when interpreting results from any source.

Knowing what is being measured and how well it is being measured

This section covers issues of how well an instrument matches the entity it is intended to measure. It brings in the concepts of reliability and validity, and applies the concept of validity in the particular context of using illness-based instruments as indicators for respondents' status with respect to infection and disease.

Reliability

The reliability of an instrument can be thought of in terms of stability, or the extent to which it produces the same result when used again for the same subject (Streiner and Norman, 1989). It is therefore concerned with individual data sources, but adequate reliability of each data source is necessary before issues of combining sources can be considered.

Stability is normally assessed by using the instrument two or more times on each member of a sample of individuals, ideally a population-representative sample. The instrument may be used by two or more different observers (interviewers and technicians, for example), and/or in two or more different settings, or just twice with these conditions not changing, depending on the aspect and context of reliability that is to be assessed. Stability for an instrument that classifies individuals into two or more distinct classes can be assessed by the percentage agreement, or by the κ coefficient, which corrects for the random component in the percentage agreement (Streiner and Norman, 1989). Filippi et al. (1997) looked at inter-observer variability between lay reporters and physicians asking the same questions about various gynaecological symptoms with a time gap of up to a week. The κ statistics indicated reasonable agreement, best for symptoms of prolapse and worst for menstrual period problems; one can see in Example 1 that women tended to report more to the physician.

κ is defined, with the same instrument used twice on each member of the sample, as follows; the results from the measurement are tabulated thus:

	First application		
Second application	Positive	Negative	Total
Positive	a	b	$a+b$
Negative	c	d	$c+d$
Total	$a+c$	$b+d$	n

Then

$$\kappa = \frac{P_0 - P_E}{1 - P_E}$$

where

P_0 = proportion of cases in the sample where both applications of the instrument agree; this is $(a + d) \div n$

P_E = proportion of cases in the sample where agreement would be expected purely by chance; this is $\{(a + c) \times (a + b)/n + (b + d) \times (c + d)/n\} \div n$.

Ranges of κ of less than 0.4, 0.4 to 0.6, 0.6 to 0.8 and above 0.8 have been proposed by Landis and Koch (1977) to indicate poor to fair, moderate, substantial and almost perfect agreement, and these are commonly used. However, κ should be used and interpreted with caution. Given a certain underlying level of observer performance and agreement, its value estimated in repeated observations depends on the underlying (true) prevalence (Thompson and Walter, 1988); this is particularly important if the prevalence is close to 0 per cent or to 100 per cent. If the two observers' results show different overall prevalence (i.e. one tends to classify 'positive' more frequently than the other, as in Example 1), then the maximum value of κ clearly cannot be 1, and the ranges that denote reasonable agreement may be lower (Kraemer and Bloch, 1988). Thus, the ranges of Landis and Koch (see above) should only be applied when the prevalence is in the middle range and the two observers show roughly the same percentages positive. Finally, κ calculated when the observations are scored on a graded scale of more than two grades tends to be lower, and the more grades in the scale the stronger this effect (Maclure and Willett, 1987).

Validity of instruments

Validity is concerned with the extent to which the instrument measures the state it is intended to measure. There are various types of validity, and various qualitative and quantitative measures to assess it. This section discusses the concept of true state before addressing these different forms.

Gold standards and the true state

In a simplistic sense, the *true state* is what we are trying to find out. This idea is most useful for the entities that can be most precisely defined in 'external' or 'objective' terms, and these tend to be entities earlier in the list in Table 14.2. However, the concept should not be abandoned for those lower in the list.

Some instruments perform better in finding a true state. The instrument that does this best (and no instrument does it perfectly) can be taken as providing the *gold standard* for the entity. Other instruments can then be assessed in relation to this instrument.

A true state depends on an accurate and complete definition. This is clear for infections, clinical diseases and impairments. For a clinical disease or an impairment, case definition may be simple. The existence of a well-described condition (for example, third degree prolapse or genital warts) is an example of a simple true state. However, many clinically defined diseases cannot be simply described as they depend on the existence of a number of changes and symptoms that together constitute the disease. It is not essential that all symptoms are present (see, for example, the definition of reproductive tract infections in Filippi et al., 1997). Nevertheless, the true state must be based on the essential features of the disease.

The concept of true state is more challenged for illness because the measurement instruments, and the questions being asked, to some extent define what the true state is. There is a potential trap here. Intelligence has humorously been defined as what intelligence tests measure. This, of course, is not true of intelligence, but the implied circularity should be avoided for definitions of illness as well. Instruments that address illness should be founded on questions that are reviewed for their validity (see below) and fit with a consensus view of the illness entity that is to be measured. It is also necessary to bear in mind that replies about symptoms mediated by cultural constructs or by personal characteristics (such as age and social class) may be highly specific to the community being studied. In-depth understanding of local concepts and terminology is important in creating questions and understanding data and results from their use (see Koenig et al., 1998).

With disability, generally with loss of functional capacity, and with handicap, one is on surer ground because it is easier to specify the aspects of functional capacity and social functioning that can constitute a true state. Loss of these must be seen in the full context of the person. For example, lengthy menstrual periods create more handicap in a society where a menstruating woman may not prepare food (see Chapter 13). In this case, the true state is specific to this kind of society.

The different forms of validity of an instrument

There are a variety of classifications of 'validity' as applied to a measurement instrument. The three definitions that principally concern us are as follows.

- *Face validity* is concerned with whether the instrument appears to be directed towards what it is intended to measure. It is the simplest way of looking at validity. Assessing it is basically a matter of judgement, based on expert and informed opinion. If there is a clear concept of a true state, then it is concerned with the correspondence of the instrument to the true state.

- *Criterion validity* is concerned with how well the instrument gives results that correspond to those of a gold standard. It is, therefore, often of greater relevance for entities early in the progression. The most straightforward example is the validation of laboratory tests.
- *Content validity* applies to instruments that have several components, such as a clinical protocol or a series of questions that together give the result, such as a scoring scale or a verbal autopsy algorithm. An instrument has adequate content validity if it covers all relevant (and measurable) aspects of the entity to be measured. This means that there must be appropriate item(s) to address each of these without excessive redundancy of items tending to reproduce the same information; deciding this is also a matter of expert judgement.

All instruments must have adequate face validity. Those that address entities with well-defined true states must have as good criterion validity as possible, as for example with the continuing refinement of laboratory tests for various infectious agents. An instrument that has several different components, such as a clinical protocol for diagnosis of a disease, a questionnaire module for an illness construct or one for a depression scale should have adequate content validity.

Sensitivity and specificity

This section is confined to entities that are described simply by whether they are present or not, and for which there are good gold standards.

Assuming that the instrument has adequate face validity, it can be assessed for criterion validity by selecting a sample of women with prevalence of the entity not too close to 0 per cent or to 100 per cent, then asking them the questions in the instrument and establishing their state by medical examination. Consider a questionnaire instrument for prolapse. The two true states are negative, no prolapse or prolapse less than the defined degree, and positive as assessed clinically. The instrument classifies women as positive and negative on the basis of their replies.

We pursue this in some detail. It is important here because a large number of the outcomes that arise in this area are reported by classifying respondents into two states. The relevant measures of criterion validity are sensitivity and specificity. Sensitivity indicates the proportion of gold standard true cases that are identified by the instrument. Specificity is the proportion of gold standard 'non-cases' that are correctly measured as such by the instrument.

These measures are now defined more exactly. This is done in terms of mathematical formulae, as in many textbooks, then numerically, taking data from Example 1 cited earlier (the Istanbul survey), with symptoms indicative of reproductive tract infection from the interview in the clinic compared with medical diagnosis also in the clinic. The medical diagnosis is the gold-standard. We note that the example is one of using an illness, symptoms indicative of reproductive tract

Table 14.4. Classification of results for an instrument under review and a gold standard

Instrument result	Gold standard (true state)		Total
	Positive	Negative	
Positive	a	b	$a+b$
Negative	c	d	$c+d$
Total	$a+c$	$b+d$	n

infection, as a measure of a disease, reproductive tract infection. The proportion of women classified as positive and negative by the gold standard and by the instrument are presented in Table 14.4 and numerically, in the example in Table 14.5.

The subjects for whom the instrument gives a positive result, but the gold standard a negative result, are called 'false positives'. They are b in Table 14.4 and 253 in the example in Table 14.5. Those for whom the instrument gives a negative result, but the gold standard a positive result, are called 'false negatives'. They are c in Table 14.4 and 56 in Table 14.5.

Sensitivity, as a percentage, is

$$100 \times a/(a+c)$$

This is the percentage of those with a diagnosed reproductive tract infection $(a+c)$, who were found to have one on the basis of the questions, a.

In the Istanbul data, it is

$$100 \times 82/138 = 59\%$$

Thus, rather more than half (59 per cent) of the medically defined cases were identified by the interview questions, and the remainder (41 per cent) were not.

Specificity, as a percentage, is

$$100 \times d/(b+d)$$

and is the percentage among those without a diagnosed reproductive tract infection $(b+d)$, who were found not to have one on the basis of the questions, d.

In the Istanbul data, it is

$$100 \times 302/555 = 54\%$$

Thus, close to half (54 per cent) of those not diagnosed with a reproductive tract infection were indicated as negative by the interview questions, and almost as many (46 per cent) of those without a diagnosis reported symptoms suggestive of a reproductive tract infection.

Table 14.5. Classification of questionnaire results according to medical diagnosis: reproductive tract infections, Istanbul

	Diagnosis		
From interview	Positive	Negative	Total
Positive	82	253	335 (48)
Negative	56	302	358
Total	138 (20)	555	693 (100)

Figures in brackets are percentages.

For an instrument to perform reasonably well in relation to a gold standard, sensitivity and specificity together must exceed 100 per cent. If their sum is exactly 100 per cent, the association between the instrument and the gold standard, in the data series in question, is not statistically significant (mathematically, the value of χ^2 without continuity correction is 0), which means that there is no evidence in these data to support any association between results from the instrument and the gold standard. In the above example, they add to 113 per cent, and although the association is statistically significant ($\chi^2 = 8.5$, $P = 0.004$), the association is not strong. Another measure of association is the odds ratio (here 1.75 and again not large).

Other reports of using questionnaire instruments in relation to reproductive infection also show low sensitivity and specificity combined, often adding to little more than 100 per cent (or even adding to less), with weak associations. Sadana (2000) lists a number of results from different studies. Kaufman et al. (1999) list results from a number of infections and questions from a study in rural Yunnan, China. Kaufman et al. (1999) also show results from using simple clinical signs for specific infections, which also show weak associations. There was more success with simple tests for the gold standard of two of the infections (trichomonas and candida). For other diseases, such as prolapse and menstrual disorders, performance can be better (Sadana, 2000). Bang et al. (1989) cross-tabulated 'any symptom' with 'any disease', with sensitivity 59 per cent and specificity 90 per cent. There were relatively few (8 per cent) without any disease.

Instrument-measured prevalence and its deviation from the gold standard prevalence

False positives and false negatives pull in opposite directions. False positives tend to build up the instrument-measured prevalence to be higher than the gold standard prevalence, while false negatives tend to reduce it. If by chance they are similar in number, then the discrepancy between the two types of prevalence will be small.

But it must be stressed that this happens only if the particular values of sensitivity, specificity and true prevalence happen to combine together to make this occur, which can be a matter of luck.

In the Istanbul example, the two are not near each other. There were 253 false positives (37 per cent of the total sample of 693) and 56 false negatives (8 per cent of the total sample). The discrepancy is therefore 37 per cent minus 8 per cent (i.e. 29 per cent), which implies that 29 per cent must be taken off the symptom prevalence to give the diagnoses prevalence. The difference between the symptom and diagnoses prevalence in Table 14.5 is 48 per cent minus 20 per cent, or 28 per cent. Apart from rounding, these are the same.

False positives tend to be more numerous if the prevalence is low and the specificity is not very high. False negatives tend to be more numerous if the prevalence is high and the sensitivity not very high.

The first effect – that of false positives – can be more subtle. It can be seen at its most extreme in an imaginary population for which the true prevalence, though unknown, is zero, so the entity is not present in the sample at all. If an instrument with reasonably high specificity of, say 90 per cent, is applied in a survey, the expected value of the survey prevalence (instrument measured, symptom-based) is 10 per cent, and every person found positive is actually a false positive. If the same instrument also has high sensitivity and is applied to a population sample with a true prevalence of 5 per cent, it will give a prevalence approaching 15 per cent (depending on the sensitivity), so that most of those found positive will be false positives. It is not uncommon for serious outcomes to have low prevalence, and thus for this over-estimation to happen. For instance, in many populations, individual STIs have prevalence below 10 per cent. Instruments with specificity of the order of 90 per cent will produce substantial numbers of false positives.

In the Istanbul example, the discrepancy between symptom-based and diagnosis-based prevalence was large. The two values were 48 per cent and 20 per cent, so the symptom-based results over-stated the true prevalence by a factor of 2.4.

An example of testing for syphilis shows that prevalence can be overestimated even when the specificity is high.

Example 3

Delport and van-den-Berg (1988) found the sensitivity and specificity of the rapid plasma reagin (RPR) test for syphilis in a series of women attending an antenatal clinic to be 92.8 per cent and 96.3 per cent. Despite these high values, if this test was to be used to establish the prevalence in a population with prevalence 5 per cent, it would give an estimated prevalence of 8.2 per cent. It would overstate the true value by a factor of approximately 1.6.

Assuming constancy of sensitivity and specificity

In Example 3, it may be reasonable to use sensitivity and specificity to correct prevalence estimates in a new, different survey since the questions and testing procedures are objectively defined. However, caution is necessary even here. Brenner and Gefeller (1997) comment on the assumption that sensitivity and specificity are independent of the prevalence. They point out that most classifications of disease status are based on a continuum of traits from clear absence to clear presence. Whether explicitly or implicitly, a 'yes/no' categorization is based on a 'cut-off' somewhere on this scale. However, the centre and spread of the scale varies with prevalence, so the way the instrument classifies also depends on prevalence. This argument can be applied to certain tests for infective microbes, which tend to be more numerous in positive cases when prevalence is higher, thus leading to higher sensitivity.

It is more complicated for questionnaire instruments that measure symptoms and illness. Because perception of illness has a strong cultural component, it is not safe to assume that the sensitivity and specificity for a set of questions will remain stable across populations or across time for indicating a disease. Additionally, perception of illness may also be related to prevalence of the illness, if a high general level of prevalence has led to it being regarded as a common problem and therefore 'a part of life'.

Discrepancies of sensitivity and specificity are illustrated in the following example.

Example 4

In community-based studies in Istanbul, Turkey (Filippi et al., 1997) and Giza, Egypt (Zurayk et al., 1995), the same type of symptoms were evaluated in community surveys of parous women of reproductive age. Taking the symptoms for reproductive tract infections of vaginal discharge, in Giza qualified as 'not of her nature' and in Istanbul as 'abnormal', and the symptom for prolapse, as a sensation of heaviness or protrusion in Giza and the pelvic organs being down in Istanbul, the sensitivity and specificity against a clinical diagnosis in each case were:

- Reproductive tract infections, Giza, 14% sensitivity, 88% specificity.
  - Istanbul, 49% sensitivity, 58% specificity.
- Prolapse, Giza, 36% sensitivity, 76% specificity.
  - Istanbul, 18% sensitivity, 96% specificity.

The differences between the two locations are considerable. This is partly due to variation in the exact questions and variation in the clinical diagnoses (Filippi et al., 1997). Also, the best combinations of questions, for optimal sensitivity and specificity in each location, were different, and results from these are not quoted here for the sake of uniformity. But these effects are unlikely to be very large, and it is reasonable to conclude that much of the discrepancy is due to the ways these illnesses construct 'work' in the two societies, and that these seem to be different.

These arguments and this example suggest that there should be considerable scepticism to using measures of sensitivity and specificity as 'transportable' between different settings and different studies.

If disease is an outcome of principal interest, then the ideal is therefore always to include the disease or infection related instruments (lab tests and/or clinical examination) in a survey, if this can be done. The cost can be substantially higher, and whether it is possible depends on local circumstances; in particular, response rates may fall (Koenig et al., 1998) to an extent that this also may jeopardize the interpretation of the results. But where this is not possible, for whatever reason, there will be considerable problems in including disease as an outcome in the study. Questions about symptoms and illness are of use in their own right so long as the illness constructs they address are (also) outcomes of interest.

What does this imply for combining information from different sources? The context here has been using questionnaire-based instruments to give information about clinically defined entities that would ideally be determined by laboratory and clinical methods. Another context is using clinical examination for specific signs to give information about associated infections, but the results of Kaufman et al. (1999) suggest this is scarcely more successful. This is not so much aimed at combining data sources as attempting to simplify survey procedures by confining them to questionnaire instruments or simplified clinical instruments. For the forms of gynaecological morbidity considered here, this does not seem to be successful (cf. Koenig et al., 1998; Sadana, 2000). There are too many respondents for whom the two sources give different answers. However, it begs the separate question as to how to combine results when both instruments have been used. We shall return to this issue later in the section on Combining Data from Different Sources.

If the prevalence is low, possible design strategies are carrying out the disease assessment on all those with positive symptoms from the questionnaire, and a random sample of those who are symptom-negative. This is effectively a case-control study, with 'cases' being those with *illness*, not disease. It is important to ensure an adequate sample size among the illness-negatives, and given that the illness-positives will miss some disease-positives, the sample size must be adequate also to generate enough disease-positives in that group. Because the overall sample represents those with and without disease to a different extent, an adjustment is needed to reconstruct the overall prevalence of disease.[1] Analysis of associations of disease status with risk factors or consequences must of course be based on the cases for which disease status is ascertained, on an appropriate case-control basis.

---

[1] A weighted average is required to allow for the under-representation of the illness-negative stratum.

Case ascertainment and misclassification

Prevalence is based on the total of positive cases; another aspect of the performance of an instrument is how well it correctly identifies positives and also negatives on an individual-by-individual basis. If this is poorly done, there is severe misclassification. This has serious implications for data analysis. As discussed earlier, prevalence and incidence rates will be unreliable. Attempts at establishing associations between variables, by cross-classification, correlation analysis or regression analysis, will suffer from much reduced power. Statistical testing of the associations far too frequently will indicate lack of evidence through a non-significant result, and even when associations are demonstrated with statistical significance, their strength will be greatly underestimated.

As with the adjustment of prevalence measures, mentioned above, problems are likely to be severe when questionnaire instruments are used to obtain information regarding infection and disease.

The relevant parameters for indicating misclassification are the positive and negative predictive values.

The positive predictive value (PPV): in terms of Table 14.4, as a percentage, this is

$$100 \times a/(a+b)$$

$(a+b)$ is the number of individuals found positive by the instrument, so the PPV is the percentage of these who are really positive by the gold standard. If it less than 100 per cent, then some of those found positive are false positives. In the Istanbul example of the symptom 'vaginal discharge' indicating a reproductive tract infection, it is 82/335, or 24 per cent; this means that about three-quarters of the women reporting the symptom did not have a reproductive tract infection.

The negative predictive value (NPV): in terms of Table 14.4, as a percentage this is

$$100 \times d/(c+d)$$

It is the proportion of the individuals who are found negative by the instrument, who are also negative by the gold standard. If it is less than 100 per cent, then some of those found negative are false negatives. In the Istanbul example, it is 302/358, or 84 per cent, so one-sixth of the women who reported not having symptoms did actually have a reproductive tract infection.

In the Istanbul example, this represents a great deal of misclassification; altogether 45 per cent of the women were misclassified one way or the other. In a statistical analysis, using data gathered using only the questionnaire instrument to investigate associations of reported morbidity with other factors, and then to deduce that the results apply to medically defined morbidity would be unwise. The results would be useful, however, for conclusions based on illness and ill health.

In Example 3, of the RPR test for syphilis, in a population with a true prevalence of 5 per cent, the PPV is 60 per cent. This means that 40 per cent of the individuals in a survey identified as having syphilis would not actually have it. This again would weaken any statistical analysis based on the data. The NPV, on the other hand, is 99.6 per cent. This indicates that false negatives are very unlikely to be a problem in this example.

Misclassification rates tabulated

The expected percentage of a sample misclassified follows the formula shown in footnote 2.[2] Table 14.6 lists the overall percentages misclassified for selected sensitivity and specificity values based on this formula.

Both sensitivity and specificity have to be high to avoid considerable misclassification. In the last row of Table 14.6, misclassification is noticeably lower, but both sensitivity and specificity at 90 per cent represents a level of overall validity that is most unlikely to be reached by questionnaire instruments as indicators of disease.

These results apply to both types of misclassification, false positives and false negatives, combined. The balance between the two varies according to the formula. The overall level of misclassification does not depend on prevalence if sensitivity and specificity are the same, but the balance varies. Except in this case, and except where the sensitivity is high, overall misclassification is more common when the prevalence is close to 50 per cent. Many of the gynaecological diseases of interest here are common or moderately common.

Combining data from different sources

The principal theme in the previous section has been the assessment of disease using illness entities based on questionnaire data. It has emerged that there are distinct difficulties in doing this; it is not recommended, and if it is carried out, care is needed in interpreting results. The argument has been made that it is more relevant and revealing to consider disease and illness (and the other entity groups) as separate in their own right so that data on each one throws a different light on the picture of morbidity as a whole.

This implies that a survey that does not include a clinical component cannot adequately address issues of disease as opposed to illness. Certain diseases and illnesses may coincide with each other (for example, prolapse or menstrual irregularity), and differences between clinical and questionnaire assessment may be largely

---

[2] $\dfrac{(100\text{-sensitivity}) \times \text{prevalence}}{100} + \dfrac{(100\text{-specificity}) \times (100\text{-prevalence})}{100}$

The first part of this formula gives the percentage misclassified as false negatives and the second the number misclassified as false positives.

Table 14.6. Misclassification in terms of sensitivity, specificity and prevalence (%)

Sensitivity	Specificity	Prevalence				
		5	10	20	40	60
50	50	50	50	50	50	50
	70	31	32	34	38	42
	90	12	14	18	26	34
70	50	49	48	46	42	38
	70	30	30	30	30	30
	90	11	12	14	18	22
90	50	48	46	42	34	26
	70	29	28	26	22	18
	90	10	10	10	10	10

differences of degree. But, generally, this will not be the case. It is then important to distinguish the different types of outcome in the results.

Example 5

Bhatia et al. (1997) show results from eight different outcomes derived from clinical and questionnaire instruments, and present each of them and their associations with various determinants, covering socio-economic factors and contraceptive-related factors, separately. The results show distinctly different associations for each of the outcomes. One particular association, commented on by the authors, was that of bacterial vaginitis (laboratory detected) with tubectomy, an association not observed with vaginitis clinically observed.

Another example is the association between psychiatric disability and gynaecological morbidity. Example 2 approaches this with the association between a disease (vaginal candidiasis) and subsequent psychological indicators. Here, the sources are diagnosis by medical assessment and questionnaires for psychological assessments. Patel and Oomman (1999), quoted earlier, present the hypothesis that women who report gynaecological symptoms but show no medically diagnosed morbidity are a significant group, with this combination associated with mental ill health. Here, what may be taken as 'misclassification' is a fruitful source of information. In general terms, the characteristics of a group with contradictory classifications may be important.

   When results from different instruments addressing different but related entities disagree and lead to misclassification or inconsistent classification, it is useful to

Table 14.7. Reasons for discrepancies between symptom reports and medical diagnosis

Possible explanation for difference	Comments
Symptoms reported without medical diagnosis	
Inadequate questionnaire	Technical deficiency
Symptoms are not specific enough	Inadequate content validity
Replies to questions incorrect, by chance	Random error
Diagnosis is wrong, by chance	Random error
Symptoms or disease of short duration and assessments separated in time	Study design deficient in this respect
Illness is distinct	Conceptually important
Medical diagnosis positive without symptoms reported	
Inadequate questionnaire	Technical deficiency
Respondent does not consider symptoms 'reportable' (worth reporting/wish to report)	Cultural aspects of illness and perception
Respondent not aware of symptoms as a problem	Cultural aspects of illness and perception
Replies to questions incorrect, by chance	Random error
Diagnosis is wrong, by chance	Random error
Symptoms or disease of short duration and assessments separated in time	Study design deficient in this respect
Does not have symptoms to report	Disease asymptomatic

consider possible reasons. We return to the context of using questionnaire results to indicate disease, and list possible reasons in Table 14.7.

Some of the reasons mentioned in Table 14.7 point to possible deficiencies in the study. Random error should not be a source of large-scale discrepancies with a large enough sample size. The cultural reasons suggest a need for understanding gained from qualitative work. Reports of illness that are distinct from the medically-defined disease may indicate a marker for other conditions (cf. Patel and Oomman, 1999, quoted earlier). It also may be a determinant for disability or handicap, even in the absence of the medically-defined disease, and important for these reasons. Under the second heading, medically diagnosed disease in the absence of symptoms or reported symptoms may indicate a burden of disease that is likely to remain untreated.

This distinction between disease determined clinically and illness ascertained via reported symptoms must always be borne in mind when interpreting results, and the need to match the instruments used to the disease or illness entities of interest will always remain important.

Factors to be considered when interpreting results from different data sources

In the final section, we return briefly to other issues that may arise when interpreting results from the analysis of data from these studies. Box 14.2 lists some basic issues that are important to bear in mind for understanding the meaning of results.

Box 14.2. Principal factors to be borne in mind when interpreting results from a quantitative study

1. *What population is represented?*

   Data analysis is usually based on a sample from a population. What population is represented by the sample? It is likely that the instruments will have different performance characteristics in different populations. For example, a symptom-based instrument that works well to detect infections in a clinic population may work less well in the general population. What the population is, and the sampling method (see below) also affect the external validity of the results (Greenberg and Daniels, 1993).

2. *How well has the sample been selected?*

   This consideration is a sequel to the last one. It is a general caveat for all interpretation, since severe biases will arise with poor sampling.

3. *Can one expect misclassification bias?*

   This question encapsulates many of the conclusions of this chapter, and is most relevant when instruments used 'cross the boundary' between entities (as in using questionnaire instruments to give data relevant to clinically defined entities). It is, however, also relevant whenever an instrument may lead to misclassification, such as when the instrument has limited reliability.

4. *Has the study adequate power?*

   This is a question of the sample size in relation to the objectives of the data analysis. When misclassification is a problem, in addition to the biases mentioned under 3, it will lead to a loss of power. It is essential that all estimates be given with confidence intervals and all associations subjected to statistical tests.

5. *Is the statistical analysis and the choice of results appropriate?*

   The principal message in this chapter is that in an interpretation of statistical results where the outcome is based on the use of one particular instrument, such as a questionnaire item for perceived morbidity, the first interpretation should always be in terms of the entity that the instrument addresses directly. Further interpretation, in terms of other correlated entities, must be made with care because of misclassification. In particular, when the statistical analysis has yielded information on associations, from regression models or otherwise, there is likely to be bias in the measures of these other associations, and this bias can go either way (see, for example, Hennekens and Buring, 1987).

Summary and conclusions

Data are gathered by applying instruments in a survey or other contexts. These instruments are questionnaires, procedures for carrying out tests (laboratory or clinical tests) and for making clinical assessments.

The data from these instruments tell us about the various conditions of the respondents, categorized into groups of entities. These are current infection, disease, impairment, illness, disability, handicap, quality of life and 'being at risk'. Each entity is best measured by a particular instrument, or combination of instruments.

The objectives of any investigation must focus on the entities to be measured, the choice of instruments then being governed by this. The interpretation depends crucially on the definitions of the entities measured.

Illness covers the symptoms for self-perceived health and morbidity asked in questionnaire interviews. This varies with place, social condition, culture and other factors. Illnesses have only a partial connection with the corresponding diseases (which are biomedically defined); although a particular disease may biomedically lead to a particular symptom, whether a respondent reports the symptom can be mediated by these other factors.

A particular area of interest here is whether illness and symptom reports can be taken as indicators of, or proxies for, gynaecological disease. It appears that this can be done only to a limited degree in this field, in general with considerable uncertainty. This is because the sensitivity and specificity are generally low, and because it is not safe to assume one can 'transport' these measures from one setting to another and use them to correct prevalence estimates.

Misclassification can be expected to be severe when symptom reports are used to indicate disease. This cannot be corrected, and leads to considerable bias in estimating associations with risk factors and consequences, with consequent problems of interpretation. For validity and safety in interpretation, data on disease must be measured by medical assessment.

It is concluded that entities in the areas of disease and illness should always be considered as logically separate. The measurement of each should be considered as distinct within the study, and the reasons for measuring each should be clear. It is complementary to know both; disease and illness are both relevant to understanding reproductive health as a whole.

REFERENCES

Bang RA, Bang AT, Baitule M et al. (1989) High prevalence of gynaecological diseases in rural Indian women. *Lancet*, 1(8629): 85–88.

Beaglehole R, Bonita R, Kjellström T (1993) *Basic epidemiology.* Geneva, World Health Organization.

Bhatia JC, Cleland JC, Bhagavan L (1997) Gynaecological morbidity in south India. *Studies in family planning,* **28**(2): 95–103.

Brenner H, Gefeller O (1997) Variation of sensitivity, specificity, likelihood ratios and predictive values with disease prevalence. *Statistics in medicine,* **16**: 981–991.

Bowling A (1997) *Measuring health: a review of quality of life measurement scales.* Buckingham, Open University Press.

Bulut A, Yolsal N, Filippi V et al. (1995) In search of truth: comparing alternative sources of information on reproductive tract infection. *Reproductive health matters,* **6**, 31–39.

Bulut A, Filippi V, Marshall T et al. (1997). Contraceptive choice and reproductive morbidity in Istanbul. *Studies in family planning,* **28**(1): 35–43.

Delport SD, van-den-Berg JH (1988) On-site screening for syphilis at an antenatal clinic. *South African medical journal,* **88**(1): 43–44.

Diallo M, Ghys P, Vuylsteke B et al. (1998) Evaluation of a simple diagnostic algorithm of *Neisseria gonorrhoeae* and *Chlamydia trachomatis* cervical infections in female sex workers in Abidjan, Côte d'Ivoire. *Sexually transmitted infections,* **74**(Suppl. 1): S106–S111.

Filippi V, Marshall T, Bulut A et al. (1997) Asking questions about women's reproductive health: validity and reliability of survey findings from Istanbul. *Tropical medicine and international health,* **2**(1): 47–56.

Greenberg RS, Daniels SR eds. (1993) *Medical epidemiology.* East Norwalk, Connecticut, Appleton and Lange (Prentice Hall).

Harwood RH, Prince M, Mann A et al. (1998) Associations between diagnosis, impairments, disability and handicap in a population of elderly people. *International journal of epidemiology,* **27**: 261–268.

Hawkes S, Morison L, Foster S et al. (1999) Reproductive-tract infections in women in low-income, low-prevalence situations: assessment of syndromic management in Matlab, Bangladesh. *Lancet,* **354**: 1776–1781.

Helman CG (1990). *Culture, health and illness,* 2nd edn. London, Wright.

Hennekens CH, Buring JE (1987) *Epidemiology in medicine.* Boston, Little Brown.

Irving G, Miller D, Robinson A et al. (1998) Psychological factors associated with recurrent vaginal candidiasis: a preliminary study. *Sexually transmitted infections,* **74**: 334–338.

Kaufman J, Yan LQ, Wang TY et al. (1999) A study of field-based methods for diagnosing reproductive tract infection in rural Yunnan Province, China. *Studies in family planning,* **30**(2): 112–119.

Koenig M, Jejeebhoy S, Singh S et al. (1998) Investigating women's gynaecological morbidity in India: not just another KAP survey. *Reproductive health matters,* **6**(11): 84–97.

Kleinman A (1995) *Writing at the margin.* Berkeley, University of California Press.

Kraemer HC, Bloch DA (1988) Kappa coefficients in epidemiology: an appraisal of a reappraisal. *Journal of clinical epidemiology,* **41**(10): 959–968.

Landis JR, Koch GG (1977). The measurement of observer agreement for categorical data. *Biometrics,* **33**: 159–174.

Maclure M, Willett WC (1987) Misinterpretation and misuse of the kappa statistic. *American journal of epidemiology,* **126**(2): 161–169.

Morré S, van Valkengoed I, Moes R et al. (1999) Determination of the *Chlamydia trachomatis* prevalence in an asymptomatic screening population; performance of the Lcx and COBAS Amplicor in urine specimens. *Journal of clinical microbiology*, **17**: 3092–3096.

Murray CJL, Chen LC (1992) Understanding morbidity change. *Population and development review*, **18**(3): 481–503.

Patel V, Oomman N (1999) Mental health matters too: gynaecological symptoms and depression in South Asia. *Reproductive health matters*, **7**(14): 30–38.

Sadana R (2000) Measuring reproductive health; review of community-based approaches to assessing morbidity. *Bulletin of the World Health Organization*, **78**(5): 640–654.

Streiner DL, Norman GR (1989) *Health measurement scales: a practical guide to their development and use*. Oxford, Oxford University Press.

Thompson WD, Walter SD (1988) A reappraisal of the kappa coefficient. *Journal of clinical epidemiology*, **41**(10): 949–958.

Tiefer L (1995) *Sex is not a natural act and other essays*. Boulder, CO, Westview Press.

Trollope-Kumar K (1999) Symptoms of reproductive tract infection – not all they seem to be. *Lancet*, **354**: 1745–1746.

World Health Organization (1980) International classification of impairments, disabilities and handicaps. Geneva, World Health Organization.

World Health Organization (1992) *The International Statistical Classification of Diseases and Related Health Problems*, 10th revision. Geneva, World Health Organization.

Younis N, Khalil K, Zurayk H et al. (1994) *Policy series in reproductive health, no. 2*. Cairo, Population Council.

Zurayk H, Khattab H, Younis N et al. (1995) Comparing women's reports with medical diagnoses of reproductive morbidity conditions in rural Egypt. *Studies in family planning*, **26**(1): 14–21.

15

Turning research into action

Ruth Dixon-Mueller

Grecia, Costa Rica

What can we learn from research on gynaecological infections and other disorders that will be most useful to sexual and reproductive health programmes and policies? In this final chapter we consider how the research methods discussed in the preceding chapters can be linked to the informational requirements of educators, service providers, policy makers, and other reproductive health advocates and practitioners. The purpose is to encourage researchers to think ahead about what planners will need to know if they are to design appropriate interventions. The chapter is organized around a series of questions addressed to the research process itself. It begins with the most basic question of all: What do we need to know about reproductive tract infections and related gynaecological problems, and why do we need to know it?

Framing the question: what do we need to know, and why?

The notion of 'framing the question' refers to how the fundamental purpose of the research is defined. Under whose auspices is it being conducted, and what is its justification? Is it intended for the advance of basic epidemiological or demographic knowledge, such as documenting the prevalence of particular diseases in a particular population that has not yet been studied? Is it to compare methods for collecting health-related and background information, such as self-reports, clinical and laboratory analyses, in-depth interviews, surveys, focus groups? Is it to establish correlations that could lead to the identification of causal factors? Is it to test specific hypotheses, supply deep descriptions, assess attitudes and practices, or measure trends and variations?

Each of these approaches to basic research has implications for the design of policies and programmes. If the connections are not clearly spelled out, however, others must decide how to translate the research into action. More applied approaches, which integrate the quest for solutions into the elements of the research design itself, are typically tailored to a particular setting, a particular problem, a particular institution. A health clinic may conduct a needs and knowledge assessment of women in the community, for example, in order to expand its sexual and reproductive health services. An NGO may collect information on women's perceptions of their overall physical and emotional health in order to identify problem areas that the organization could address programmatically. Researchers concerned about harmful practices may collect basic prevalence data with the simultaneous purpose of assessing the possible acceptability of a variety of interventions. A multi-faceted study in rural northern Ghana, for example, is intended 'to develop a community-informed approach to the eradication of female circumcision in a traditional setting. The research is guided by the hypothesis that specific actions and activities [which are described in some detail] can reduce the prevalence of female circumcision' (Nazzar et al., 1999:7).

Whether the research leans more to the basic or to the applied end of the continuum, the interconnections are unavoidable. Answering the question of what is to be studied, inevitably leads to the question of, Why? Similarly, answering the 'Why' question helps to justify the 'What'. According to social science research guidelines published by WHO, 'A pragmatic approach to health research necessitates identifying research questions which are likely to contribute to action or change' (Campbell et al., 1999:7). Thus, research aimed at 'identifying . . . reproductive health problems by measuring the magnitude and nature of reproductive/sexual behaviour and reproductive ill-health, and identifying its determinants and consequences' is connected with research aimed at 'improving and supporting intervention programmes which attempt to prevent or treat reproductive health problems . . . and understanding, informing and influencing the policy, legal or social arena in which reproductive health concerns arise' (Campbell et al., 1999:7).

This book deals primarily with the biomedical and social measurement of gynaecological problems and their causes, consequences and correlates. Such investigations have clear potential for informing programmes and policies, as the examples in Table 15.1 suggest.

Once the research question is precisely framed (that is, the objective of the research is articulated and its importance justified), then the process of deciding on a study design that can turn research into action begins.

Designing the research: who is to be studied, and how?

The purpose here is not to describe the many possible approaches to sampling, data collection, measurement and analysis (for an excellent review see Campbell et al., 1999), but rather, to stress the importance of selecting a plan that is tailored to the informational needs of those who are most likely to use the data. In this sense, the design follows logically from the answers to the 'What' and 'Why' questions

Table 15.1. Examples of research questions and implications for action

WHAT do we need to know? (Topic of inquiry)	WHY do we need to know it? (Planned intervention)
The prevalence of diagnosed infections in particular populations and subgroups	Inform policy makers, design appropriate services, train providers, equip laboratories
People's knowledge of and experiences with a variety of health care providers	Identify and overcome barriers to service utilization, including quality of care
Women's perceptions of what is 'normal' and 'abnormal' pelvic discomfort	Develop culturally appropriate methods for diagnosis, treatment and education
Practices of personal hygiene, including management of the menses	Promote practices and products that will improve hygiene, reduce infections
The quality of technical care offered by particular reproductive health providers	Reduce risks and improve effectiveness through better training and supervision
Sexual behaviour of persons at risk; practices, partnerships, negotiation	Identify pathways of transmission of infections and design educational campaigns
Women's experience of morbidity and mortality resulting from unsafe abortion	Promote a national policy favouring safe and legal abortion; train and equip providers

posed in the preceding section. Here we address the 'Who' and the 'How' of the research.

Service providers, service users and the general population (including male and female adolescents, married and unmarried adults, older people and specific socio-economic groups) are all potential grist for the mill in a community-based sexual and reproductive health study.

Although it may be tempting to launch directly into a full-scale sample survey of the at-risk population to identify the nature and prevalence of gynaecological problems, it is useful first to undertake a community or district 'mapping' of formal and informal providers of health information and services. At the top of the list are those family planning and antenatal service providers in the public and private sector (gynaecologists, nurses, paramedics) who routinely talk with clients and perform pelvic examinations. Others include general physicians, pharmacists, midwives, herbalists, street peddlers of folk or 'modern' medicines (e.g. antibiotics), and indigenous healers, such as spiritualists, who may be consulted on matters of menstruation, sexual difficulties, childbirth, infertility, genital infections and related problems.

The purpose of this preliminary work is, first, to document the range of providers already in place and the types of information and services they offer; second, to gain an understanding from the providers' point of view of the nature, prevalence, causes, cures and prevention of the gynaecological disorders they treat; and third, to ensure (if possible) their cooperation with the study and avoid possible backlash if they feel threatened. The support of health care providers and educators will be crucial to the success not only of the research project but of most actions that are likely to follow, such as staffing and equipping facilities, retraining personnel or undertaking public information campaigns. For these and other reasons, researchers should be familiar with the location, *modus operandi* (including the quality of care) and particular vested interests (money, power, prestige) of those who are currently serving (however well or poorly) the population or subgroup to be studied.

Who among the population is to be selected? The definition of the sampling frame and the method of drawing from it depend in part on the interests of the organizations or agencies responsible for implementing the recommendations that may follow. A national-level family planning programme with clinics throughout the country, for example, or an antenatal clinic in a large maternity hospital, may decide to integrate into its services a programme of diagnosis, treatment and counselling in sexually transmitted infections (STIs) and other reproductive tract infections such as cervical cancer. In these cases, systematic random samples could be drawn for study from the population of women (and their partners) who are current programme clients (e.g. every *n*th woman presenting within the time frame), which facilitates interviewing, examination and testing. Note, however, that such findings cannot be generalized beyond this client group. If inferences are to be made to a broader population, such as all women of reproductive age in a geographically circumscribed area, or to all adolescents between the ages of 10 and 19 years, or to post-menopausal women, then the sampling frame must consist of this entire community and every eligible person should have an equal chance of being selected.

Less systematically representative samples are useful for exploratory work, such as engaging in 'body mapping' exercises or eliciting people's perceptions in focus groups. Convenience samples, such as young mothers waiting in a crowded health centre or secondary school students in a classroom, or purposive samples selected according to desired demographic categories (married and single, male and female, adolescent and adult, low and moderate income) or occupational categories (factory workers, street traders, prostitutes) or social categories (members of a women's club who are asked to bring a neighbour), can all contribute information and interpretations that feed into the more formal aspects of the research process.

The 'How' questions are far more numerous than the 'Who'. The relative strengths and limitations of various qualitative and quantitative research methods have been outlined in some detail in Chapters 11, 12 and 13. In general, quantitative methods (such as standardized questionnaires) are best suited to well-defined, carefully worded topics addressed to large, scientifically representative samples, the results of which are amenable to statistical analysis and inference to the population from which the sample is drawn. Qualitative methods such as in-depth interviews, direct observations, focus groups, mapping exercises, case studies and personal narratives are useful for exploratory, open topics addressed to small, selected samples, the analysis of which is typically thematic and illustrative. Each method has its advantages in soliciting a particular type of information. In their study of people's knowledge and attitudes toward STIs in Argentina, for example, Ramos and Gogna (1997) found that men typically did better in focus groups where they enjoyed talking about the culture of sex and STIs, whereas women revealed more in private interviews about topics they were reluctant to discuss in the presence of others. Different approaches extract different portraits of 'reality', each of which is significant in its own right in providing information for programmes and policies.

Oomman and Gittelsohn (Chapter 12) point out that the use of qualitative methods permits flexibility, iteration (a sequencing in which each stage informs the next), triangulation (the use of different techniques to collect information on the same topic) and contextualization (a detailed analysis of the social setting in which data are gathered). Ideally, one would combine the advantages of both quantitative and qualitative approaches by using them sequentially and interactively, as Pelto and Cleland (Chapter 13) suggest. This sequential process permits adjustments to be made in the way questions are asked (between a pilot test and a larger survey, for example, or between successive rounds of interviews), in the topics covered and in the people involved. Most important for our purposes, it allows for feedback from key individuals and institutions who have a stake in interpreting the results and/or designing and implementing interventions. Rather than presenting the end users with a finished product when the research is done, the research team incorporates their views (where possible and relevant) in the research process itself.

Working within the community: where will the study take place, and who needs to be involved?

In their review of practical and ethical issues relating to the clinical testing of microbicides, a consortium of scientists and women's health advocates affirmed that 'genuine community involvement is essential to ethically and scientifically sound research' (Heise, McGrory and Wood, 1998:37). Given that virtually all STIs (if not reproductive tract infections or other reproductive morbidities) can be prevented (although not all can be cured), the issue of community involvement becomes particularly salient. Programmes need to be designed with prevention in mind, not just diagnosis and treatment. The focus on prevention will almost always require significant behavioural changes among individuals at risk and in the practices of health and family planning personnel across the entire spectrum of formal and informal health care services.

Ideally, research on reproductive tract infections and other gynaecological morbidities would be initiated by, or in collaboration with, key organizations or members of the community for which the findings can serve as decision-making tools. Administrators of primary health or family planning programmes, women's groups, community development associations, social welfare programmes, secondary schools and other organizations involved in some aspects of health education or service delivery all have a stake in identifying problem areas and proposing solutions. The idea is to make sure that organizations and individuals on whom effective implementation depends are involved from the beginning in planning the research proposal so that it serves their needs. If the research initiative comes from outside the community, the investigating team's first task would be to identify and recruit sponsoring agencies and collaborators in a genuine research partnership.

Just as for the selection of a sample of individuals within a population, the selection of communities within a district or region requires a clearly defined sampling frame and a justification. Communities may be selected randomly with the use of cluster sampling such that each has an equal (or at least known) probability of being included, in which case statistical inferences can be made to all such communities within the sampling frame. A community may be selected purposively because it is considered 'typical' of some district or regional characteristic ('typical low-income urban', 'typical rural', 'typical Chinese or Malay settlement'), or because it is unique in some significant way. This latter category might include a centre of long-distance trading, for example, in which the constant movement of people through an economic and sexual marketplace creates conditions favourable to the transmission of STIs such as HIV/AIDS. Or it may be selected because it is convenient: it is where the researchers or the sponsoring agency are already located.

Additional considerations are likely to modify the selection of communities, however, such as their geographical and cultural accessibility to the research team (e.g. linguistic or religious compatibility); the quality, location and availability of facilities and personnel for conducting needed clinical examinations and laboratory analysis; and the cooperation of key groups and individuals whose public endorsement (if not formal permission) may be required. These might include district administrators, health officials, mayors or village committees, councils of elders, influential landowners, religious leaders, and others such as teachers or local women's groups whose cooperation or lack of it could spell the success or failure of the entire project.

The manner in which the research question is articulated to community leaders (and others whose formal permission is required) and to potential study participants is also important. Although researchers may in fact wish to investigate only a narrow range of gynaecological problems for some purpose of their own, they may have to present the project to the community as a study of 'women's health' or 'family health' or 'infertility' in order to make it acceptable. They may even have to include diversionary inquiries in the survey that are not actually intended for analysis. One way around this ethical dilemma, of course, is to design a study that is, indeed, addressed to a broader range of topics. Another is to offer health services to participants even though such examinations are not part of the research agenda itself, such as treatment for sick children and other family members (see Bang and Bang, Chapter 7, and Bhatia et al., 1997).

What will the community gain from the research? Ideally, it will receive some follow-up benefits that will be in place long after the research team has departed. If this is not feasible, however, there are still benefits to be gained from the research process itself if key community members become active collaborators in its formulation, design, implementation and interpretation. The careful selection of paid interviewers and other experts such as gynaecologists or midwives from the community under investigation is not only critical to the project's success but also a means of winning the community's cooperation. Together with the presence of outside experts, visitors and the resulting publicity, the project can also offer considerable prestige to the community, provide multiple opportunities for learning and stimulate a demand for improved services from existing health and family planning centres.

Dealing with the ethics of individual participation: what issues are likely to arise, and how will they be handled?

Any research project that involves outsiders coming into a community to study the habits of its residents and to ask questions about even simple matters such as the age, sex and relationship of all persons living in a household or compound is bound to raise suspicions about the motives of the investigators. Even the inquiries of insiders can raise doubts. 'Why is my neighbour (or the health visitor, or the teacher?) asking me these questions? What will she do with the information I am giving her?'

When we consider that the questions discussed in this book are among the most personal and indeed provocative that can be asked ('Do you have vaginal discharge? Does it have a strong odour? Do you have discomfort during intercourse? How many different sexual partners have you had in the past year? Does your current partner have other partners that you know of? Male or female? Does he visit prostitutes?') and that, in addition, the woman may be asked to submit to a pelvic examination and to contribute samples of blood, urine or vaginal secretions for analysis, it is clear that what she is being asked to do is breathtaking in its prospects of vulnerability and betrayal. A woman's safety and security may be severely compromised if she is discovered to have an infection that is sexually transmitted. In cultures where such infections are called the 'woman's disease', she will almost certainly be blamed for her condition and face the threat if not the actuality of disgrace, desertion, divorce or physical or emotional abuse from her husband and other family members. In the Buenos Aires study of cultural attitudes, for example, both men and women agreed that it was better not to ask or talk about sensitive problems such as STIs with one's partner because of the interpersonal conflicts that were likely to arise. 'The breakdown of the marriage, violent reactions, disappointment ("it will never be the same") and the "destruction of the family" were some of the catastrophic consequences imagined . . . Only a few considered the need for dialogue, mutual understanding and compassion' (Ramos and Gogna, 1997:8).

It is essential that the ethical issues involved in the research be addressed as fully as possible at the outset, throughout the planning phases, and during the entire process of investigation, analysis, reporting and follow-up. What ethical questions may be raised in gaining the consent of participants, for example? Of offering (or not offering) counselling, treatment and other follow-up? Of informing (or not informing) sexual partners about a STI? Of permitting a pregnant woman with a disease that threatens her newborn to refuse treatment?

Let us consider first the question of random sampling for the purposes of assessing disease prevalence. If the statistical purity of the sample is to be protected, then participation must be maximized to prevent bias. Studies with very low refusal rates are typically considered successes in this regard. But how can we be sure that participation is genuinely voluntary? Lessons from national family planning campaigns in some countries have revealed that overzealous recruiters or health workers sometimes pressured women to accept intrauterine contraceptive devices, implants or sterilization in order to meet their programme targets and that women may not have been fully informed about what is going to happen to them. These lessons clearly need to be applied to the investigations discussed here.

Researchers will need to plan ahead as to how they will deal with issues of informed consent and the right to refuse. In some cultures, the permission of a male household head or female elder will be required before the interviewer can gain access to anyone inside. This does not imply consent of the woman herself, however, who should be informed that she can refuse to participate, decline to answer any question, stop the interview, or refuse or terminate a physical examination even if someone else has instructed her to cooperate. Confidentiality of answers and examination results must also be assured, especially with regard to parents or in-laws who gave permission for her to be examined and insist they have a right to know, and with regard to the general comportment of the research team.

The ethical issues arising in the course of diagnosis, counselling and treatment are even more complex. The woman has a right to know the results of her examination. An incorrect clinical or laboratory diagnosis not only reduces the validity of the scientific findings but produces false positive and false negative reports, either one of which has serious ethical consequences when the woman receives wrong information. One must also consider the question of whether a woman has the right *not* to be informed of the results if she does not want to know them. There is the question of the researchers' obligations to notify her husband or non-marital partner(s) of an infection that may be transmitted by or to him or to a foetus or newborn. And what if the woman and/or her partner refuses treatment? Where do the rights of the participant conflict with the responsibilities of the researchers, and how can they be reconciled?

The question of incentives for participation can be a tricky one, especially if participants expect some form of compensation. Family planning programmes that once relied on incentive payments to 'acceptors' and 'motivators' have mostly abandoned the practice as a result of widespread criticism that such incentives, no matter how small, are potentially coercive among those who are too poor to refuse any gift. In the studies discussed here, however, the assurance of being listened to, carefully examined and competently treated at no cost should be a sufficient incentive for participation, especially where an environment of trust has been built up over a number of months of contact between households and the research team. Sometimes a small gift may be appropriate, such as the packages of soap and biscuits that were given to women in the Egyptian study following their participation, and at their own suggestion (see Khattab, Chapter 7). In the Ugandan study of sexually transmitted infections, bars of soap and health consultations were given to all household members regardless of their participation (see Serwadda and Wawer, Chapter 7). In this way no one is placed in the position of having to decide to participate or not based on the promise of some gift or payment.

Establishing the distribution of reproductive tract infections and other gynaecological problems: who has what, according to whom, and why is it important?

If there is one thing that the collection of population-based research on reproductive tract infections has demonstrated, it is that information obtained from women's self-reports of symptoms represents one level of reality, information from clinical examinations of these same women by trained medical personnel represents another, and information obtained from laboratory analysis of specimens (vaginal and anal swabs, blood and urine samples) represents quite another. The reasons for obtaining such disparate results from the three approaches are extensively discussed in Chapter 14. Consider these findings from an investigation of the prevalence of reproductive tract infections in a rapidly urbanizing area of Istanbul, Turkey (Bulut et al., 1995: 31):

> This study . . . compared the reliability of self-reporting, clinical diagnosis and laboratory examinations for determining the extent of reproductive tract infections in 696 women. It found that a physician diagnosed an infection in more than half the women who did not report a problem spontaneously, and in only two-thirds of those who did report a problem. According to the laboratory examination, less than a fifth of those reporting a problem had an infection, while 76 per cent of those who did not recognize they had a problem in fact had one. Worse still, of the women that the physician diagnosed as not having an infection, 69 per cent actually had one.

Who is wrong, and who is right? Everyone and no one. From the perspective of the women themselves, what is important is how they feel and what they are worried about. From the perspective of the examining physicians, what is important is what they identify as a medical problem in the pelvic examination. And from the perspective of the laboratory, what is important is what the microscope reveals to the technician. The lack of reliability applies not only across categories, but also within categories. One woman reports as abnormal a pain or a discharge that another considers not worth mentioning. Clinical examiners differ among themselves in their expectations of what to look for and how to interpret what they find. Laboratory technicians and the tests they use are unreliable in some settings and for some infections, generating false positives and false negatives along with true ones with equal confidence.

Each approach has its advantages and limitations, depending on 'What' exactly one wants to know, and 'Why'. Women's spontaneous self-reports tend to be subjective, culturally constructed and often unspecific. General terms such as 'weakness' or 'dizziness' represent intermixtures of physical and emotional conditions that are difficult to identify precisely. In their study of women living in poverty in Bombay, for example, Ramasubban and Singh (1997) found that virtually all women complained of an overwhelming weakness that was best described as 'feeling physically ill all the time, and of wanting to lie down and sleep and to never get up' (Ramasubban and Singh, 1997:8). Self-reported symptoms tend to be poor predictors of actual disease status, particularly with regard to STIs, which are so often asymptomatic. Studies suggest that the reliability of self-reports can be improved by using standardized checklists of symptoms together with their perceived severity, adapted to local terminologies and augmented with other conditions or terms obtained from focus group sessions and discussions with formal and informal providers (see Cleland and Harlow, Chapter 11 for a review). The lack of specificity should not be taken as a devaluation of self-reports, however, for when properly done they are the true conveyors of how women think and talk and feel about their bodies and their lives.

Clinic-based gynaecological examinations have also been shown to be poor predictors of disease status, in part because symptoms are often not apparent and in part because of differences in training and perceptions of examiners. However, clinical examinations can be useful for diagnosing some types of infection such that clients with visible symptoms can be treated before undergoing an invasive procedure such as insertion of an intrauterine contraceptive device, abortion, sterilization, diagnostic D&C (dilatation and curettage) or assisted delivery. Such examinations can also identify other problems, such as uterine prolapse, tears or cuts in the vaginal wall, scarring from genital cutting, evidence of abrasion or burning of the vaginal walls from the use of vaginal substances, or signs of cervical infection, the latter which may sometimes be efficiently dealt with in a single 'see and treat' visit (Bishop et al., 1995). Ideally, the clinical examination will be accompanied by a medical/behavioural history that repeats the symptom checklist of self-reports and inquires further into behaviours and practices that may put someone at risk of disease (recent change of sexual partners, husband recently returned from work elsewhere) even if symptoms are not apparent. The reliability of clinical reports can be improved by the use of standard checklists used by the examiner with indications of site and severity (see Elias, Low and Hawkes, Chapter 8). Despite, or even because of, their variability, however, findings of clinical examinations are useful for identifying training and supervision needs of clinical personnel. Counsellors or interviewers who accompany women to the clinical examination could also observe and provide feedback on the quality of care, particularly with regard to the empathetic treatment of clients. This component is itself an 'intervention' in raising medical examiners' awareness of the anxieties and discomfort that virtually all women experience in this situation.

As the chapters by Meehan et al. (Chapter 10) and Marshall et al. (Chapter 14) attest, the ultimate demonstration of reproductive tract infection/STI status comes from an array of laboratory tests that require biological specimens for analysis, such as blood, urine, vaginal or rectal swabs, saliva or semen (for infertility studies). Like pelvic examinations, these procedures may be considered unpleasant, offensive or taboo; in some cultures, body substances are endowed with spiritual meanings and their loss is dangerous; in others, the giving of blood, in particular, may be considered highly suspect. A considerable investment of time, patience and understanding may be required by the research team before participants agree to such procedures, the most exhaustive of which is revealed in Serwadda and Wawer's (Chapter 7) off-hand comment that 'In the Rakai study [in Uganda], after 6 years in the study community it was possible to collect blood.' A very strong sense of mutual trust is clearly essential for the performance of this phase of the research.

Properly conducted with 'gold standard' methods, such tests are the most reliable means we have for determining whether a person has a reproductive tract infection. The tests provide important feedback for clinicians in their hypothesis testing, confirming or challenging their observations or intuition. Moreover, precise estimates of the prevalence of STIs and other reproductive tract infections in the population at large or within particular subgroups are essential for creating baseline data, establishing trends and variations, attracting the attention of local and national policy makers responsible for estimating health service needs and distributing resources, designing training programmes for health professionals at all levels, developing strategies for integrating reproductive tract infection diagnosis and treatment in primary health care centres, maternal and child health programmes and family planning clinics, deciding on particular treatment regimens, and devising educational and counselling programmes. In Chapter 8 on clinical diagnosis, Elias et al. propose that, at a minimum, investigators should include laboratory tests for gonorrhoea, *C. trachomatis*, *Trichomonas vaginalis*, candidiasis, syphilis and bacterial vaginosis. The adoption of routine testing for particular reproductive tract infections in health programmes would, in turn, depend on its feasibility (including the cost of the tests and other resources required); the probability of finding the condition in a particular population (e.g. syphilis among pregnant women; prevalence data are useful for this); the treatability of the condition (cost and feasibility); and the urgency or seriousness of the condition, especially if left untreated (e.g. progression to pelvic inflammatory disease, transmission to partner, foetus or newborn).

Are all three approaches necessary in a community survey? Certainly there are advantages in doing all three, not only in comparing the outcomes but in the learning opportunities they provide, especially for clinicians. Each, as we have seen, presents a different overall portrayal of the distribution of complaints and of infections and other gynaecological problems in a population. Of particular interest, however, is the analysis on a case-by-case basis of the discrepancies between self-reports of symptoms or complaints, clinical examinations and laboratory analyses.

Consider, as a simple model, a set of fourfold tables in which a particular condition of interest is either present or absent as reported by the woman herself, by the clinical examiner, and by the laboratory technician. If a woman reports a problem such as heavy or odorous vaginal discharge that is confirmed by the examiner and diagnosed as an infection by the laboratory, then the consistencies are clear, the woman is probably motivated to seek treatment, and the appropriate solution will be at hand. Similarly, if she reports no problem and none is identified, then the matter ends there. Of special interest, however, are those cases where the woman reports no problem, nor does the clinician, but the laboratory tests diagnose an infection. Such asymptomatic women can represent a major health risk to themselves and to others, yet in the ordinary course of events they will not seek treatment or be singled out for it. There is a clear and urgent need to come up with disease-specific estimates of asymptomatic carriers if routine screening or prophylactic treatment (based on some probability that the woman is a carrier) is contemplated.

Similarly, there are cases in which the clinician diagnoses (and treats) a problem that the laboratory does not confirm, in which case the woman has been over-treated. There are cases in which the clinician does not diagnose a problem but later tests reveal its existence, in which case the woman would have been undertreated by the clinician. And there are cases in which the woman reports a problem but neither the clinician nor the laboratory analysis identifies it as a recognizable infection, in which case the woman is likely to feel anxious or frustrated or annoyed with the health system and to seek help elsewhere. It would be very helpful if researchers could follow up on these possibilities by re-interviewing women, clinicians and perhaps technicians on each class of discrepancy to uncover the patterns of causes and consequences of the different diagnoses. This is an excellent opportunity for reproductive health providers to help interpret results and suggest possible modifications of procedures, as suggested earlier; and for women to comment on the discrepancies between what they feel and what the examinations and tests have revealed.

Listening to explanations: how do people interpret symptoms and their causes?

Just as women's self-reports of health problems may tell us little about their actual disease status, clinical and laboratory results tell us little if anything about how women experience health or illness, how they interpret symptoms and their causes, and how they go about preventing or treating infections and other gynaecological problems. Yet one cannot think of designing an intervention strategy to diagnose, cure and prevent reproductive tract infections without understanding what perceptions people commonly hold of why they have what they have and what they do about it.

Attributions of causality are imbedded in culturally constructed views of health and illness. Ailments that in one belief system are attributed to bacteria or a virus or tubal scarring are attributed in another to God's will or to evil spirits, to breathing night air, eating wrong foods, violating a taboo or some other force. In a study of five villages in Tamil Nadu in southern India, for example, women and men who reported genital symptoms such as discharge identified 'excessive body heat' more than any other factor as the cause. It follows that eating 'cooling' foods and resorting to other cooling treatments such as herbs or oil baths were considered to be logical treatments whereas changes in sexual behaviour were not (Santhya and Dasvarma, 1998). On the other hand, when asked about sources of genital infections in general, that is, in the world 'out there', people were more likely to point their finger at 'those bad women' or at 'those who behave immorally'. Ironically, it is this shared social perception that may have inhibited husbands and especially wives from talking to one another about their symptoms (Santhya and Dasvarma, 1998).

As part of a seamless whole, it is inevitable that treatment-seeking behaviour (if any) will be determined in large part by culturally or personally defined attributions of causality such as these. Eating cooling foods to treat discharge is just one example. Women may insert various cleaning substances in their vaginas, buy patent medicines from street vendors, consult health workers in the local clinic, visit a private doctor (who may or may not be qualified), or present herself at the out-patient services of a public or private hospital. She might also consult a spiritualist or make offerings at a shrine or submit to a local 'healer' who may make things worse instead of better. Harmful practices such as the gishiri cut, for example (which can result in fistula), are in some settings considered treatments for conditions such as delayed onset of first menstruation, failure to conceive or even hysteria (Kisekka, 1992; Wall, 1998). In cases such as these, the treatment (based on a misplaced cause) compounds the problem, setting in motion an ever-worsening sequence of gynaecological distress.

Focus group discussions will often elicit a multiplicity of causes or explanations for certain conditions, thus making it even more difficult for people to decide on prevention or treatment. The men interviewed by Ramos and Gogna (1997) in Buenos Aires, for example, attributed STIs not only to sexual contact with 'bad women' but also to bodily weakness, mental depression, poor nutrition, hard work, low self-defences, lack of personal care and unhygienic surroundings. Interestingly, however, they said that the best avoidance strategy was to choose their sexual partners carefully, and the best cure was a simple one – an injection of antibiotic. Indiscriminate use of antibiotics becomes, in some cases, both a prevention strategy and a cure, thus raising the likelihood that subsequent infections will be more difficult to treat (see Olukoya and Elias, 1996).

Listening to people's explanations of symptoms helps us to construct a model of perceived causality and corresponding treatment-seeking behaviour among population subgroups that can then be matched with the treatment-offering and client-seeking behaviour of formal and informal providers. How good is the fit? How do potential clients weigh factors such as efficacy, familiarity, cost, confidentiality and accessibility in choosing treatments and providers? We know that where women consider problems such as excessive menstrual bleeding, genital discharge or pain during intercourse to be their normal lot in life, they are unlikely to seek any treatment at all. Moreover, the tendency of women to place their own health needs below those of their children and other family members affects the calculus of care. Power relationships and patterns of discrimination within the household will have an impact on interpersonal communication about illness and on the utilization of services, depending on who decides about health care (e.g. woman head of household, husband, mother-in-law) and who pays for services. As Jejeebhoy and Koenig (Chapter 3) point out, limitations on women's autonomy, especially in cultures practising female seclusion, pose additional barriers to a woman's ability to act on her own behalf and need to be addressed programmatically. But even when problems are clearly identified and treatment is possible, clients' fears of formal clinic or hospital settings can inhibit utilization, even in settings where the need is great and the facilities are close by.

Research that reports on women's (and men's) treatment-seeking behaviour for specific conditions is especially useful in understanding the calculus that people use. For programme personnel and policy makers, it is certainly important to know what proportion of women with symptoms such as reproductive tract infections or pelvic inflammatory disease seek treatment and where (e.g. in a government hospital, primary health centre, through a private doctor or a traditional healer) (see Bhatia and Cleland, 1995, reporting on their study in Karnataka, India). What such reports do not usually show is the multiplicity of treatments and their sequencing, as when a woman who fears she may be pregnant tries an assortment of herbs and other remedies to 'bring on the period' before seeking menstrual regulation or abortion services. Often these delays cause serious consequences that need to be addressed through public information programmes and the training of health workers and private providers, such as midwives and pharmacists.

Collecting information about related behaviours and conditions: what else do we need to know, and why?

The conceptual framework presented by Jejeebhoy and Koenig (Chapter 3) offers a number of ideas for collecting additional information relating to the possible causes, correlates and consequences of reproductive tract infections and other gynaecological disorders. Taking complete contraceptive and reproductive histories together with descriptions of the conditions under which procedures were performed is essential for establishing connections between iatrogenic disorders and delivery practices, abortion or attempted abortion, intrauterine contraceptive device insertions, sterilization and other invasive procedures. Because infections from these causes are mostly avoidable, appropriate interventions can then be designed to investigate and raise the technical level and hygienic standards of such procedures in maternity centres and family planning clinics, among other sites.

In addition to contraceptive and reproductive histories, sexual histories that include information on age and circumstances of first intercourse; characteristics, number and changes of partners; the frequency and nature of sexual contacts (including practices such as oral and anal sex, forced intercourse, use of sexual aids); the woman's capacity to negotiate pleasurable sex and to avoid physical or emotional abuse; and the nature of protection used (if any) against STIs and unwanted pregnancies, is essential for understanding the social dynamics of sex and gender in which behavioural interventions to reduce disease transmission may be needed (Aral, 1992; Dixon-Mueller, 1993; Tsui, Wasserheit and Haaga, 1997). To the extent possible, sexual histories should also be taken from the woman's current male partner (if any), because his behaviour may place her at risk even if she is monogamous. As Mbizvo and Bassett (1999) point out, 'for most women, the risk of HIV relates not to her personal sexual behaviour, but to the behaviour of their partners and husbands'. In addition, of course, men have their own sexual and reproductive health needs that should be identified and addressed programmatically, as Hawkes and Hart (Chapter 4) emphasize.

Simple medical histories of the woman and of her children and other family members (e.g. checklists that require only an 'ever had' or 'have had within the last three months' response) can be useful in establishing connections between reproductive health and general health status. 'Just as [a condition such as] weakness impacts upon reproductive health (bearing children in a state of anaemia, lowered immunity and therefore greater susceptibility to infection including of the reproductive tract), it also has its roots in specific reproductive episodes (problematic pregnancies and deliveries, sterilization)' (Ramasubban and Singh, 1997:2). Identifying problems in the population such as diabetes, anaemia, high blood pressure or malaria by piggybacking on the reproductive health survey provides important information for setting health service priorities when separate health surveys are not feasible. Finally, information about the immediate environment of the household and neighbourhood – those physical, economic and social characteristics that threaten the health of people who reside there or intensify their anxieties about family survival and security – help to identify problems that may need to be addressed as part of a community-wide approach to improving the health and well-being of all of its members.

Using research to inform programmes and policies

The social and biomedical research agenda required to create a solid basis for policy and programme interventions in the prevention, diagnosis and treatment of reproductive tract infections and related gynaecological disorders is both vast and complex (see, for example, Germain et al., 1992; International Women's Health Coalition, 1991; Lande, 1993; Tsui, Wasserheit and Haaga, 1997). Scientists participating in a seminar on the global implications of reproductive tract infections for women's health in Bellagio, Italy identified six 'basic needs' for research and action, although others could certainly be added (Germain et al., 1992):

- Prioritize prevention and control of reproductive tract infections on national and international public health agendas.
- Integrate information, screening and services for STIs and endogenous infection into ongoing health and family planning programmes already serving women in the general population.
- Increase investments in training, supervision and basic supplies to minimize procedure-related infections in these health and family planning programmes.
- Increase attention to partner notification and services in STI programmes.
- Undertake carefully selected research to develop products for the prevention, detection and treatment of disease; to enhance understanding of the behavioural factors that promote infection; and to delineate cost-effective programmatic actions.
- Modify public policies on education, employment and legal rights to foster women's ability to protect their sexual health, and to enable women and men to be caring, responsible and respectful in sexual relationships, thus reducing the risk of infection.

The purpose of this concluding section is to suggest some ways in which research of the type described in this volume can help to fulfil policy and programmatic needs such as those listed. The intent is not to turn researchers into activists, for each activity (although dependent on the other) requires different skills. Rather, it is to encourage researchers to think about how they can turn their research findings into *tools for action* by analyzing and presenting the data in accessible ways. We are speaking here of life 'beyond the scientific journals', that is, of materials that people working in the field (in hospital training programmes, neighbourhood clinics, village health centres, house-to-house visits, schools and the media) as well as policy makers and administrators may find useful.

Presenting findings to national and international audiences

Scientific journals will find their way to some members of this audience, but how can the research results be presented to others in a clear and visually stimulating way that does not require an advanced degree in epidemiology or statistics? Audiences at the national level include health ministries, government offices of population or women's affairs, national associations of physicians and nurses/midwives, attorneys, family planning associations, associations of social workers and women's organizations. Each offers a forum for the presentation of findings to influential people, tailored of course to the specific interests and capacities of each group. Key data points can be highlighted, arguments summarized, and (most important) a list of proposed actions presented that point out what the specific agency or organization being addressed (and its members in their individual capacity) can do. National associations of obstetricians and gynaecologists can be urged to press for decriminalization of abortion, for example, and to adopt more liberal policies in their own practices and institutions so that safe and early termination of unwanted pregnancies becomes a routine component of women's health care (Brazier, Rizzuto and Wolf, 1998). Health ministries can be urged to integrate reproductive tract infection services into primary health care and maternal and child health services, and to develop pilot programmes of how this can best be done. Women's organizations can place reproductive health on their national and local agendas and create educational programmes for their members. Printed fact sheets together with ideas for action and lists of contacts and other resources could facilitate a process of coalition-building for action.

At the international level, data on the prevalence and consequences of STIs and other reproductive tract infections have already served to move the policy agenda forward, for example in highlighting the issue in the Programme for Action at the International Conference on Population and Development in Cairo in 1994. Presentations to multilateral and bilateral funding agencies, foundations and other donors have helped to put reproductive tract infections and other aspects of sexual and reproductive health on the policy and programme map in many countries. Indeed, many of these same agencies and organizations, such as WHO, UNICEF, the World Bank and the UN Population Fund, together with private donors, such as the Ford Foundation and the Rockefeller Foundation in the US, have funded some of the research and symposia that have helped to produce the policy changes.

Talking to state, district and local groups

In their account of the Uganda STIs project, Serwadda and Wawer (Chapter 7) emphasize that 'the community and civic leaders expect investigators to disseminate the results of the research findings [to them]'. They suggest that the findings be discussed with and reviewed first by district health officers and then by local leaders and committees before community meetings are held, and before outsiders such as the scientific and local media are informed.

Although the range of actions possible at the district and local levels may be circumscribed to some extent by national laws, policies and institutions, there is much that can be done at this level to identify gaps and problems in the delivery of reproductive health care, to set up mechanisms for overseeing the quality of care, and to mobilize local leadership among health and family planning providers, educators, community representatives and women's groups. NGOs based at the state and local level could play an important role in this regard. Again, the key issue is to

prepare data sheets summarizing the most vivid and relevant of the research findings together with discussion points that could provoke ideas for programmatic
interventions.

Preparing training materials for providers

The educational and training needs of providers should become clear in the course
of the research, such that informational materials and practical guidelines can be
prepared for practitioners such as physicians and medical students, practising
nurses and those in training, midwives, paramedics and social workers (counsellors) in health and family planning clinics (Helzner and Roitstein, 1995), pharmacists and others practising in the public or private sectors. Such materials, where
appropriate, would include guidelines for diagnosis and testing, taking medical histories (together with contraceptive, reproductive and sexual histories), performing
clinical examinations, doing laboratory analyses, maintaining high standards of
pregnancy, delivery and abortion care under aseptic conditions, counselling clients
of family planning, primary health, and maternal and child health services (and
their male partners) and other areas as such needs are identified. It is clear that
guidelines will be necessary for diagnosing and treating men as well; considerable
thought should be put into how and where this can best be done. Ideally, training
materials would address both the technical and social aspects of service delivery,
identify correct and incorrect practices, and confront some of the traditional beliefs
about prevention, causality and transmission that emerge in the qualitative work
of the research.

Preparing informational materials for outreach workers and community members

Outreach workers, such as health educators and teachers, could be prepared with
findings from the research to address community members directly with messages
relating to the prevention of STIs and other reproductive tract infections that
require changes in personal behaviours and community norms. Tsui et al. (1997)
stress the need for interventions that would increase knowledge of the symptoms,
signs and consequences of STIs; encourage delay in initiation of sex among adolescents of both sexes (including the arranged marriages of young girls); promote
partner communication and monogamous relationships or condom use where relevant; and identify sources of quality care for suspected infections. In addition, one
would want to identify common misperceptions, warn against certain ineffective
'cures' or harmful practices as revealed in the research, and stress the seriousness of
the consequences of untreated reproductive tract infections. Posters, illustrated
booklets, comic books, discussion points, teaching exercises, informational videos
and talks by local providers could all be helpful in dispelling dangerous misconceptions and clarifying appropriate courses and locations of treatment. Language,

messages, terminology, drawings and other presentations should be pretested to make sure they are comprehensible to the intended audiences.

Feeding ideas and research results to the media

Newspapers, popular magazines, radio and television programmes, and other communication media are valuable resources for informing people about reproductive health and discussing sexual behaviour in a lively way. Efforts could be made to cultivate contacts with the media and to propose story or programme ideas (e.g. topical magazine columns, episodes of widely watched tele-novellas) and even to write or produce them. Journalists or producers could be invited to the research sites, provided with easily summarized research findings, and interview women who participated in the study, plus health care providers, community leaders and members of the research team.

Using entertainment as a means of informing hard-to-reach groups

Most communities offer public entertainment from time to time: fiestas, melas, community fairs with food, entertainment, sports, children's games and other diversions. This is an excellent place to set up a booth with easy-to-read informational handouts, hold contests that test people's knowledge, and perform topical skits or create songs and dances that make fun of sex and men's power over women (see, for instance, Capoor and Mehta, 1995 on adolescent fairs in India). Skits in which men's and women's roles are reversed can point out the extremes of accepted behaviour in an amusing way, as when a wife forbids her husband to leave the house or threatens to beat him when he complains that he is too tired to have sex. The theme of treatment-seeking behaviour that involves comical exchanges with a series of uninformed relatives or neighbours (each with different ideas of what to do or take) and self-promoting quacks, each of whom worsens the woman's condition, can lead to the 'correct' resolution when a visiting health worker sets the client straight and takes her to the clinic. Humour can be an effective means of breaking through barriers of misinformation and taboos.

Sexuality education and group counselling

Material on the causes, correlates, consequences, symptoms and treatments of STIs and other reproductive tract infections in both women and men, along with information on protection against unwanted pregnancy, safe and unsafe sexual practices, and sexual pleasure and responsibility, should clearly be incorporated into sexuality education programmes in schools. Research findings can provide important data on attitudes and behaviours that are useful not only for schools but also for group counselling sessions offered by adult education programmes, health centres or NGOs. Groups in need of special information would include out-of-school male and female adolescents, couples about to be married, married women in their prime childbearing years, unmarried sexually active women, post-menopausal women, and married and unmarried men (including those with same-sex contacts) in groups or with their partners. Other special interest groups could be based on the workplace, such as men serving in the armed forces, young women and men working in factories, market women, commercial sex workers (female and male) and long-distance truck drivers. Aside from the general messages relating to STIs and other reproductive tract infections, special messages regarding prevention can be designed for each group that address the particular risks that each may face.

With respect to addressing men's sexual and reproductive health needs, Hawkes and Hart (Chapter 4) raise the question of how best to integrate men's services into the existing health care system. Can men be persuaded to go to services tradition-ally seen as being a female domain, such as family planning clinics or primary health care systems that are predominantly a site of maternal and child health ser-vices? Can services be adapted to their needs? If not in these sites, then where? In addition, the relative merits of women-only, men-only, and mixed or couple ser-vices need to be considered in each locale and perhaps even on a case-by-case basis. Some critics (for instance, Sciortino, 1998) have pointed out that women-only approaches may not empower women sufficiently to act on their own behalf when confronted directly with the power relationships of their families and communities. Women often want programmes also directed at their husbands. In turn, of course, men may feel far more comfortable talking about sexuality and personal health problems with other men. Couple-oriented approaches also need to be considered as a means of encouraging communication and joint treatment, addressing gender inequalities and working toward behavioural changes in relationships as a whole.

Finally, there is much that governments can do – politically, administratively and judicially – to create a positive policy and programme environment with regard to the control of reproductive tract infections. They can institute public health campaigns similar to those informing populations about cholera or other diseases and allocate public health resources to prevention, diagnosis and treat-ment (Ronald and Aral, 1992; Tsui, Wasserheit and Haaga, 1997). They can set medical standards for safe childbearing and ensure that facilities and regulations throughout the country provide for safe and accessible contraception, abortion and sterilization. Also they can create a legal and policy framework that supports more equitable and equal relations between women and men by instituting and enforcing laws penalizing violence against women, sexual harassment, rape and child abuse; by ensuring girls' and women's full legal rights at the time of marriage, during marriage and at its dissolution; and by promoting equality in inheritance, property rights, education and employment, among other areas. Targeted biomed-ical programmes can contribute substantially to the reduction of reproductive tract infections, but ultimately it is society's treatment of girls and women that is most likely to determine their effectiveness.

REFERENCES

Aral SO (1992) Sexual behavior as a risk factor for sexually transmitted disease. In: Germain A et al., eds. *Reproductive tract infections: global impact and priorities for women's reproductive health.* New York, Plenum Press.

Bhatia JC, Cleland J (1995) Self-reported symptoms of gynecological morbidity and their treatment in south India. *Studies in family planning,* **26**(4): 203–216.

Bhatia JC, Cleland J, Bhagavan L et al. (1997) Levels and determinants of gynecological morbidity in a district of south India. *Studies in family planning,* **28**(2): 95–103.

Bishop A, Wells E, Sherris J et al. (1995) Cervical cancer: evolving prevention strategies for developing countries. *Reproductive health matters,* **6**: 60–71.

Brazier E, Rizzuto R, Wolf M (1998) *Prevention and management of unsafe abortion: a guide for action.* New York, Family Care International.

Bulut A, Volsal N, Filippi V et al. (1995) In search of truth: comparing alternative sources of information on reproductive tract infection. *Reproductive health matters,* **6**: 31–39.

Campbell O, Cleland J, Collumbien M et al. (1999) *Social science methods for research on reproductive health.* Geneva, World Health Organization.

Capoor I, Mehta S (1995) Talking about love and sex in adolescent health fairs in India. *Reproductive health matters,* **5**: 22–36.

Dixon-Mueller R (1993) The sexuality connection in reproductive health. *Studies in family planning,* **24**(5): 269–282.

Germain A, Holmes KK, Piot R et al. (1992) *Reproductive tract infections: global impact and priorities for women's reproductive health.* New York, Plenum Press.

Heise LL, McGrory CE, Wood SY (1998) *Practical and ethical dilemmas in the clinical testing of microbicides: a report on a symposium.* New York, International Women's Health Coalition.

Helzner JF, Roitstein F (1995) HIV/STD prevention in family planning services: training as a strategy for change. *Reproductive health matters,* **5**: 80–88.

International Women's Health Coalition (1991) *Reproductive tract infections in women in the Third World: national and international policy implications.* New York, IWHC.

Kisekka MN (Ed.) (1992) *Women's health issues in Nigeria.* Zaria, Nigeria, Tamaza.

Lande R (1993) Controlling sexually transmitted diseases. *Population reports,* Series L, no. 9. Baltimore, Johns Hopkins School of Hygiene and Public Health, Population Information Program.

Mbizvo, MM, Bassett MT (1999) Men and their roles and responsibilities in gynaecological morbidities. Paper presented at the Meeting of the Consultative Group on Guidelines for Research on Reproductive Tract Infections/Gynaecological morbidity, Geneva, 1999. (Unpublished.)

Nazzar A, Reason L, Adongo P et al. (1999) Community-based strategic planning: utilizing social research to develop a culturally appropriate program for female genital mutilation prevention in a traditional area of northern Ghana. Paper presented at the annual meetings of the Population Association of America, New York, March.

Olukoya AA, Elias C (1996) Perceptions of reproductive tract morbidity among Nigerian women and men. *Reproductive health matters,* **7**: 56–65.

Ramasubban R, Singh B (1997) Gender, reproductive health and weakness: experiences of slum dwelling women in Bombay, India. Paper presented at the Seminar on Cultural Perspectives on Reproductive Health, Rustenburg, South Africa, 16–19 June. Liege, Belgium, International Union for the Scientific Study of Population.

Ramos S, Gogna M (1997) Health, gender and sexuality: how does culture shape STDs? Paper presented at the Seminar on Cultural Perspectives on Reproductive Health, Rustenburg, South Africa, 16–19 June. Liege, Belgium: International Union for the Scientific Study of Population.

Ronald A, Aral SO (1992) Assessment and prioritization of actions to prevent and control reproductive tract infections in the Third World. In: Germain A et al., eds. *Reproductive tract infections: global impact and priorities for women's reproductive health*. New York, Plenum Press.

Santhya KG, Dasvarma GL (1998) Spousal communication on reproductive illness: a case study of rural women in Southern India. Paper presented at the Seminar on Gender Inequalities and Reproductive Health, Campos de Jordao, Brazil, 16–19 November. Liege, Belgium, International Union for the Scientific Study of Population.

Sciortino R (1998) The challenge of addressing gender in reproductive health programmes: examples from Indonesia. *Reproductive health matters*, **6**: 33–43.

Tsui AO, Wasserheit JN, Haaga JG (Eds) (1997) *Reproductive health in developing countries: expanding dimensions, building solutions*. Washington, D.C., National Academy Press.

Wall LL (1998) Dead mothers and injured wives: The social context of maternal morbidity and mortality among the Hausa of northern Nigeria. *Studies in family planning*, **29**(4): 341–359.

Appendix A

Notes on contributors

Rani Bang and Abhay Bang founded and jointly manage the Society for Education, Action and Research in Community Health (SEARCH), a non-governmental organization that provides community-based health care in 150 villages in Gadchiroli, a remote rural district in Maharashtra, India. They have been instrumental in identifying and addressing, with community participation, important public health problems that are of concern to the community they serve. Their work also involves the conduct of research and the design and implementation of health programmes that are acceptable at community level. Their activities – addressing gynaecological morbidity in rural women, pneumonia in children and neonatal care in villages for example – have been recognized in national and international public health agendas. Drs Rani and Abhay Bang are members of India's National Commission of Population and have received numerous awards including the Gold Medal from the Indian Council of Medical Research, the Mahatma Gandhi Award for humanitarian service and three literarey awards. Drs Rani Barn and Abhay Bang received their medical education (MD) in India and a masters in public health from Johns Hopkins University, Baltimore, USA.

Aysen Bulut is Head of the Department of Family Health, Institute of Child Health, Istanbul University, Turkey. After graduating from medical school at Hacettepe University, Ankara, in 1976, she specialized in public health. She received a diploma in population research from the Sociology Department of Exeter University, UK in 1984. She became a professor in 1996 and has worked extensively in the areas of quality of care in reproductive health, measurement and evaluation of health interventions, medical education and sexual education for youth in Turkey. She has also served as a consultant in Swaziland, Jordan, The Sultanate of Oman and Azarbaijan.

John Cleland is Professor of Medical Demography, London School of Hygiene and Tropical Medicine where he has served since 1988. Before joining the School he spent many years working for the World Fertility Survey based in London, a pioneering survey research organization that conducted fertility and family planning surveys in over 40 developing countries. His special interests include fertility and family planning in developing countries, the determinants of infant and child mortality and, more recently, he has focused on risk behaviours in connection with the HIV pandemic. In the 1990s, he studied women's obstetric and gynaecological morbidity in Karnataka State, India. The current focus of his work is on health-seeking behaviour and health expenditures by adult women on their own ailments and the role of private practitioners.

Ruth Dixon-Mueller was formerly Professor of Sociology at the University of California, Davis, and Senior Research Associate in Demography at the University of California, Berkeley, USA. She is currently an independent consultant in population and reproductive health, and is the author of *Population Policy and Women's Rights: Transforming Reproductive Choice* (1993).

Christopher Elias is president of PATH (Program for Appropriate Technology in Health), an international, non-profit NGO in the US dedicated to improving health, particularly the health of women and children. Prior to joining PATH, Dr. Elias was a Senior Associate in the International Programmes Division of the Population Council where he served as the Country Representative in Thailand, managing reproductive health programmes in Thailand, Myanmar, Cambodia, Yunnan, and the Lao PDR. In conjunction with the Population Council's Centre for Biomedical Research and New York-based International Programmes Division staff, he helped to co-ordinate efforts to develop and test woman-controlled vaginal microbicides. Dr. Elias also worked with the Population Council in New York, where he co-ordinated global research activities concerning sexually transmitted infection and HIV/AIDS for the Robert H. Ebert Programme for Critical Issues in Reproductive Health and Population. Dr. Elias received his MD from Creighton University, completed postgraduate training in internal medicine at the University of California, San Francisco, and received a Masters in Public Health from the University of Washington, USA, where he was a fellow in the Robert Wood Johnson Clinical Scholars Programme.

Véronique Filippi, PhD, is a lecturer in reproductive epidemiology and demography at the London School of Hygiene and Tropical Medicine. She has research interests in the measurement of reproductive and maternal morbidity in developing countries, aspects of safe motherhood in Africa, learning from adverse events in health services and improving quality of care through audit.

Joel Gittelsohn, PhD, MSc, Associate Professor, Department of International Health, Johns Hopkins University, USA, is a medical anthropologist who specializes in the use of qualitative and quantitative information to design, implement and evaluate health and nutrition intervention programmes. Dr. Gittelsohn integrates qualitative and quantitative approaches to understand better culture-based beliefs and behaviours regarding dietary patterns, and how these factors influence the success or failure of dietary and lifestyle modification strategies. He has refined and tested methods to assess food intake and intra-household food distribution in different cultures, including the direct, structured observation of behaviour. He applies these methods and interventions to the prevention of obesity and diabetes among different indigenous and ethnic groups, to nutrient deficiencies of Nepalese children and women, and to improve infant feeding in diverse settings, such as The Gambia, Hartford (CT, USA) and Peru. He is currently working on chronic disease interventions among children of the White Mountain and San Carlos Apache (obesity prevention), the Ojibwa-Cree (diabetes prevention), African–American church-going women (cardiovascular disease prevention) and children and adults in the Republic of the Marshall Islands (obesity and undernutrition prevention). He has also conducted qualitative studies on reproductive decision-making in Zimbabwe and tobacco use among African–American and white teens in Baltimore City, USA.

Ronald H. Gray MD, MSc, is Professor, Department of Population and Family Health Sciences, Johns Hopkins School of Hygiene and Public Health, USA, with joint appointments in the Departments of Epidemiology and International Health; and Director of the STD Core in the JHU NICHD-sponsored Population Centre. Since 1994, Dr. Gray has been co-principal investigator of the Rakai Project in Uganda. He was co-investigator on the Rakai STD Control for AIDS Prevention Study, and co-principal investigator on the Maternal Infant Supplementary Study (MISS) nested within the latter. He is co-principal investigator on the Rakai Cohort continuation (CHER) study and the Rakai Molecular Epidemiology Research Study (MER) funded by the Walter Reed Army Institute of Research/Henry M. Jackson Foundation, USA; and principal investigator on an NICHD R01 on the effects of HIV on fertility.

Dr. Gray has also been principal investigator on numerous international epidemiological studies of reproductive and perinatal health, including cohort studies of reproductive outcomes associated with in utero or lactational exposure to steroid contraceptives (Thailand); studies of low birth-weight, prematurity and perinatal mortality (Sudan, India, Brazil and Pakistan); multi-centre prospective studies of pregnancy outcome associated with timing of conception (Chile, Colombia, Ecuador, Italy, US); prospective endocrinological research on lactational infertility (Philippines and US); WHO multinational contraceptive clinical trials and studies of pelvic inflammatory disease and genital tract cancer; and on retrospective and prospective investigations of reproductive health among male and female workers in semi-conductor manufacturing. Dr. Gray has assisted in the initiation of innovative data and sample collection methodologies in community-based epidemiological trials in developing country settings, and has collaborated in developing statistical analyses for complex cluster randomized community trials.

Siobán Harlow is Associate Director of the International Institute and Associate Professor of Epidemiology at the University of Michigan, Ann Arbor, USA. Her research focuses on the life circumstances and biological processes of unique relevance to women's health, with a primary interest in the epidemiology of menstrual function. Major contributions of this research include one of the first epidemiological studies of the determinants of the duration of menstrual bleeding, one of the most comprehensive studies published to date on patterns and determinants of dysmenorrhoea, and the first study of ethnic differences in the menstrual bleeding characteristics conducted in the US. She has recently defined a lifespan approach to understanding the nature of variation in menstrual function throughout the reproductive lifecourse. Currently, in a project originally funded by the Burroughs Wellcome Fund and in collaboration with Oona Campbell of the London School of Hygiene and Tropical Medicine, London, UK, she has presented evidence of the growing impact of menstrual dysfunction in developing countries on women's health and daily functioning, and articulated the importance of addressing menstrual dysfunction in reproductive health programmes.

Graham Hart is Associate Director of the MRC Social and Public Health Sciences Unit, University of Glasgow, UK, and is Head of the Unit's programme of research on sexual and reproductive health. He has published widely on the subject of sexual risk behaviour for HIV and other sexually transmitted infections.

Sarah Hawkes is a physician and researcher specializing in strategies for the control of reproductive tract infections in low-income areas. Her PhD in this topic was conducted in the Matlab area of rural Bangladesh where she spent three years working for the International Centre for Diarrhoeal Disease, Bangladesh. She is currently a Programme Associate in Reproductive Health research at the Population Council in New Delhi, India.

Shireen J. Jejeebhoy has recently joined the Population Council's India office. Until early 2002, she worked at the UNDP/UNFPA/WHO/World Bank Special Programme of Research, Development and Research Training in Human Reproduction, Geneva, Switzerland. Her work focuses on adolescent sexual and reproductive health in a number of developing countries. Earlier, she worked in India as an independent researcher in the field of reproductive health. Her recent research interest has been applied social science research in reproductive health issues, and female autonomy and gender issues. She has published extensively in areas relating to women's education and reproductive behaviour, women's autonomy in India, and adolescent sexual and reproductive health. She holds a PhD in demography from the University of Pennsylvania, USA.

Hind Khattab is Chairperson the Egyptian Society for Population Studies and Reproductive Health, and a Founding Member of the Reproductive Health Working Group. She holds a PhD in population anthropology from the University of North Carolina, USA, and has worked in the areas of applied anthropology, social science research, health education and counselling. She has over four decades of experience in research and projects, ranging the broad span of family planning and maternal and child health; reproductive health; health, population and development; women's involvement in community development; health education; and the impact of labour migration on family structure and emergency obstetric care. She has taught at the Social Research Centre, The American University in Cairo and the Institute of Statistics, Cairo University, Egypt. She has served as consultant to a number of organizations, including WHO, UNICEF, FHI, Ford Foundation, UNFPA, European Union, IPPF, Red Cross/Red Crescent, AVSC, and the Ministry of Health and Population, Egypt. She has authored over 25 publications, including several on women's reproductive health in Egypt.

Michael Koenig is currently an Associate Professor in the Department of Population and Family Health Sciences at the Johns Hopkins University School of Public Health, Baltimore, USA. Prior to this, he worked with both the Population Council in Bangladesh and the Ford Foundation in India on family planning and reproductive health programmes. His research interests focus upon applied social science research on family planning and reproductive health issues, and community-based programmes to address health needs.

Jane Kuypers has a PhD in medical microbiology from the University of Wisconsin, USA, and has worked for the past 10 years as a research scientist in the Department of Pathology at the University of Washington, Seattle, USA. Since March 2001, she has been Director of Extraction Services for Qiagen Genomics, Inc. in Bothell, Washington, USA. Formerly Director of the DNA Probe Laboratory, she has conducted laboratory testing in support of large epidemiologic research studies on HPV, HIV and other sexually transmitted infections.

Nicola Low is a clinical epidemiologist specializing in sexually transmitted infections. Her main research interests are in the epidemiology and prevention of bacterial sexually transmitted infections, ethnicity and sexual health, study design and systematic reviews and meta-analysis. She is currently a Senior Lecturer in Epidemiology and Public Health Medicine at the University of Bristol, UK.

Tom Marshall is a medical statistician working in the London School of Hygiene and Tropical Medicine, UK, where he works with groups concerned with the maternal health and public health interventions. His statistical work brings him in contact with a wide range of projects and topics in reproductive health and related areas, and he has an interest in survey methods, including measurement issues in surveys and asking questions about morbidity, and problems of inference relating to episode length from cross-sectional data.

Mary P. Meehan, BSc (Med Tech), ASCP, MSc, is Research Associate, Heilbrun Centre for Population and Family Health, Mailman School of Public Health, Columbia University, New York, USA, and Laboratory Coordinator, Rakai Project, Uganda. Ms. Meehan has been the Rakai Project Laboratory Coordinator since 1997, when she participated in the STD (sexually transmitted diseases) Control for AIDS Prevention Trial. Ms. Meehan, who is resident in Uganda, oversaw all laboratory activities for the community-based trial, which collected, processed and tested serological, urine, vaginal swab and genital ulcer swab samples from over 14 000 persons per year. The study also followed close to 3000 pregnant women and their infants, and examined the effects of HIV and STD control and prevention on maternal-infant health and placental pathology. Ms. Meehan is highly experienced in the oversight and quality control required to ensure adequate field and laboratory procedures in large, complex data and sample collection studies. Prior to her work with Rakai, Ms. Meehan was a medical technologist in the virology, immunology and blood banking laboratories at Johns Hopkins University in Baltimore, USA, and a Blood Bank Medical Technologist in St. Thomas, US Virgin Islands.

André Meheus, Professor, MD, PhD, graduated as MD from the University of Ghent, Belgium. He studied tropical medicine (Institute of Tropical Medicine, Antwerp, Belgium), medical statistics and epidemiology (University of Brussels, Belgium) and occupational health (University of Ghent). In 1969 he became assistant in the Department of Social Medicine and Hygiene, University of Ghent, and from 1971 to 1974 he was responsible for public health teaching and training at the National University in Butare-Rwanda, Central Africa. In 1974 he moved to the Department of Epidemiology and Social Medicine at the University of Antwerp as senior lecturer, became Associate Professor in 1978 and Professor in 1986. From 1987 to 1993 he was the Programme Manager at the World Health Organization, Geneva, Switzerland, of the Programme for Sexually Transmitted Diseases and Treponematoses (WHO/VDT); in 1993 he resumed his post as professor and head of the Department of Epidemiology and Social Medicine in Antwerp. In the late 1960s, his research interests focused on the epidemiology of ischemic heart disease and chronic non-specific lung disease. Since the early 1970s, his research in developing countries has focused on the epidemiology and control of infectious diseases, in particular sexually transmitted infections, including HIV/AIDS. He has published more than 250 scientific articles and books on subjects of public health, preventive medicine and infectious disease control, is a member of the editorial board of the major sexually transmitted infections and AIDS journals and the expert panel for venereal diseases and treponematoses of the World Health Organization. He is an adviser on international public health for multilateral and bilateral agencies.

Nandini Oomman is an independent health researcher. She has focused her work for over a decade on social science research in women's health. Nandini has worked with the Rockefeller Foundation, New York until recently and is currently an Associate in the Department of Population and Family Health Sciences at the Johns Hopkins University School of Public Health, Baltimore, USA.

Pertti J. Pelto is a medical anthropologist with a Doctorate from the University of California, Berkeley, USA. He is currently Professor Emeritus (retired) from the University of Connecticut, USA. Since 1989 he has been involved in projects of technical assistance for community-based research in India. He took up residence in Baroda, Gujarat in 1995, and has been living in India since then. Dr. Pelto's activities in India and other countries of South Asia are focused on capacity building in research on reproductive health issues, with special emphasis on qualitative data-gathering methods. Many of the projects he advises are involved in research and interventions directed to HIV/AIDS. His activities in workshops and site visits to NGOs and other research groups have been funded under a programme grant from Ford Foundation, currently administered at the University of North Carolina, USA.

Thomas C. Quinn, MD, MSc, is Senior Investigator and Head of the Section on International AIDS Research in the Laboratory of Immunoregulation at the National Institute of Allergy and Infectious Diseases, USA. Since 1981, he has been at the Division of Infectious Diseases at Johns Hopkins University School of Medicine (USA) where he is a Professor of Medicine. He also has adjunct appointments in the Department of International Health, and the Department of Immunology and Molecular Microbiology in the Johns Hopkins School of Hygiene and Public Health. He currently directs the Johns Hopkins School of Medicine P3 HIV/AIDS Research Facility and the International STD Research Laboratory.

Dr. Quinn's investigations have involved the study of the epidemiological, virological, and immunological features of HIV infection in Africa, the Caribbean, South America and Asia. In 1984, he helped establish the interagency project called Projet SIDA in Kinshasa, in the former Zaire (now Democratic Republic of the Congo), which was the largest AIDS investigative project in sub-Saharan Africa. Dr. Quinn has been involved in laboratory investigations that have helped define the biological factors involved in heterosexual transmission and perinatal transmission, the natural history of HIV infections in developing countries, and the identification and characterization of unique strains of HIV-1 infection.

Immunological studies have included the changes in T-cell phenotypes and cytokines in patients with HIV infection and other endemic tropical diseases such as malaria and tuberculosis. Dr. Quinn has been involved in HIV clinical and epidemiological investigations in 25 countries, with current projects in Uganda, South Africa, Zimbabwe, the Democratic Republic of the Congo, Ethiopia, India, China, Thailand, and Brazil. He has been an Advisor/Consultant on HIV and sexually transmitted infections to the World Health Organization, UNAIDS and the US Food and Drug Administration. He is a member of editorial boards of six journals focusing on infectious diseases, AIDS and sexually transmitted infections, and has published widely.

David M. Serwadda, MB, ChB, Msc, M.Med, MPH, is Associate Professor, Institute of Public Health, Makerere University, Kampala, Uganda. His main area of interest is infectious disease epidemiology. He has spent the last 15 years in population-based studies working on the evaluation of innovative HIV intervention and studying the dynamics of HIV and sexually transmitted infection in rural populations in Uganda.

Mary E. Shepherd, MS, is a Research Associate in the Department of Infectious Diseases, Johns Hopkins University School of Medicine and a PhD candidate in the Department of Population and Family Health Sciences, Johns Hopkins University School of Hygiene and Public Health, Baltimore, USA.

Maria J. Wawer, MD, MHSc, FRCP(C), is currently Professor of Clinical Public Health, Heilbrun Centre for Population and Family Health, Mailman School of Public Health, Columbia University, New York, and Adjunct Professor of Public Health, Johns Hopkins School of Public Health, USA. Dr. Wawer has almost two decades of experience in the design and implementation of international reproductive health research and programmes. She has worked in over 15 countries in Africa, Asia and Latin America. In the 1980s, Dr Wawer assisted with the implementation of family planning operations research studies in, among other countries, Brazil, Niger and Burkina Faso. In 1988, along with Drs Serwadda and Sewankambo, Dr Wawer initiated the Rakai Project in Uganda, with a principal focus on HIV, other bacterial and viral sexually transmitted infections and maternal–infant health. Within the Rakai Project, she has helped develop complex epidemiological studies and community-based HIV prevention trials, which incorporate intensive home-based sample and data collection procedures, for the study of HIV/sexually transmitted disease epidemiology, behavioural and other risk factors, and prevention. Dr. Wawer had also conducted HIV research in Thailand, and has served on numerous international HIV research-related advisory boards.

Janneke van de Wijgert, PhD, MPH, MSc, is currently Programme Associate in the Reproductive Health Programme of the Population Council, New York, USA. Prior to this, she has held several positions, including Programme Director and co-founder of the UZ-UCSF Women's Health Programme, Harare, Zimbabwe; Post-Doctoral Researcher at the University of California, San Francisco, USA; and Visiting Lecturer at the University of Zimbabwe Medical School, Harare. Her recent work includes microbicides development and testing, assessing the impact of HIV prevention interventions and studying the role of traditional vaginal practice and reproductive tract infections in HIV transmission. She received her Ph.D. in epidemiology from the University of California, Berkley.

Huda Zurayk is a biostatistician, whose research interests are in the area of population and health. She has focused on reproductive health issues while working as a Senior Associate in the Population Council's regional office for West Asia and North Africa in Cairo, Egypt, and serving as Coordinator of the regional Reproductive Health Working Group. She is currently Professor and Dean of the Faculty of Health Sciences at the American University of Beirut.

Index

Note: page numbers in *italics* refer to figures, tables and boxes. Numbers with suffix 'n' refer to footnotes